Personality Characteristics of
Patients With Pain

Personality Characteristics of
Patients With Pain

edited by
Robert J. Gatchel
and
James N. Weisberg

American Psychological Association
Washington, DC

First printing March 2000
Second printing December 2000

Published by
American Psychological Association
750 First Street, NE
Washington, DC 20002

Copies may be ordered from
APA Order Department
P.O. Box 92984
Washington, DC 20090-2984

In the U.K., Europe, Africa, and the Middle East, copies may be
ordered from
American Psychological Association
3 Henrietta Street
Covent Garden, London
WC2E 8LU England

Typeset in Times Roman by EPS Group Inc., Easton, MD

Printer: Port City Press, Inc., Baltimore, MD
Cover Designer: Lynne Komai, The Watermark Design Office,
  Alexandria, VA
Technical/Production editor: Eleanor Inskip

The opinions and statements published are the responsibility of the
authors, and such opinions and statements do not necessarily represent
the policies of the APA.

Library of Congress Cataloging-in-Publication Data

Personality characteristics of patients with pain / editors, Robert J.
  Gatchel and James N. Weisberg.
      p.   cm.
    Includes index.
    ISBN 1-55798-646-0 (hardcover)
    1. Pain—Patients—Psychological aspects.   2. Pain—
  Psychological aspects.   3. Patients—Attitudes.   I. Gatchel,
  Robert J., 1947–   II. Weisberg, James N., 1963–
  RB127.P476   2000
  616′.0472′019—dc21

                                                     99-052773

British Library Cataloguing-in-Publication Data
A CIP record is available from the British Library.

Printed in the United States of America

To the individuals who helped me most in my growth as a psychologist: Jim Geer, who initially stimulated my interest in psychology as an undergraduate at the State University of New York at Stony Brook; Peter Lang, who served as my inspirational graduate research mentor at the University of Wisconsin; Andy Baum, who helped to significantly blossom my interest in health psychology; and Maurice Korman, who has provided me with a nurturing academic environment within which to freely pursue my professional development.

R.J.G.

To my wife, Shelby, and my sons Justin and Drew for their unselfish support and encouragement. Also in memory of Timothy C. Toomey, mentor, colleague, and friend, who contributed much to the field of pain, as well as my professional and personal development.

J.N.W.

CONTENTS

List of Contributors   ix

Preface   xi

Introduction   3

Part I: Early Approaches to the Study of Personality and Pain
  Chapter 1. *History of Psychoanalytic Ideas Concerning Pain*   25
    Harold Merskey
  Chapter 2. *Psychometric Testing: The Early Years and the MMPI*   37
    Richard C. Robinson

Part II: Advances in Personality Testing in Patients With Chronic Pain
  Chapter 3. *Assessing Personality With the Millon Behavioral Health Inventory, the Millon Behavioral Medicine Diagnostic, and the Millon Clinical Multiaxial Inventory*   61
    Neil Bockian, Sarah Meager and Theodore Millon
  Chapter 4. *Nonpathological Factors in Chronic Pain: Implications for Assessment and Treatment*   89
    James B. Wade and Donald D. Price
  Chapter 5. *The MMPI-2 and Chronic Pain*   109
    William W. Deardorff

Part III: Nonpathological Personality Characteristics of Pain
  Chapter 6. *Relationship of Pain-Coping Strategies to Adjustment and Functioning*   129
    Douglas E. DeGood
  Chapter 7. *Locus of Control in the Patient With Chronic Pain* . . .   165
    Janette L. Seville and Amy B. Robinson
  Chapter 8. *Extraversion–Introversion and Chronic Pain*   181
    Jennifer M. Phillips and Robert J. Gatchel
  Chapter 9. *Perceived Optimism and Chronic Pain*   203
    John P. Garofalo

Part IV: Personality Disorders and Chronic Pain
  Chapter 10. *Studies Investigating the Prevalence of Personality Disorders in Patients With Chronic Pain*   221
    James N. Weisberg

Chapter 11. *How Practitioners Should Evaluate Personality to Help Manage Patients With Chronic Pain* 241
Robert J. Gatchel

Chapter 12. *Personality and Pain: Summary and Future Perspectives* 259
James N. Weisberg, Jeffrey R. Vittengl,
Lee Anna Clark, Robert J. Gatchel, and
Amy A. Gorin

Author Index 283

Subject Index 299

About the Editors 311

CONTRIBUTORS

Neil Bockian, PhD, Assistant Professor, Illinois School of Professional Psychology

Lee Anna Clark, PhD, Associate Provost for Faculty, University of Iowa

William W. Deardorff, PhD, West Coast Spine Institute, Los Angeles, California

Douglas E. DeGood, PhD, Department of Psychiatric Medicine, University of Virginia Health System, Charlottesville; Augusta Pain Management Center, Fishersville, Virginia

John P. Garofalo, PhD, University of Pittsburgh Cancer Institute

Robert J. Gatchel, PhD, Elizabeth H. Penn Professor of Clinical Psychology and Professor of Psychiatry and Rehabilitation, University of Texas, Dallas.

Amy A. Gorin, MA, PhD Candidate, Department of Psychology, State University of New York at Stony Brook

Sarah Meager, BPhil, Institute for Advanced Studies in Personology and Psychopathology, Coral Gables, Florida

Harold Merskey, DM, Professor Emeritus of Psychiatry, University of Western Ontario, London, Canada

Theodore Millon, PhD, DSc, Dean, Institute for Advanced Studies in Personology and Psychopathology, Coral Gables, Florida

Jennifer M. Phillips, PhD, Fellow, Department of Family Resources and Human Development, Arizona State University

Donald D. Price, PhD, School of Dentristry, University of Florida, Gainesville

Amy B. Robinson, PhD, Assistant Professor of Psychiatry, Dartmouth Medical School, Lebanon, New Hampshire

Richard C. Robinson, PhD, Department of Psychiatry, University of Texas Southwestern Medical Center at Dallas

Janette L. Seville, PhD, Assistant Professor of Psychiatry, Dartmouth Medical School, Lebanon, New Hampshire

Jeffrey R. Vittengl, PhD, Department of Psychology, University of Iowa

James B. Wade, PhD, Director, Psychological Assessment, MCV Family Counseling Center, Richmond, Virginia

James N. Weisberg, PhD, Assistant Professor of Clinical Psychiatry and Behavioral Sciences, State University of New York, Stony Brook.

PREFACE

Pain is extremely prevalent. It is estimated that 70 million Americans will experience some form of acute, recurrent, or chronic pain each year and that 10% of the population will report the presence of pain at least 100 days in a year. Moreover, a great deal of suffering is experienced by patients and their families as a result of this pain. Unfortunately, traditional pain management procedures, such as surgical and pharmacological interventions, have not been totally successful for dealing with this significant health care problem. As a result, there has been a growing interest in the role of psychosocial and personality factors in the experience of and adaptation to pain. Indeed, one truly frustrating aspect of pain management for many clinicians is dealing with certain personality characteristics of patients who experience pain. A significant challenge for health care professionals is found in dealing with the personality attributes of those patients. For example, some patients with neurotic tendencies are hypersensitive about minor pain and discomfort long after the tissue pathology has been resolved. Patients who have long-standing depressive personalities can seem hopeless about the course of their pain and can take an inactive, helpless approach rather than an active role in their treatment. Patients who have clear-cut personality disorders, such as a borderline personality disorder, sometimes demand immediate attention or request unnecessary medication and can respond in a threatening or angry fashion when their demands are not met—immediately alienating them from treatment staff.

To deal with such "personality difference" challenges, pain treatment specialists have attempted to develop and refine approaches to better assess and explain personality factors in patients who have pain. Although there is no research consistently demonstrating a link between a *specific* personality type and the development of chronic pain disability, there can be no doubt that, on the basis of their experiences, patients develop unique ways of interpreting information and coping with pain and stress. Such patterns will affect their perceptions of and responses to the presence of pain. If the patterns are maladaptive, then one would expect the patients to have more difficulty in coping with pain. Individuals who have personality disorders *in general* can be expected to display an inability to cope successfully with a major stressor, such as chronic pain. In addition, viewing personality disorders from a slightly different perspective—one influenced by developmental vulnerabilities, premorbid styles, and dimensionality—rather than simply finding the "cause" of the chronic pain, can help clinicians and patients alike.

Research has been unable to isolate a primary, preexisting "pain personality." Indeed, there is no one consistent "pain-prone personality syndrome." Rather, recent work has begun to demonstrate that patients have predisposing personality–psychosocial characteristics that differ from one patient to the next and that can be exacerbated by the stress of coping with pain. There has been a resurgence in the evaluation of personality characteristics attendant to the realization that it is important to account for such factors to provide the most effective treatment of these patients. A major redirection has been to abandon the attempt to isolate a specific "pain-prone personality'' and instead to develop methods for assessing personality and coping characteristics in general. The object is to help treatment staff better understand specific characteristics and how they affect the pain treatment process. Part of the new direction has been to attempt to develop novel approaches to personality assessment. Several issues are beginning to receive more attention: Should a categorical approach or a dimensional approach to personality disorder assessment be used? What are the important factors that mediate the relationship between a personality characteristic and pain? Do specific clusters of personality characteristics predict response to treatment? These questions are stimulating exciting clinical research in the field. This text provides a comprehensive review of the advances in the field of personality and pain and highlights the important future directions of this field.

Our intention is to provide the most comprehensive information on the current understanding of how personality characteristics affect all aspects of pain and its management. The contributors were selected for their stature as respected clinical investigators in the field. The text has been written for specialists in applied pain assessment and management and for those involved in clinical pain research. As such, it should be of use not only to health care professionals but also to those who are receiving advanced training in undergraduate courses, graduate school, internships, and residencies. It will provide readers with practical approaches to important, everyday clinical concerns and issues that arise when dealing with the vagaries of personality and psychosocial issues displayed by patients experiencing pain.

Of course, a text of this type is not possible without the help of many talented people. All of the contributors were diligent in providing outstanding ''state-of-the-art'' chapters in a timely fashion. We thank the various reviewers of the chapters who graciously gave freely of their time and enhanced the quality of the chapters: Tim Ahles, Gerald Casenave, Cindy Claassen, Robert Dworkin, John Herman, Rod Hetzel, Francis Keefe, Erin Owen-Salters, Arthur Stone, Ray Tait, Sally Tarbell, and Robert Trestman. We also acknowledge the help and support we received from the American Psychological Association publications staff, particularly Susan Reynolds. Finally, once again, the timeliness in the preparation of the text for publication was greatly aided by the unselfish and professional efforts of Carol Gentry.

Personality Characteristics of
Patients With Pain

INTRODUCTION

Robert J. Gatchel and James N. Weisberg

As reviewed earlier (Gatchel, 1999), the search for an understanding of and ability to control pain has been a significant human pursuit since earliest recorded history. Descriptions of pain treatment have been found in Egyptian papyri dating back to 4000 B.C. In ancient China, almost 2000 years ago, acupuncture therapy was used for pain reduction. Temporomandibular joint disorder was recognized by Hippocrates (400–300 B.C.), who speculated about its origins and treatment. Hippocrates also proposed one of the earliest temperamental theories of personality. He posited that four bodily fluids (what he called *humors*)—blood, black bile, yellow bile, and phlegm—were responsible for specific personality or temperament types, as well as for various physical and mental illnesses. Galen (A.D. 130–200) elaborated on the four-humor theory by proposing specific associations between the humors and temperament: An excess of yellow bile was associated with a choleric temperament; an excess of black bile was associated with a melancholic personality; an excess of blood was associated with a sanguine personality; and an excess of phlegm was associated with a phlegmatic personality. Indeed, that theory was quite popular until only a few centuries ago, and it provides an excellent example of how physical and biological factors were viewed through the ages as significantly interacting with, and in fact, affecting the personality or psychological status.

This view of the potential interaction between the mind and body, however, began to be replaced with a more "dualistic" perspective during the Renaissance, when it became regarded as unscientific to view the mind (or the soul) as influencing the body. A new science emerged in which the body was explained by its own mechanisms. Such a viewpoint initiated a trend toward a *biomedical reductionist* approach, which argued that constructs such as the mind or soul were not needed to explain physical function or behavior. Indeed, in 1644, René Descartes (1596–1650) conceptualized pain as a specific type of activity in the sensory nervous system. He imagined the pain system as a "straight-through" channel from the skin directly to the brain. In his analogy, the pain system is like the bell-ringing mechanism in a church: If someone pulls the rope at the bottom of the tower, the bell rings at the top. He proposed, therefore, that a flame applied to the hand sets particles in the hand into activity, and that motion is transmitted up the arm and neck into the head, where it activates something like an alarm system. The individual feels the pain and responds to it. Descarte's purely deductive theory of pain physiology, although lacking any empirical evidence, unfortunately influenced the study and management of pain for the next few centuries.

As pointed out by Melzack and Wall (1965), a much more formal model of this pain process was proposed by von Frey in 1894, called the *specificity theory of pain*. This theory proposed that sensory receptors were responsible for the transmission of

---

The writing of this chapter was supported in part by National Institutes of Health grants R01 DE 10713 and K02 MH 01107 awarded to the first author.

specific sensations, such as pain, touch, pressure, and warmth, and the various receptors had different structures that made them sensitive to different types of stimulation. Thus, pain was perceived as having a specific central, as well as peripheral, set of mechanisms—similar to those that operate for other bodily senses.

At about the same time, Goldschneider was proposing an alternative perspective, called the *pattern theory of pain* (Melzack & Wall, 1965). Goldschneider posited that pain sensations were the result of transmission of nerve impulse *patterns* that were produced and coded at the peripheral stimulation site and that the differences in the patterning and quantity of peripheral nerve fiber discharges produced differences in the quality of sensation. Goldschneider's theory assumed that the experience of pain was the result of the central nervous system's coding of nerve impulse patterns and not simply the result of a specific connection between pain receptors and pain sites.

Although initially accepted by the scientific community, the above two theories were found insufficient to explain pain, even though there was some level of support proposed for each (Baum, Gatchel, & Krantz, 1997). More important, though, various reported findings could not be accounted for by either theory. The strict mechanistic, dualistic approach to medicine began to mellow somewhat because of the initial psychoanalytic work of Sigmund Freud (1856–1939) in Europe. Freud emphasized the potential interaction of psychological and physical factors in various disorders. This psychoanalytic or psychodynamic perspective also was applied to the area of pain. It should be noted that in their comprehensive review of psychodynamic psychotherapy with patients with chronic pain, Grzesiak, Ury, and Dworkin (1996) provided an insightful historical overview of psychodynamic themes that appear to be present in the experience of chronic pain. They noted that "over the years, a number of psychoanalytic theorists have addressed the problem of pain and suffering. It is well known that there is neither a unified theory of psychoanalysis nor a standard approach to conducting psychodynamic psychotherapy" (p. 155). They highlight the important psychodynamic themes that are useful to consider in the treatment of chronic pain. These include: (a) the significance of early developmental experiences influencing a patient's experience of pain and illness; (b) the empirically demonstrated association between childhood sexual and physical abuse experiences with chronic pain; (c) somatoform disorders, and abnormal illness behaviors; (d) unadmitted and unaccepted feelings of anger, helplessness, depression, and loss; (e) *alexithymia*—the inability to label or communicate effectively experiences commonly found in individuals with psychophysiological, addictive, or posttraumatic conditions; and (f) chronic pain and suffering viewed as punishment for past transgressions. Thus, in the psychoanalytic orientation, "We consider the phenomenon of pain as a crystallized dynamic conflict to be one of the most important of the psychodynamic themes that are relevant in psychotherapy with chronic pain patients" (Grzesiak et al., 1996, p. 161). This particular perspective is also advocated by Bellissimo and Tunks (1984). Of course, Freud (1895; 1966) hypothesized the symbolic significance of physical pain earlier. He stimulated much of the subsequent clinical interest in the psychosomatic underpinnings of pain.

Although there was a great deal of disenchantment with the psychoanalytic principles that were developed to explain pain, there was no doubt that psychological factors, such as anxiety, can significantly affect the pain experienced from a noxious stimulus. Bonica (1953) had pointed out the various shortcomings of both of the earlier purely mechanistic models of pain. Moreover, by the 1950s, the strict bio-medical reductionist and dualistic approaches began to lose popularity, being replaced by the growth and acceptance of an integrated, more holistic approach to health and illness. The trend toward a comprehensive *biopsychosocial* approach to illness that was occurring in medicine in general was paralleled by a similar approach to the understanding and treatment of pain. Beginning with the pioneering work of Beecher (1956), which demonstrated the importance of how the psychological state of a person can affect the perception of pain, numerous studies have shown the important role of psychological factors in pain perception (see Gatchel, 1999).

The next major theory to operate on the acceptance of the importance of a close interaction between psychological and physiological processes and pain was that of Melzack and Wall (1965), who introduced the *gate-control theory of pain*. This theory accounted for the many diverse factors involved in pain perception. Its major contribution was the introduction to the scientific community of the importance of central nervous system *and* psychological variables in the pain perception process. It highlighted the potentially significant role of psychosocial factors in the perception of pain (Melzack, 1993). It should be noted that the physiological processes involved in the gate-control model initially were challenged, and it was suggested that the model was incomplete (e.g., Nathan, 1976; Schmidt, 1972). As research accumulated after the original formulation of the model in 1965, particular aspects of the hypothesized mechanisms were disputed, and they required revision and reformulation (Nathan, 1976; Wall, 1989). For all that, the gate-control model has proved quite resilient in the face of recent scientific data and theoretical challenges, to the point that it still provides the most heuristic perspective of the wide range of pain phenomena encountered in medical settings today. A more refined model will evolve over time as understanding of pain neurophysiology, neurotransmission, and endogenous opioids increases.

The most current heuristic approach to pain is the biopsychosocial perspective, which assumes that pain is a complex, subjective phenomenon that consists of a host of factors, each of which can contribute to the interpretation of nociception as pain. Pain is experienced uniquely by each person. The complexity of pain is especially evident when it persists over time, as a range of psychological, social, and economic factors can interact with physical pathology to modulate a patient's report of pain and subsequent disability (Turk, 1996). Obviously, the biopsychosocial perspective of pain highlights the potentially significant role of psychosocial factors, including personality, in the pain perception process. As is reviewed in subsequent chapters, there is a great amount of research implicating the important role of personality in pain perception, which can have important clinical implications for treatment.

The remainder of this introduction is an overview of many of the topics and issues discussed in greater detail elsewhere in the text. As a starting point, we review evidence that highlights the importance of evaluating personality traits and disorders to more reliably predict the development of chronic pain. Trait and personality disorders have much to offer in this prediction process. We summarize the psychological tests and methods that can provide a reliable and standardized means of assessing personality traits and disorders in patients with pain. Such characteristics appear to significantly influence the course and treatment of chronic pain, and accounting for them is likely to improve pain treatment. We end this introduction with a discussion of the pros and cons of personality trait and disorder screening in early acute stages of pain.

MMPI "Pain Profile" Studies

As a result of the gradual acceptance of the gate-control theory of pain, copious research has attempted to isolate the psychological characteristics of patients with chronic pain. For example, the Minnesota Multiphasic Personality Inventory (MMPI) has been used widely to delineate these characteristics. In chapter 2 of this volume the author reviews much of this early clinical research. To summarize, the early work attempted to differentiate *functional* from *organic* pain. Among the earliest studies was one done by Hanvik (1951) in an evaluation of patients who were then considered to have either chronic pain with an organic cause or to have a functional pain disorder. We should point out that the earlier traditional biomedical reductionist view of pain assumed that every "real" report of pain originated from a specific physical, or organic, cause. If such a cause could not be found, then the pain was viewed as functional—the result primarily of psychological factors. Even though such an organic–functional distinction has, fortunately, been replaced with the more comprehensive biopsychosocial model (e.g., Turk, 1997), Hanvik's investigation provided the basis for numerous subsequent studies evaluating the psychological profiles of patients with chronic pain.

Hanvik isolated 25 items on the MMPI to differentiate the organically and functionally disordered groups. He pointed out that the functionally disordered group had elevations on Scales 1, 2, 3, 4, 7, and 8 (Hypochondriasis, Depression, Hysteria, Psychopathic Deviance, Psychosthenia, and Schizophrenia, respectively) and that the "Conversion V" pattern (1, 2, 3 elevated, with 2 lower than 1 and 3) was present. The organically disordered group displayed this Conversion V pattern as well, although to a lesser degree.

Further research has demonstrated inconsistency in replicating the initial results, and most investigations have been unable to support Hanvik's conclusions (e.g., McCreary, Turner, & Dawson, 1977; Sternbach, Wolf, Murphy, & Akeson, 1973). In the study by Sternbach and colleagues, the MMPI profiles of a group of patients with acute low back pain (pain present for less than 6 months) were compared with those of a group of patients with chronic low back pain (pain present for more than 6 months). Results indicated significant differences between the two groups on the first three clinical scales (Hypochondriasis, Depression, and Hysteria). The combined elevation of these three scales is often called the *neurotic triad* because it is commonly found in individuals with neurosis who are experiencing a great deal of anxiety. The results indicated that, during the early stages of pain, major psychological problems did not occur; however, as the pain became chronic, psychological changes were observed. The changes most likely resulted from the constant discomfort, despair, and preoccupation with pain that comes to dominate the lives of such patients. This can produce concurrent behavioral–psychological problems along with the original nociception, or tissue damage, itself.

Sternbach (1974) subsequently challenged the utility and validity of drawing a functional–organic dichotomy in assessing chronic pain. Rather, he viewed chronic pain as a complex psychophysiological behavior pattern that cannot be divided into distinct psychological and physical components. This perspective is embraced today, with the widely accepted biopsychosocial conceptualization of chronic pain (Engel, 1977; Turk, 1997).

It should be noted that, although there have been additional efforts to identify various "pain profiles" with the use of the MMPI, such studies have been strongly criticized (e.g., Main & Spanswick, 1995). As Gatchel and Epker (1999) have reviewed, results from such studies have been variable and inconsistent. One controversy attending the use of the MMPI with chronic pain populations is the frequent overlap of symptoms of a particular disorder and items on the MMPI. Positive responses to symptoms of a chronic pain disorder can lead to an erroneous estimate of psychopathology. For example, Pincus, Callahan, Bradley, Vaughn, and Wolfe (1987) isolated 5 items on the MMPI that reflect both the presence and the severity of rheumatoid arthritis. Each item codes on Scales 1 and 3 (Hypochondriasis and Hysteria, respectively), and 3 of them also code on Scale 2 (Depression). If positive responses to these 5 items are not included, the T scores for the 3 scales decline 4.10 points. Such findings in the population with rheumatoid arthritis suggest that similar confounding exists for other chronic pain populations.

Developmental Course of Chronic Pain

In the field of psychosomatic medicine, the search for specific personality and psychosocial factors that predispose individuals to problems with chronic pain has always been a major focus of attention. For example, clinical investigators have attempted to identify specific disorder personality types (such as the "migraine personality"), as well as a more general "pain-prone personality" (Blumer & Heilbronn, 1982). Overall, however, these efforts have received little empirical support and have been challenged extensively (e.g., Gatchel, 1991; Turk & Salovey, 1984). Indeed, part of the problem with attempts to uncover a "pain personality" is that patients with pain often present with a variety of problems that differ depending on the period during which they have been experiencing pain. For example, in the study by Sternbach and colleagues (1973), patients with chronic pain reported significantly more psychological distress—as evidenced by their higher elevations on the first three MMPI scales—than did patients with acute pain. Thus, early reports of pain are not associated with reports of major psychological distress. However, an increase in the duration of the pain often results in an increase in the report of psychological disturbance. These changes likely result from the sustained physical discomfort, emotional despair, and preoccupation with the pain that becomes a focus in these patients' lives.

Gatchel (1991, 1997) has proposed the occurrence of such changes along the developmental course of chronic pain. A three-stage model is proposed: Stage 1 is associated with emotional reactions such as fear, anxiety, and worry as a consequence of the perception of pain during the acute phase. Pain or hurt is usually associated with harm, so there is a natural emotional reaction to the potential for physical harm. If the pain persists past a reasonable acute period of time (2–4 months), this leads to the progression into Stage 2. This stage is associated with a wider array of behavioral–psychological reactions and problems, such as learned helplessness–depression, anger–distress, and somatization, that are the result of suffering with the now chronic nature of the pain. The hypothesis is that the form these problems take depends primarily on the premorbid or pre-existing personality–psychological characteristics of the individual, as well as on the patient's current socioeconomic–environmental conditions. Thus, for an individual with a premorbid problem with depression who is seriously affected economically by the loss of employment due to the pain and disability, depressive symptomatology will be greatly exacerbated during this stage. Similarly, an individual who had premorbid hypochondriacal characteristics, and who receives a large amount of secondary gain for remaining disabled, will most likely display a great deal of somatization and symptom magnification.

This model does *not* propose that there is a primary pre-existing "pain personality." It is assumed there is a general *nonspecificity* in terms of the relationship between personality–psychological problems and pain. This is in keeping with research that has found no such consistent personality syndrome. Moreover, even though there is a relationship usually found between pain and specific psychological problems, such as depression (Romano & Turner, 1985), the nature of the relationship between the two variables remains inconclusive. Some, but not all, patients develop depression secondary to chronic pain. Others show depression as the primary syndrome, of which pain is a symptom. In addition, the factors that mediate the relationship between the two are largely undefined (Turk & Rudy, 1988). In the present model, it is assumed that patients bring with them predisposing personalities and psychological characteristics, which differ from one patient to the next, and that the characteristics are exacerbated by the stress of attempting to cope with the chronic pain. Indeed, the relationship between stress and exacerbation of mental health problems has been documented (Barrett, Rose, & Klerman, 1979).

This conceptual model proposes that the persistence of behavioral–psychological problems leads to progression into Stage 3, which can be viewed as the acceptance or adoption of a "sick role," which excuses patients from normal responsibilities and social obligations. This can become a potent reinforcer for not becoming "healthy." The medical and psychological "disabilities" or "abnormal illness behaviors" (Pilowsky, 1978) are consolidated during this phase. Moreover, if compensation issues are present, these too can serve as a disincentive for becoming well again because compensation is a critical factor in the persistence of disabilities (Beals, 1984). Interacting with the above stages is the physical *deconditioning syndrome* (Mayer & Gatchel, 1988), which is manifested as a significant decrease in physical capacity (strength, flexibility, and endurance) attendant to the disuse and resultant atrophy of the injured area. There is usually a complex interactive process between the physical deconditioning and the three stages. For example, physical deconditioning can "feed back" to reduce emotional well-being and self-esteem (Gatchel, 1988; Gatchel, Baum, & Krantz, 1988). This can lead to further psychological sequel. Conversely, negative emotional reactions, such as depression, can significantly feed back to physical functioning by, for example, decreasing the motivation to get involved in work or recreational activities and thereby further contribute to physical deconditioning.

On the other side, attempts to find a purely physiological basis for chronic pain have not yet met with success. Even though there have been advances in our knowledge of sensory physiology, biochemistry, and anatomy, as well as the development of potent analgesic medications and other innovative surgical and medical interventions, pain relief remains elusive for many patients. Yet the search continues. Hopkin (1997) provides a review of how research on pain mechanisms and pathways has continued to expand over the past few years. Such research could help explain how the nervous system senses, interprets, and responds to pain. It is not likely, however, that a completely effective pain management program could be developed solely on the basis of a better understanding of the physiological bases of pain. There is still a great deal of basic research being done to find the "magic bullet" medication or an underlying physiological mechanism that could be modified. And even if such a cure were found, there is still the probability that there would be individual differences in response to a new medication or procedure along with variations in side effects and the like. So the need for a comprehensive pain management program will still be important.

As an example of how a variety of psychosocial factors must be considered in the equation, a study by Gatchel, Polatin, and Mayer (1995), found that the best predictor of patients with acute low back pain who subsequently developed chronic pain disability consisted of a *psychosocial disability factor.* The factor included the interaction of self-reported pain and disability, a high score on the MMPI Hysteria scale, gender, and workers' compensation–personal injury insurance status. They found no significant differences between patients who developed chronic pain (defined as preventing them from returning to work at 1 year) and those who did not develop chronic pain (able to return to work at 1 year) on physician ratings of the severity of the initial back injury or in the physical demands of the patients' jobs. Such results again highlight the fact that chronic pain disability reflects not only the presence of some physical symptomatology, but that personality–psychosocial characteristics contribute significantly in the identification of injured workers who could develop chronic low back pain disability. In fact, some investigators argue that only a very small amount of the total disability phenomenon in someone complaining of back pain can be attributed to physical impairment (Waddell, Main, & Morris, 1984). Physical findings, such as radiographic results, have not been found to be reliable indicators of low back pain (Mayer & Gatchel, 1988). Most cases of low back pain are ill defined and physically unverifiable—often classified as "soft-tissue injuries" that cannot be visualized or confirmed on physical examination. Even the correlation between radiography-documented disk-space narrowing and disk-rupture level in proven disk herniation is less than 50% (Pope, Frymoyer, & Anderson, 1984). Moreover, in a well-controlled magnetic resonance imaging study by Jensen, Brant-Zawadzki, Obuchowski, et al. (1994), significant spinal abnormalities were found in patients who were not experiencing back pain.

Thus, when viewed individually, clinical, physiological, and radiographic findings alone have not been good indicators of chronic pain or predictors of the development of chronic pain. Again, such findings highlight the importance of assuming the more heuristic biopsychosocial perspective of chronic pain in which a clinician must be astute enough to account for the unique interactions of these different variables to develop an accurate and comprehensive understanding of a patient with chronic pain. This, of course, does not rule out the importance of individually assessing each of these and other factors. However, it does imply that one should view each finding as a separate piece of the puzzle that must be considered in the context of the whole picture for *each* patient (Figure 1). The

Patient 1

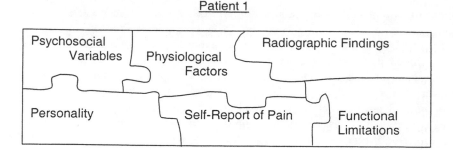

Patient 2

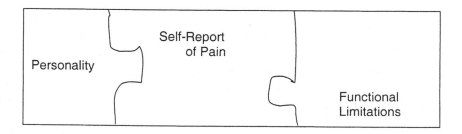

Patient 3

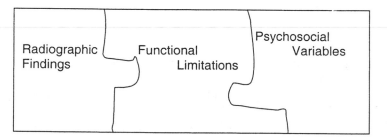

Figure 1.   The various pieces of the pain puzzle that must be considered for different pain patients.

ability to identify the complete picture from one piece of the puzzle is largely an impossibility for clinicians who work with the great percentage of patients who experience chronic pain. It is necessary to integrate all of the pieces of the puzzle to treat chronic pain. Unfortunately, this takes time and patience, and there is a paucity of data to support the well-accepted contention that all must be accounted for, not only in treatment, but in preventing acute pain from developing into a chronic pain disability. In chapter 11 of this volume the author proposes a method to help practitioners to better evaluate the pieces of the puzzle, including personality, to best manage patients with chronic pain.

Prospective Prediction of the Development of Chronic Pain

We turn now to the important question of whether one can predict which patients with pain are at greater risk for developing chronicity. Although personality factors have always been assumed to be important, an understanding of the temporal–causal relationship between pain and personality remains undiscovered. Gatchel and Epker (1999) provide a review of this issue. One approach to examining the influence of personality on the development of chronic pain involves a prospective evaluation of personality traits and disorders and in following individual patients longitudinally to observe which of them develop chronic pain. Most studies in this area have focused on the MMPI to predict the outcome of conservative treatment or invasive intervention. As of this writing, only a few prospective studies have been conducted, presumably because of the large number of participants needed for an initial evaluation to obtain a sample group that is large enough to provide statistically significant or clinically meaningful data.

Prospective MMPI Studies to Predict Chronic Pain

Bigos and colleagues (1991) collected a variety of physical and psychosocial measures (including the MMPI) from more than 3000 employees at a Boeing aircraft manufacturing plant. Two-hundred-seventy-nine of these employees developed acute back problems during the 4-year study period. Overall, MMPI score elevations were lower than those found in studies of patients with chronic pain. Individuals who scored in the upper quintile on the Hypochondriasis scale were two times more likely to develop back pain than were individuals with the lowest scores on the same scale. Additionally, the Psychopathic Deviant and Schizophrenia scales, as well as Hanvik's Low Back scale (Hanvik, 1951), differentiated those who developed acute low back pain from those who did not.

In another predictive study, Hansen, Biering-Sorensen, and Schroll (1995) administered the MMPI to 397 Danish men and women at ages 50 and 60 and asked questions about the presence or absence of back pain during each subsequent 10-year interval (50–60 years and 60–70 years). Results indicated that MMPI scale elevations on the Hypochondriasis, Depression, and Hysteria scales at ages 50 and 60 were associated with low back pain during the subsequent decade. In addition, elevated MMPI scores at age 60 were associated with back pain from age 50 to 60. Although there were several methodology problems, the results are interesting in that they suggest a relationship between specific personality traits and the development of pain complaints (Weisberg & Keefe, 1997). Unfortunately, there was no attempt to document or control for the participants' physical status. Patients having more physical findings might simply be more prone to focus on their somatic complaints. Second, the researchers did not try to explain observed changes in the MMPI over time in the sample. Thus, the study does not provide a definitive test of which came first, the back pain or the MMPI elevations. Most important, although the MMPI scores of patients with low back pain were statistically significantly higher than were those of patients without back pain, the scores were still within the normative range ($T < 70$) and therefore not clinically significant.

If we consider the lack of prospective MMPI studies, we ought to be surprised to find any that have used structured clinical interviews to assess both clinical psychopathology (Axis I) and personality disorders (Axis II) of the Diagnostic and Statistical Manual of Mental Disorders (DSM-IV, 4th ed.; American Psychiatric Association, 1994). The study described below used the Structured Clinical Interview for *DSM-III-R* (SCID and SCID II; Spitzer, Williams, Gibbons, & First, 1988).

Prospective Studies Using Personality Disorder Interviews to Predict Chronic Pain

Gatchel and colleagues (1995) systematically compared the ability of the MMPI, the SCID (Axis I), and the SCID II (Axis II) (Spitzer et al., 1988) to predict subsequent pain and disability status of patients with low back pain. Four-hundred-twenty-one patients were recruited within 6 weeks of pain onset and were administered a variety of tests, including those listed above. All of the patients were contacted at a 1-year follow-up, at which time their job status was classified as working–in school, not working due to pain, or not working–unrelated to pain. Data analyses determined the degree to which scores on the MMPI and SCID measures predicted disability at follow-up. Patients who initially scored higher on the MMPI Hysteria scale were much more likely to be disabled from work than were patients who scored low on this scale. Other predictors related to treatment outcome included gender, presence of workers' compensation or personal injury claim, and initial score on a pain and disability measure. Regression analyses revealed that the MMPI scores combined with these other predictors correctly classified outcome for more than 90% of patients treated. Gatchel and colleagues (1995) found that major psychopathology, such as depression and substance abuse, did not precede disability, but that it developed after pain became chronic. Although this study did not report the SCID II results on personality disorders, it is important because it supports other research that the chronicity of pain disability results in Axis I psychopathology (depression and anxiety), rather than the psychopathology causing the chronic pain disability. As a result, Gatchel and colleagues point out the need for early psychosocial intervention to prevent disability from occurring. They also encourage further study to determine the specific emotional and psychosocial events that follow injury that can result in chronic disability (Gatchel et al., 1995).

Personality Measures to Predict Treatment Response

Gatchel and Epker (1999) provide a comprehensive review of studies evaluating various psychosocial variables that could be used to predict response to a range of pain management treatments, including invasive procedures, conservative approaches, and multidisciplinary pain treatment programs. In this section, we focus primarily on those personality factors.

MMPI Studies

Several studies have examined whether standardized psychological tests can predict the outcome of both conservative and invasive pain treatments. Several *retrospective* studies have used the MMPI to predict the outcome of low back surgery (McCreary, Turner, & Dawson, 1979; Waring, Weisz, & Bailey, 1976; Wiltse & Rocchio, 1975) or multidisciplinary pain management programs (Moore, Armentrout, Parker, & Kivlahan, 1986).

Wiltse and Rocchio (1975) used the MMPI and other tests to determine whether they could differentiate between patients who reported pain relief after surgical intervention and those who had no symptom relief. The study's participants were 130 patients undergoing a surgical intervention that consisted of chemonucleolysis (chemical ablation of a displaced [herniated] disk). High scores ($T > 75$) on the MMPI Hysteria and Hypochondriasis scales predicted poorer surgical outcome than did scores within the normative range, 30–70. Waring and colleagues (1976) used the MMPI to evaluate 34 patients with low back pain who had been admitted to a hospital for surgical treatment. The MMPI was not predictive of surgical outcome. In fact, for patients who had a successful treatment outcome, T-scores resembled a Conversion V in pattern, but not in magnitude, of scale elevations. Surgeons' preoperative ratings of patients' physical findings and emotional readiness for surgery were the best predictors of outcome.

McCreary and colleagues (1979) conducted a retrospective study in which they examined MMPI clinical scales and the Low Back scale (Hanvik, 1951) after completion of a conservative pain management program. Patients who scored low on the Hypochondriasis scale were more likely to show improvement in two of three outcome measures (pain intensity and ability to resume activities). Patients who scored higher on the Depression scale also were more likely to have pain (pain intensity) at follow-up. There were no significant differences on the Hysteria scale with respect to any of the outcome measures. The Low Back scale discriminated those who were more likely to report pain relief and return to normal activities from those less likely to report a good outcome for the same variables.

Moore and colleagues (1986) administered the MMPI (among other tests) to 57 patients before admission to an inpatient multidisciplinary pain program and after completion of the program. In a subset of 32 patients, the MMPI also was given between 2 and 5 months before admission. All patients were men with chronic pain who were being treated at a Veterans Administration hospital. Treatment included physical and occupational therapy, cognitive–behavioral pain management, and medication withdrawal. In addition to the MMPI, outcome measures included pain severity, daily activities, mood, sleep, and sexual function. There was a nonsignificant increase in most MMPI scales from baseline to admission. This finding provided some support for the ideas that the period in which an individual is assessed affects the degree of psychopathology and that, untreated, psychological dysfunction increases over time. Moreover, the authors reported significant decreases in many MMPI scales, including Frequency, Hypochondriasis, Depression, Hysteria, Psychopathic deviate, Masculine–Feminine, Paranoia, Psychasthena, and Schizophrenia. The improvements appear to be nonspecific, however. A cluster analysis of previously identified MMPI subgroups (Bradley, Prokop, Margolis, & Gentry, 1978) revealed no significant differences in treatment outcome between the subgroups (Moore et al., 1986).

Based on the overall lack of significant differences between both empirically and clinically derived MMPI subgroups, Chapman and Pemberton (1994) attempted to evaluate differences in treatment outcome for seven subgroups derived from previously identified profiles found in MMPI interpretation manuals. Their participants were 122 men and women who participated in a 6–10-week outpatient or 2-week inpatient multidisciplinary pain program. In addition to conservative treatments— including medication withdrawal; physical, vocational, and occupational therapy; and multiple components of cognitive–behavioral pain management—patients underwent a series of lumbar sympathetic nerve blocks. There was little overall utility of the MMPI to predict treatment outcome. However, participants with either a normal MMPI profile or mild elevations ($T = 71-80$) on the Hysteria and Hypochondriasis scales reported less pain at follow-up than did participants with higher MMPI scale elevations ($T > 80$) on the same scales. The authors report no differences between those who attended the inpatient program and those who attended as outpatients. They do warn clinicians against making treatment predictions based on MMPI findings at admission, and they reinforce the need for those who work with pain patients to consider the wide array of biological, psychological, and social influences on treatment outcome.

Structured Interviews to Predict Treatment Response

In an investigation of clinical and personality disorders, Gatchel, Polatin, Mayer, and Garcy (1994) compared pretreatment SCID and SCID II diagnoses (Spitzer et al., 1988) of 152 patients who returned to work with those of patients who failed to return to work after a functional restoration program. Consistent with other studies (Fishbain, Goldberg, Meagher, Steele, & Rosomoff, 1986; Polatin, Kinney, Gatchel, Lillo, & Mayer, 1993), 58% of patients met criteria for an Axis II personality disorder. The personality disorders found most commonly in each group were paranoid personality disorder, passive–aggressive personality disorder, and borderline personality disorder. There were no significant differences between the returning and nonreturning groups on any of the personality disorders. More important, there were no significant differences in the prevalence of either Axis I or Axis II disorders between patients who successfully returned to work and those who did not.

The authors believe this study demonstrates that, if treatment addresses clinical psychiatric symptoms and personality issues alike, psychopathology need not interfere with successful outcome and return to work. Therefore, although this is just one study that has examined personality disorders as a predictor of returning to work, a few facts are important to bear in mind. First, further studies are certainly needed to corroborate or refute these findings. Second, return to work is just one measure of outcome, albeit an important one. There might have been differences in other outcome measures between persons with or without personality disorders. Last, and most important, as mentioned by the authors, it could be because personality disorders were diagnosed at the start of a rehabilitation program that patients received treatment that incorporated their personality issues. Without a personality disorder diagnosis at the beginning of treatment, this potentially important variable could have been overlooked and gone unaccounted for in treatment.

Future Directions

Both the trait and the personality disorder approaches have much to offer the field of chronic pain research. Future studies should compare personality traits in patients with chronic pain who have different personality diagnoses. Research also should compare the degree to which personality diagnosis and personality trait measures are useful in elucidating measures of pain and adjustment in chronic pain populations. These issues are discussed in chapter 12 of this volume.

Psychological tests can provide a reliable and standardized way to assess personality traits in patients with chronic pain. Of the several psychological tests applied, the MMPI has been the most widely used. Descriptive studies using the MMPI have identified common profile subtypes with diverse populations of patients who have chronic pain. Although there is a large body of research in the topic, debate continues as to the test's predictive utility.

Two factors, in particular, contribute to the discussion. First, results of predictive studies of personality traits in patients with chronic pain have been inconsistent. Although some have found a relationship between personality traits (hypochondriasis, hysteria, and depression) and treatment outcome, other studies have not found evidence for such relationships. Second, concerns have been expressed that patients who have physical findings that result from underlying disease or injury can appear to be neurotic on the MMPI because they score high on items measuring somatic focus (e.g., items on the Hysteria and Hypochondriasis scales) (Love & Peck, 1987).

Several conclusions can be drawn from our review of the literature. First, the assessment of personality can be useful in identifying personality traits and personality disorders that could influence the course and treatment of chronic pain. Pain treatment programs are likely to improve outcomes when they account for individual personality differences in treatment decisions. Second, personality disorders occur at a higher rate in the chronic pain population than in the population at large. It has long been observed that patients with chronic pain have psychiatric comorbidity that includes clinical symptoms, such as depression and anxiety, and personality traits and disorders; however, a causal relationship between personality traits or disorders and chronic pain has yet to be established. Many scholars and researchers have posited that some personality traits, such as histrionic, dependent, and depressive, predispose an individual to the development of chronic pain disorders. More recently, however, there is increasing evidence that the occurrence of an acute episode of pain and the resulting physical, emotional, and psychosocial consequences could account for various forms of psychopathology often observed in the chronic pain population. These diagnoses include the depressive and anxiety disorders on Axis I and the high rate of personality disorders on Axis II—most commonly, the dependent, histrionic, and passive–aggressive personality disorders.

Although it is incompatible with the concept of a "long-standing, lifelong pattern" required for the *DSM* diagnosis of personality disorders, Weisberg and Keefe (1997) propose elsewhere a diathesis–stress model of personality disorders in chronic pain. In this model, traits that normally are controlled by an individual's defensive structure become exacerbated by the stress of acute pain and subsequent psychosocial stressors and, when poorly managed, can result in a personality disorder. One study (Vittengl, Clark, Owen-Salter, & Gatchel, 1999) appears to support the Weisberg and Keefe diathesis–stress model.

Vittengl and colleagues (1999) reported dimensional personality characteristics and categorical personality disorders (*DSM-III-R*) in patients with chronic pain (*n* = 125) and control patients (*n* = 75). A subset (*n* = 56) was assessed both before and 6 months after treatment in a functional restoration program. Measures included the MMPI, SCID II, and the Schedule for Nonadaptive and Adaptive Personality (SNAP: Clark, 1993), a 375-item, multiple-choice instrument that assesses 3 temperament dimensions and 12 personality dimensions (see Vittengl et al., 1999). Results of the SCID II were similar to results from other structured-interview studies. Compared with the control group, the patients with chronic pain demonstrated a higher frequency of 8 personality disorders (paranoid, schizotypal, narcissistic, borderline, avoidant, dependent, passive–aggressive, and self-defeating). In the subset of patients assessed before and after treatment, paranoid, obsessive–compulsive, passive–aggressive, and self-defeating personality disorders decreased significantly from their pretreatment diagnoses. Overall, the results of Vittengl's group demonstrate greater stability of dimensional personality traits before to after treatment (MMPI and SNAP) than of categorical personality disorders assessed with the SCID II. The authors cite regression to the mean and the "arbitrary nature" of diagnostic cutting points inherent in categorical diagnoses as possible explanations for the differences seen before and after treatment. A third explanation, not cited by the authors, is that of our previously hypothesized diathesis–stress model of personality disorders (Weisberg & Keefe, 1997). After treatment that has as its primary goals increased function and coping, stress likely decreases, and individuals who met criteria for personality disorders before treatment continue to have similar traits, although not to the extent required for a categorical diagnosis. Only large-scale, prospective studies similar to that of Bigos and Battie (1987) will shed light on the causal nature of these difficult conditions.

Personality Disorder Screening in the Early Stages of Pain: Pros and Cons

Pain treatment professionals must be astutely aware that, when evaluating pain patients, especially those with acute pain, there are practical drawbacks to the assessment process. The tests are often time-consuming and can be disturbing for patients to complete, and the psychological assessment often reinforces patients' convictions that their physicians believe their pain is imaginary. An effort must be made to convince patients that the reason they are asked to take a particular assessment battery is to provide an overall picture of general psychophysiological functioning, not to label them with any particular mental disorder. There is a pervasive misperception regarding psychological evaluation—and about psychologists in general—that has developed because so many patients in the past were told their pain was not real. It is imperative that patients be educated about the role of psychological assessment services in any treatment program. (Chapter 11 in this volume reviews the practical issues of personality assessment.)

We note here that we find it useful to use the term *behavioral medicine evaluation* instead of *psychological evaluation* in our first encounters with patients. This helps defuse some of the misperceptions about the evaluation process, and it can reinforce to patients the medical nature of the assessment. We emphasize with our patients that one reason for the behavioral medicine evaluation is that, as with treatment of any chronic medical condition, various pain syndromes can lead to pressures and changes of lifestyle that most people find unpleasant, at the very least. Unplanned and unwanted lifestyle changes can lead to stress, so patients feel worse than they ever anticipated, and the stress actually can interfere with physical recovery. We explain this in terms of a cycle in which pain and the changes it brings lead to stress, which leads to increased pain, which leads to increased stress, and so on. This "pain–stress cycle" is then pointed out to the patients as important to deal with (see Figure 2). We also explain that the behavioral medicine evaluation focuses on stress-related issues that are intertwined with the actual pain problem. Of course, for ethical reasons, we must then reveal that the evaluation involves the assessment of psychological issues that are related to pain. By this time, though, the preparation of patients makes them less resistant to the idea of having a psychological evaluation.

We also try to avoid using the terms *psychological problems* and *psychopathology* whenever possible. Rather, we use the terms *stress, behavioral medicine,* and so on, which have more neutral connotations. Most patients are relieved when these terms are used, and consequently they are more open to the evaluation process. Indeed, the lay public is generally familiar with the notion of stress and does not interpret it with any negative psychiatric connotations. Thus, in presenting the evaluation as means to assess stress factors that could be interacting with their pain, patients are frequently quite receptive and understanding of the purpose. Therefore, a great deal of education of the patient is needed before the psychological assessment to reduce resistance to undergoing such an evaluation.

A focus on the "somatic" aspects of the evaluation such as the psychophysiological evaluation (biofeedback) if conducted, and on the role of stress and its physiological counterpart, tension, in pain perception, usually helps patients to engage in the evaluation process more easily. As presented in chapter 12 of this volume, a stepwise approach to evaluation is recommended, in which the administration of each new assessment battery is predicated on the results of the previous assessment

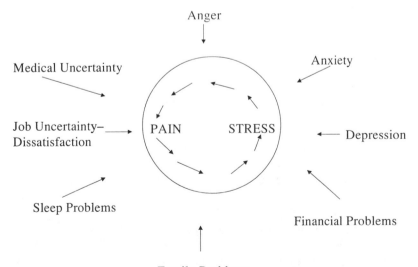

Figure 2. The pain–stress cycle, emphasizing the interaction of stress-related issues and the actual pain problem. It is helpful to draw patients' attention to this cycle.

test. In this way, the patient is not completely overwhelmed by a massive amount of psychological tests.

One important positive aspect of personality disorder screening in the early stages of pain is the potential for preventing the development of a chronic pain disability. Indeed, early detection to prevent chronic disorders is now recognized as a high-priority clinical research area (Human Capital Coordinating Committee, 1996). As Linton and Bradley (1996) have cogently pointed out, although cost reduction is often used as an argument for early intervention programs, there has been a paucity of adequate analyses reported in the literature. Goossens and Evers (1997) have similarly noted this paucity in the area of low back pain. However, the few studies that have been reported clearly suggest such savings (as cited by Linton & Bradley, 1996).

Mitchell and Carmen (1990) presented preliminary findings from a multicenter trial (involving more than 3000 patients with acute soft-tissue and back injuries). Two groups of patients were compared: those who received early intensive intervention and those who received standard treatments at other facilities. During a 5-month follow-up, it was found that there was a savings each month of roughly $1 million to $1.5 million in lost wages and health care costs. In a follow-up evaluation of 542 patients, Mitchell and Carmen (1994) found that the early intensive intervention produced projected savings of $5000 per patient. Linton and Bradley (1992) also report cost savings of an early intensive intervention with back pain patients. As Linton and Bradley (1996) concluded in their review of the literature, the current data suggest that it is possible to prevent the development of chronic disability:

> However, if this goal is to be met, we need to continue to make bold attempts—both clinically and scientifically—to provide effective secondary prevention measures. Research to date has provided a very good beginning, but the details have yet to be worked out. If the promise of prevention is to be fully realized, these details are urgently needed. (p. 454)

Summary and Conclusions

This introduction to the text highlights the importance of evaluating personality traits and disorders to more reliably predict the development of chronic pain and to influence its course and treatment. Such an evaluation provides an important missing link in establishing the most valid and comprehensive assessment–treatment methods for patients who are disabled by pain. As noted, there is no unequivocal evidence for the perspective that there is a primary, pre-existing "pain-prone personality." Rather, the assessment of personality can be useful in identifying various traits and disorders that can significantly affect the course and treatment of chronic pain. Pain treatment programs are likely to improve outcomes when they account for various individual personality differences presented by patients.

Traditional psychological tests, such as the MMPI (now the MMPI-2), can provide a reliable, standardized way to assess personality traits in patients with chronic pain. Various other such tests are reviewed in the text. Recent data suggest that there is more stability to be had from a dimensional approach to assessing personality traits (by the use of the MMPI and the SNAP, for example) than can be offered by a categorical approach (such as that provided by the SCID).

As noted in the Preface, there is growing interest in the role of psychosocial and personality factors in the experience of and adaptation to pain. The goal of this volume is to provide readers with comprehensive information that will support their understanding of the way personality characteristics affect all aspects of pain and its management.

The text is organized into four parts. Part I provides a review of the earliest attempts to elucidate the function of psychosocial–personality factors in the pain process—psychoanalytic perspectives and the early years of psychometric testing, especially the use of the MMPI. The encouraging findings of these early attempts subsequently led to major advances in the personality testing of patients with chronic pain. These are covered in Part II. Part III highlights some nonpathological factors associated with pain perception and treatment outcome (such as locus of control, extraversion–introversion, perceived optimism, and coping strategies). Part IV is a discussion of more specific areas of personality disorders in chronic pain and their clinical implications. It concludes with a summary and a look into the future of the area of personality and pain.

Even though each chapter reviews one or two specific personality assessments or constructs, it is worth pointing out that one must avoid the overly simplistic viewpoint that there is a single, simple measure of personality that can capture important characteristics of all patients with pain. Rather, each patient is unique, and health care professionals should administer the best array of tests to best elucidate a patient's personality characteristics and their effects on pain expression and management.

Almost two decades ago, in commenting about the field of personality psychology, I stated

> The task of understanding personality and predicting [is] very complex. Many variables—person, situation, their interaction, the type of data collected—have to be simultaneously considered. If the field of personality psychology is to advance, such complexity will have to be embraced and dealt with. (Gatchel & Mears, 1982, p. 489)

This is still true today, especially in the area of identifying the personality characteristics of patients with pain.

References

American Psychiatric Association. (1994). *Diagnostic and statistical manual of mental disorders* (4th ed.). Washington, DC: Author.

Barrett, J. F., Rose, R. M., & Klerman, G. L. (Eds.). (1979). *Stress and mental disorder*. New York: Raven Press.

Baum, A., Gatchel, R. J., & Krantz, D. (1997). *An introduction to health psychology* (3rd ed.). New York: McGraw-Hill.

Beals, R. (1984). Compensation and recovery from injury. *Western Journal of Medicine, 140,* 233–237.

Beecher, H. K. (1956). Relationship of significance of wound to the pain experienced. *Journal of the American Medical Association, 161,* 1609–1613.

Bellissimo, A., & Tunks, E. (1984). *Chronic pain: The psychotherapeutic spectrum*. New York: Praeger.

Bigos, S. J., & Battie, M. C. (1987). Acute care to prevent back disability. Ten years of progress. *Clinical Orthopaedics & Related Research, 221,* 121–130.

Bigos, S. J., Battie, M. C., Spengler, D. M., Fisher, L. D., Fordyce, W. E., Hansson, T. H., Nachemson, A. L., & Wortley, M. D. (1991). A prospective study of work perceptions and psychosocial factors affecting the report of back injury. *Spine, 16*(1), 1–6.

Blumer, D., & Heilbronn, M. (1982). Chronic pain as a variant of depressive disease: The pain-prone disorder. *Journal of Nervous and Mental Disease, 170,* 381–406.

Bonica, J. J. (1953). *The management of pain.* Philadelphia: Lea & Febiger.

Bradley, L. A., Prokop, C. K., Margolis, R., & Gentry, W. D. (1978). Multivariate analyses of the MMPI profiles of low back pain patients. *Journal of Behavioral Medicine, 1,* 253–272.

Chapman, S., & Pemberton, J. (1994). Prediction of treatment outcome from clinically derived MMPI clusters in rehabilitation for low back pain. *Clinical Journal of Pain, 10,* 267–276.

Clark, L. A. (1993). *Schedule for nonadaptive and adaptive personality and its disorders.* Dallas: Author.

Engel, G. L. (1977). The need for a new medical model: A challenge for biomedicine. *Science, 196*(4286), 129–136.

Fishbain, D. A., Goldberg, M., Meagher, B. R., Steele, R., & Rosomoff, H. (1986). Male and female chronic pain patients categorized by DSM-III psychiatric diagnostic criteria. *Pain, 26,* 181–197.

Freud, S. (1966). Project for a scientific psychology. In J. Strachey (Ed. and Trans.), *The standard edition of the complete psychological works of Sigmund Freud* (Vol. 1, pp. 281–397). London: Hogarth Press. (Original work published 1895)

Gatchel, R. J. (1988). Clinical effectiveness of biofeedback in reducing anxiety. In H. L. Wagner (Ed.), *Social psychophysiology and emotion* (pp. 197–210). Chichester, England: Wiley & Sons.

Gatchel, R. J. (1991). Early development of physical and mental deconditioning in painful spinal disorders. In T. G. Mayer, V. Mooney, & R. J. Gatchel (Eds.), *Contemporary conservative care for painful spinal disorders* (pp. 278–289). Philadelphia: Lea & Febiger.

Gatchel, R. J. (1997). Biofeedback. In A. Baum, C. McManus, S. Newman, J. Weinman, & R. West (Eds.), *Cambridge handbook of psychology, health and medicine* (pp. 197–199). London: Cambridge University Press.

Gatchel, R. J. (1999). Perspectives on pain: A historical overview. In R. J. Gatchel & D. C. Turk (Eds.), *Psychosocial factors in pain: Critical perspectives* (pp. 3–17). New York: Guilford Press.

Gatchel, R. J., Baum, A., & Krantz, D. (1988). *Introduction to health psychology* (2nd ed.). New York: McGraw-Hill.

Gatchel, R. J., & Epker, J. T. (1999). Psychosocial predictors of chronic pain and response to treatment. In R. J. Gatchel & D. C. Turk (Eds.), *Psychosocial factors in pain: Critical perspectives* (pp. 412–434). New York: Guilford Press.

Gatchel, R. J., & Mears, F. (1982). *Personality: Theory, assessment, and research.* New York: St. Martin's Press.

Gatchel, R. J., Polatin, P. B., & Mayer, T. G. (1995). The dominant role of psychosocial risk factors in the development of chronic low back pain disability. *Spine, 20*(24), 2702–2709.

Gatchel, R., Polatin, P., Mayer, T., & Garcy, P. (1994). Psychopathology and the rehabilitation of patients with chronic low back pain disability. *Archives of Physical Medicine and Rehabilitation, 75,* 666–670.

Goossens, M. E. J. B., & Evers, S. M. A. A. (1997). Economic evaluation of back pain interventions. *Journal of Occupational Rehabilitation, 7,* 15–32.

Grzesiak, R. C., Ury, G. M., & Dworkin, R. H. (1996). Psychodynamic psychotherapy with chronic pain patients. In R. J. Gatchel & D. C. Turk (Eds.), *Psychological approaches to pain management* (pp. 148–178). New York: Guilford Press.

Hansen, F. R., Biering-Sorensen, F., & Schroll, M. (1995). Minnesota Multiphasic Personality Inventory profiles in persons with or without low back pain: A 20-year follow-up study. *Spine, 20*(24), 2716–2720.

Hanvik, L. J. (1951). MMPI profiles in patients with low back pain. *Journal of Consulting Psychology, 15,* 350–353.

Hopkin, K. (1997). Show me where it hurts: Tracing the pathways of pain. *Journal of NIH Research, 9,* 37–43.

Human Capital Coordinating Committee. (1996). *Doing the right thing: A research plan for healthy living.* Washington, DC: American Psychological Association.

Jensen, M. C., Brant-Zawadzki, M. N., Obuchowski, N., Modic, M. T., Malkasian, D., & Ross, J. S. (1994). Magnetic resonance imaging of the lumbar spine in people without back pain. *New England Journal of Medicine, 331,* 69–73.

Linton, S. J., & Bradley, L. A. (1992). An 18-month follow-up of a secondary prevention program for back pain: Help and hindrance factors related to outcome maintenance. *Clinical Journal of Pain, 8,* 227–236.

Linton, S. J., & Bradley, L. A. (1996). Strategies for the prevention of chronic pain. In R. J. Gatchel & D. C. Turk (Eds.), *Psychological approaches to pain management: A practitioner's handbook* (pp. 438–457). New York: Guilford Press.

Love, A., & Peck, C. (1987). The MMPI and psychological factors in chronic low back pain: A review. *Pain, 28,* 1–12.

Main, C. J., & Spanswick, C. C. (1995). Personality assessment and the Minnesota Multiphasic Personality Inventory: 50 years on: Do we still need our security blanket? *Pain Forum, 4,* 90–96.

Mayer, T. G., & Gatchel, R. J. (1988). *Functional restoration for spinal disorders: The sports medicine approach.* Philadelphia: Lea & Febiger.

McCreary, C., Turner, J., & Dawson, E. (1977). Differences between functional versus organic low back pain patients. *Pain, 4,* 73–78.

McCreary, C., Turner, J., & Dawson, E. (1979). The MMPI as a predictor of response to conservative treatment for low back pain. *Journal of Clinical Psychology, 35*(2), 278–284.

Melzack, R. (1993). Pain: Past, present and future. *Canadian Journal of Experimental Psychology, 47*(4), 615–629.

Melzack, R., & Wall, P. D. (1965). Pain mechanisms: A new theory. *Science, 50,* 971–979.

Mitchell, R. I., & Carmen, G. M. (1990). Results of a multicenter trial using an intensive active exercise program for the treatment of acute soft tissue and back injuries. *Spine, 15,* 514–521.

Mitchell, R. I., & Carmen, G. M. (1994). The functional restoration approach to the treatment of chronic pain in patients with soft tissue and back injuries. *Spine, 19,* 633–642.

Moore, J., Armentrout, D., Parker, J., & Kivlahan, D. (1986). Empirically derived pain-patient MMPI subgroups: Prediction of treatment outcome. *Journal of Behavioral Medicine, 9*(1), 51–63.

Nathan, P. W. (1976). The gate-control theory of pain: A critical review. *Brain, 99,* 123–158.

Pilowsky, I. (1978). A general classification of abnormal illness behavior. *British Journal of Medical Psychiatry, 51*(2), 131–137.

Pincus, T., Callahan, L. F., Bradley, L. A., Vaughn, W. K., & Wolfe, F. (1987). Elevated MMPI scores for hypochondriasis, depression and hysteria in patients with rheumatoid arthritis reflect disease rather than psychological status. *Arthritis and Rheumatism, 29,* 1456–1466.

Polatin, P. B., Kinney, R. K., Gatchel, R. J., Lillo, E., & Mayer, T. G. (1993). Psychiatric illness and chronic low-back pain. The mind and the spine—Which goes first? *Spine, 18*(1), 66–71.

Pope, M., Frymoyer, J., & Anderson, G. (1984). *Occupational low back pain.* New York: Praeger.

Romano, J. M., & Turner, J. A. (1985). Chronic pain and depression: Does the evidence support a relationship? *Psychological Bulletin, 97,* 18–34.

Schmidt, R. F. (1972). The gate-control theory of pain: An unlikely hypothesis. In R. Jansen, W. D. Keidel, A. Herz, C. Streichele, J. P. Payne, & R. A. P. Burt (Eds.), *Pain: Basic principles, pharmacology, therapy* (pp. 57–71). Stuttgart, Germany: Thieme.

Spitzer, R. L., Williams, J. B., Gibbons, M., & First, M. B. (1988). *Structured clinical interview for DSM-III-R.* New York: New York State Psychiatric Institute.

Sternbach, R. A. (1974). *Pain patients: Traits and treatment.* New York: Academic Press.

Sternbach, R. A., Wolf, S. R., Murphy, R. W., & Akeson, W. H. (1973). Traits of pain patients: The low-back "loser." *Psychosomatics, 14,* 226–229.

Turk, D. C. (1996). Biopsychosocial perspective on chronic pain. In R. J. Gatchel & D. C. Turk (Eds.), *Psychological approaches to pain management: A practitioner's handbook* (pp. 3–32). New York: Guilford Press.

Turk, D. C. (1997). Psychosocial and behavioral assessment of patients with temporomandibular disorders: Diagnostic and treatment implications. *Oral Surgery Oral Medicine Oral Pathology, 83,* 65–71.

Turk, D., & Rudy, T. (1988). Toward an empirically derived taxonomy of chronic pain patients: Integration of psychological assessment data. *Journal of Consulting and Clinical Psychology, 56,* 233–238.

Turk, D., & Salovey, P. (1984). Chronic pain as a variant of depressive disease: A critical reappraisal. *Journal of Nervous and Mental Disease, 172,* 398–404.

Vittengl, J., Clark, L., Owen-Salter, E., & Gatchel, R. (1999). Diagnostic change and personality stability following functional restoration treatment in a chronic low back pain patient sample. *Assessment, 6,* 79–92.

Waddell, G., Main, C. J., & Morris, E. W. (1984). Chronic low back pain, psychologic distress, and illness behavior. *Spine, 5,* 117–125.

Wall, P. D. (1989). The dorsal horn. In P. D. Wall & R. Melzack (Eds.), *Textbook of pain* (2nd ed., pp. 102–111). New York: Churchill Livingstone.

Waring, E. M., Weisz, G. M., & Bailey, S. I. (1976). Predictive factors in the treatment of low back pain by surgical intervention. In J. J. Bonica & D. Albe-Fessard (Eds.), *Advances in pain research and therapy* (Vol. 1) (pp. 283–299). New York: Raven Press.

Weisberg, J. N., & Keefe, F. J. (1997). Personality disorders in the chronic pain population: Basic concepts, empirical findings, and clinical implications. *Pain Forum, 6*(1), 1–9.

Wiltse, L. L., & Rocchio, P. D. (1975). Preoperative psychological tests as predictors of success of chemonucleolysis in the treatment of the low back syndrome. *Journal of Bone and Joint Surgery, 57*(A), 478–483.

Part I

Early Approaches to the Study of Personality and Pain

Chapter 1
HISTORY OF PSYCHOANALYTIC IDEAS CONCERNING PAIN

Harold Merskey

The attempt to understand pain in psychological terms has a very old history, nearly as old as that of writing. One of the most striking observations comes from Jeremiah (Lamentations 1:12–13) as follows: "Is it nothing to you, all ye that pass by? Behold and see if there be any pain like unto my pain, which is done unto me, wherewith the Lord has afflicted me in the day of his fierce anger. From above he has sent fire into my bones . . . and I am weary and faint all the day." This is part of the dismay and lament of the prophet on the destruction of Jerusalem by the Babylonians in 586 B.C.E. It exemplified pain associated with sadness or depression as well as other somatic effects, like weariness and faintness due to the distressing event.

The Greeks too had a psychological method of understanding pain. The doctrine that there were five senses—sight, hearing, smell, taste, and touch—is ascribed to Aristotle who stated that touch "discriminates several qualities" and that pain was set apart from these. Aristotle like Plato classed pain with pleasure as a "passion of the soul," an expression that nowadays might be translated as "a state of feeling." Dallenbach (1939), who discussed these historical points of view, remarked that "once pain, identified with unpleasantness is set in opposition to pleasure, it transcends the limitations of the sensory field and extends into the other fields of mental life."

This need to handle pain differently from other sensory information sometimes has been discounted when seemingly specific "pain nerves" or pain mechanisms were favored as a result of discoveries in sensory physiology. Nevertheless, more sophisticated approaches to pattern theory, and later to plasticity of the nervous system, inevitably emphasized the relevance of emotional states to pain. This was particularly reinforced in the first half of the 20th century by the difficulty many doctors had explaining physically the large number of cases of pain that they were seeing (Merskey & Spear, 1967). Although the concept of hysteria has repeatedly fluctuated in its meaning and content, it has almost always involved the idea of psychological disturbances and pain as part of those disturbances.

It follows that during the 20th century the leading psychological theory of bodily symptoms was applied to pain. That theory was psychoanalysis as developed by Sigmund Freud. At the end of the 20th century, Freudian ideas are discredited and physiology has more to tell us than it did in the middle of the century about the causes of pain (Merskey, 1999). The importance of psychogenesis as an etiological factor has not disappeared completely, but it has declined significantly. One part of the decline has been the abandonment of psychodynamic theories with respect to pain. However, those theories were prominent for a long time and in this chapter I outline how they developed and what they implied.

This chapter is based in part on Merskey, H. and Spear, F. G. (1967). *Pain: Psychological and psychiatric aspects.* Material used with permission of Baillière, Tindell, and Cassell, London, United Kingdom.

This chapter's purpose is to show how Freudian ideas were introduced to the world of pain and how they evolved and decayed. In doing so, I should make my past personal position clear. My own greatly respected teacher, Erwin Stengel, was taught by Freud, something I had always appreciated and thought a bonus in my training. I was not analyzed, and by the time I started in psychiatry in Britain in the 1950s, psychoanalysis was not considered a useful therapeutic procedure. Nor were the specific details of oedipal theory and the oral, anal, and genital stages strongly believed. Defense mechanisms and repression were popular explanations at the time, as they still are, in most of psychiatry.

At the outset, I should also note that three features stand out with regard to the history of psychoanalytic or psychodynamic views about pain. First, the system of psychoanalysis constituted a bold and sustained effort to try to explain human motives and the personality features that accompany them. Second, it failed because far-reaching theories were not grounded in proper evidence, and it has taken a little more than a century for the theory to be put forward, accepted, and demolished. Third, psychodynamic theories of pain are affected equally with supposed recovered memories—now widely recognized as unproven.

Not everyone in the fields of psychiatry or psychology accepts that the demolition has occurred. This is partly because the essential work—more of which should have been done within these professions—has largely been done outside them: by historians, biographers, "Freud scholars," philosophers, and others who have looked closely at the circumstances in which Freud generated his theories, their evolution, the epistemological basis for psychoanalytic claims, the poverty of valid data, and the poor results that have attended psychoanalytic practice.

Much new information has come forward in the past three decades, but there have always been critics who pointed to the fundamental flaws in Freudian theory and who were neglected or ignored. In the end, the situation with psychoanalysis boils down to this: What is new is not good, and what is good is not original. Ideas about the influence of motive on overt behavior, and even such terms as *repression* and *the unconscious*, were present long before Freud. The framework he erected for them is no longer believable. But the purpose of this chapter is not to revisit that discussion: It is readily available in other sources. The book by Crews, *Unauthorised Freud* (1998), provides ready access to the relevant literature, and the monograph by Esterson, *Seductive Mirage* (1993), shows how an intelligent lay inquirer was able to pierce the rhetoric of Freudian arguments to demonstrate their remarkable deceitfulness and to uncover a striking lack of sound data in Freud's original writings. Why and how Freud—a man of unquestioned brilliance misled himself, and much of the rest of the world—is an unsolved problem except that it is well recognized that he was ambitious to be a great discoverer and thought he was one.

Pain and Hysteria in Psychoanalysis

When Freud was developing his ideas of hysteria it was commonplace for unexplained pains to be regarded as "hysterical." This does not mean the same as what is called a "conversion" symptom today. Hirschmuller (1989) points out that, for Breuer and Freud (1893/1974) in their archetypal original paper ("The Psychical Mechanisms of Hysterical Phenomena"), hysteria meant "any general neurosis without specific localisation'' (p. 87) as it had for the previous 50 years or more. In other words, what was called hysteria, and what are now called conversion or dissociative disorders, differed despite some overlap. In addition to nonepileptic seizures, paralysis without organic evidence, and so forth, hysteria covered a good deal of mild to moderate depression of various types; some misdiagnosed physical symptoms, such as many tics; and a fair quota of anxiety, including phobias. Freud himself was relatively lacking in psychiatric knowledge. He was primarily a neurologist, and he had not worked systematically with the major forms of psychiatric illness or bipolar disorder. He came to the topic by way of neurology, hypnotism, and private psychotherapy, but he does appear to have been the first to identify obsessive–compulsive disorders as a specific entity.

In their introductory essay Breuer and Freud (1893/1974) put forward the view that ideas that are completely absent from the patient's memory in a normal mental state, or else present only in a "highly summary form," could be revealed by hypnosis. These memories were held to be related to psychological trauma that had not been disposed of either by abreaction or by normal "associative wearing away" in consciousness. Undischarged feeling was held to be attached to the abnormal state or else the person was supposed to be afflicted with a disposition to "hypnoid states." Four of the women whom Breuer and Freud (1893/1974) described in these studies had pain as a prominent symptom. One of them, Breuer's patient Anna O., also had facial pain, although it was not initially a major part of her difficulties, which are best understood in terms of severe depression. Freud offered to explain the pain from which his patients suffered in terms of hysteria and symbolic symptom formation. Thus, in one full case history (Emmy von N.), pains in the leg were related to a long series of distressing and irritating experiences in nursing a sick brother. In discussing these limb pains, Freud argued that they were originally rheumatic muscular pains that might still partly be muscular but that also had become associated accidentally with unpleasant domestic experiences and so "were later repeated in her memory as the somatic symbol of the whole complex of association" (p. 129). He was fond of the idea that pain that was originally organic in origin could come to have psychic associations that determined its later appearance (in modern terms, this might be called *pain behavior*, based on a physical illness that has ended).

During the treatment of his patients Freud began to lay increasing stress on the way in which pain resulted from psychic conflict. In the case of Elisabeth von R., he described them as a successful conversion phenomenon that spared her from facing the conviction that she loved her sister's husband: "She repressed her erotic idea from consciousness and transformed the amount of its affect into physical pain" (p. 235). In another case, Frau Cäcilie von M., Freud reproduced and abreacted a facial neuralgia by calling up a traumatic scene, which the patient described as "like a slap in the face" (p. 251). He thought the hysterical patient was not just taking liberties with words, but reviving once more the sensations to which the verbal expression owed its justification.

Freud's views about pain in his earliest studies appear to be the following:

1. Pain is a common conversion symptom.
2. Unpleasant affect is converted to bodily pain.
3. The choice of the symptom is determined by precipitating events.

4. The pain often has symbolic meaning.
5. There is a frequent hereditary influence.
6. There is always an organic substratum, sometimes a local lesion (e.g., stiff muscles), but at the least a mnemic trace.
7. Conflict, guilt, and resentment were aspects of the illness in many of the cases described but were not stressed by Freud in relation to pain (Merskey & Spear, 1967).

Freud's later practice appears to have moved away from patients with organic complaints (Engel, 1959), probably because they stopped coming to him. In his later works he discussed pain in "Mourning and Melancholia" (Freud, 1917/1957), in "Beyond the Pleasure Principle" (Freud, 1920/1955), and in "Inhibitions, Symptoms and Anxiety" (Freud, 1926/1959), and he took the view that pain and mourning were "affective reactions to separations" thus distinguishing them from anxiety, which he regarded as a reaction to the threat of the loss of the loved object.

After Freud, many psychologically oriented writers discussed pain. Some contributions were purely theoretical or were opinions advanced on the basis of one or two cases. Several discussed phantom pain (Flescher, 1948; Gallinek, 1939; Kolb, 1954; Scott, 1948), and a few, such as Halliday (1937a, 1937b); Ellman, Savage, Wittkower, and Rodger (1942); Engel (1951, 1959); and Gidro-Frank and Gordon (1956), discussed the topic on the basis of a series of cases.

Reik (1914) gave one of the earliest reports on the psychogenesis of pain in his chapter on the couvade. This phenomenon of pseudo-labor and other symptoms in the husband of a woman in childbirth or during pregnancy remains perhaps the most striking example of pain due to ideas. The word *couvade* is thought to come from a Basque root, meaning to sit on eggs, and couvade symptoms have been widely described in various societies. Bardhan (1965a, 1965b) reported 20 cases of psychological illness among expectant Indian fathers of various social levels, including clerks, medical practitioners, senior civil servants, and military officers. Headache, heartburn, gastralgia, and localized pain all occurred. This is rather different from specific brooding. It was common in some societies to suppose that men had such pains because their wives were pregnant—but of course this need not necessarily be interpreted as due to an idea. Instead, it might be explained as a psychophysiological effect of anxiety. Nevertheless, the connection between the two ideas was often made in mining communities (P. Crann, personal communication, 1965; Dennis, Henriques, & Slaughter, 1956) and elsewhere in modern urban society, with reports by Curtis (1965) and by Trethowan and Conlon (1965) on Australian cases. The psychoanalytic explanation Reik (1914) offered was that such phenomena served primarily to protect the woman against the latent hostility and sexual aggression of the man. Perhaps so, but there was no proof.

Asymbolia and Phantom Pain

Schilder and Stengel (1928, 1931) described a somewhat different phenomenon, *asymbolia for pain*, in which some patients with brain damage did not react appropriately to noxious stimuli by withdrawal even though they could recognize the assault. The existence of this phenomenon suggested a difficulty in relating noxious stimuli to the body image. This observation has generally been regarded as a valid neuropsychological observation. It is tested clinically, for example, by showing that a patient not only does not treat noxious stimuli as painful, but fails to react when a threat—such as bringing a lighted match close to the face—is offered.

Schilder's (1931, 1935) thinking went further and led him to stress the importance of the postural model of the body with respect to pain. He had developed the idea of a body schema and attached pain to it. He also stressed the communicative value of pain, the importance of childhood experiences, quarrelsome parents and a severe father, and the relationship of sadism to genital pain. After Schilder, the problem of phantom limb pain came to be discussed in terms of body image, and Kolb (1954) suggested that the phantom phenomenon was best explained as the patient's enduring concept of his total body image. He claimed that patients with the acute painful phantom limb syndrome had overemphasized the idea of body development.

Szasz (1957) put forward the idea that phantom limb pain represented a denial of the loss of a part. Parkes (1973) suggested that the loss of a limb leads to grieving that is analogous to the mourning of the loss of a close relative. Szasz's view was challenged by Simmel (1959), who had many patients with phantom limb pain and who claimed that they were fully aware of their unpleasant affect and loss and that such mechanisms of denial might be related to the phantom and not to the loss of the limb. (Patients with phantom limbs are liable not to discuss them.)

Many authors related pain to aggression or hostility: Wittkower, Rodger, and Wilson (1941) and Weiss (1947) attributed rheumatic pain to resentment. Ellman et al. (1942); Rome (1949); Coventry (1958); and Brown, Nemiah, Barr, and Barry (1954) claimed that their clinical experience also supported this view. Holmes and Wolff (1952) offered experimental evidence in support, measuring muscle tension, but gave no quantitative details of their psychological assessments either in 65 patients or in 10 control participants. Marcussen and Wolff (1949) also induced headache experimentally in patients with migraines by precipitating anger in conditions under which the patient was unable to take action. The theory about this, however, was difficult to understand and involved an undefined concept of mental energy.

Pain, Guilt, and Aggression

The most common feature of psychoanalytic theory was to say that pain was an unconscious defense against aggression. Many authors, therefore, stressed the association of guilt, resentment, hostility, and pain, and they emphasized the symbolic significance of pain (Bostock, 1951; Brenner, Friedman, & Carter, 1949; Ellman et al., 1942; Forrer, 1962; Furmanski, 1952; Graven, 1924; Grinker & Gottschalk, 1949; Halliday, 1937a, 1937b; Knopf, 1935a, 1935b; Kolb, 1954; Lancaster, 1953; Marcussen & Wolff, 1949; Nemiah, 1953; Saul, 1935; Schilder, 1931; Seidenberg, 1947; Selinsky, 1939; Sifneos, 1956; Sperling, 1952; Szasz, 1957; Trowbridge, Cushman, Gray, & Moore, 1943; Whiskin, 1955; Wright, 1947). Hart (1947) reviewed still more, and others also argued that such patients had a tendency to seek unnecessary operations (Engel, 1959; Greenacre, 1939; Jelliffe, 1933, cited in Menninger, 1938; Menninger, 1938). Nearly all of these authors described plausible relationships between pain, guilt, and hostility, but the evidence they give is consistently anecdotal. Most report only a few cases. Those who reported more than a dozen or so are

Knopf (1935a; 1935b), Halliday (1937a; 1937b), Ellman et al. (1942), Brenner et al. (1949), Kolb (1954), and Engel (1951, 1958, 1959). None considered the question of whether the guilt, resentment, hostility, and supposed transformations of affect and libido that were frequently mentioned could occur similarly without pain being present. All of this writing was largely impressionistic and uncontrolled.

Schilder (1931) expanded the theory by suggesting that there were frequently special psychic factors determined by the existence of guilt, which gave rise to particular pains, especially when preceded by pleasure in that body part (e.g., sexual stimulation in a woman who had pain in her breast). He described two patients who might illustrate the importance of pain as a symptom. The first was a brief example of pain occurring in those parts of the body about which the patient had homosexual fantasies, and Schilder very economically suggested that the pain was a defense, a perverse fantasy, and a punishment for this fantasy. In a second case, a man complaining of pain in his genitals, it emerged during treatment that the pain was closely connected with sexual excitement, acted as a stimulant, and occurred more frequently as the analysis proceeded, weakening some of the patient's rigid sexual morality. In this case, Schilder interpreted the pains as a defense against sexuality and as a perverse sadomasochistic satisfaction.

Eisenbud (1937) provided an interesting single case study of a man experiencing amnesia and headaches. His conclusion is that the patient had anxiety aroused by his own hostility and aggression and dealt with it by developing a conversion headache associated with amnesia for the incidents in which feelings were aroused. In Eisenbud's view, unconscious hostility toward the patient's father caused symptoms of headache in response to the father's admission to hospital. The headache was relieved by going over these events under hypnosis and bringing them back after that to consciousness. Eisenbud examined his hypothesis in a series of experiments involving the hypnotic induction of so-called *artificial complexes*. Of six hostile or aggressive complexes induced, the first three led to headache. When complexes with heterosexual erotic conflicts were introduced, these were not followed by headache. Eisenbud is restrained in his discussion of the limitations of his study but considered that the repeated production and subsequent elimination of the artificial complex by bringing it into consciousness had an abreactive effect that made the patient refractory to the further induction of headache by this means. Currently, we might say that desensitization to the induction procedure occurred. This theory is based on hypnotic procedures that have now become notoriously suspect by virtue of the possibility of contamination through knowledge of the patient's interests or through implicit suggestion.

Szasz and Engel

The peak of analytic theorizing was probably reached by Szasz (1957) and Engel (1951, 1958, 1959). Szasz made a notable contribution with his discussion of the philosophy and meaning of pain, emphasizing its standing as a subjective psychological phenomenon rather than as a physical event. He presented his theory on pain and pleasure as bodily feelings and suggested that the body is perceived by the ego as an object. In this theory, pain arises as a consequence of threatened loss of or damage to the body in the same way that anxiety arises from threatened loss of an external object, at least according to analytic theory. The question of whether the symptom is to be considered organic or functional then depends on the observer's assessment of the reality of the threat to the body.

Szasz (1957) claimed that pain may be considered at three levels of symbolization. At the first level, the communications are essentially those concerning a physical symptom. The next level involves the use of pain as a communication that requests help. This level is always involved in any complaint of pain. Nevertheless, there are occasions when the second level predominates over the first, and it is important to appreciate these occasions and to respond to the cry for aid.

Communication at the third level is more complex, and Szasz (1957) seemed to mean that at this level pain can persist as a symbol of rejection if the request for help is frustrated. Then, the repeated complaint of pain can become a form of aggression and the suffering can expedite guilt. Spear (1967) argued that if Szasz was correct and if analytic theory in general is correct, patients with pain should show more overt or covert hostility. He assessed this by having staff, not informed about his theory, check off in a psychiatric unit with patients with anxiety, depression, or similar complaints whether the patients were more aggressive or more ingratiating. Heightened ingratiation was taken to imply covert hostility. Patients with pain did not differ from other patients in regard to covert hostility. Spear provided patients with a questionnaire in which responses to some of the questions would signal overt hostility and others' possibly covert hostility.

Engel (1951, 1959) provided the most widely influential discussion of psychoanalytic ideas on pain. He described (Engel, 1951) 19 women and 1 man with atypical facial pain. This is taken to be a hysterical conversion symptom, but he emphasized that they presented a "masochistic" character structure with many varieties of self-punishing behavior. He stressed the frequency in their cases of unnecessary surgery and remission of the pain at times of misfortune, or when there was other cause for suffering—whether physical or mental. Later, Engel (1959) named this type of patient "the pain-prone patient" and described more examples. He argued, as had others, that pain would serve as a warning of bodily damage; that it has a communicative function; and that it is linked with punishment, aggression, guilt, sexual feelings, and the loss of a loved object. He regarded punitive or abusive parents as very important in the development of patients who complain of pain. He emphasized the occurrence of various individual characteristics of the pain-prone patient before the onset of the pain and stated that, although one might be inclined to pass this off as a consequence of the pain, such a view is mistaken because the patients often tend to put themselves in the way of their misfortunes.

These theoretical discussions suggested that hostility is an important factor in the genesis of pain, either directly or through the guilt it produces. Engel (1951, 1958, 1959) postulated that it acts in people of a specific personality to produce pain. Szasz (1957) suggested that there is a much more complex symbolic situation in which the imminence of a threat to bodily integrity is feared. As with the earlier writers, neither Szasz (1957) nor Engel (1951, 1958, 1959) provided systematic or compelling data.

Merskey (1965) compared psychiatric patients with pain of more than 3 months' duration ("persistent pain") offered as a major presenting complaint with others who were attending the same clinic but had no complaint of pain. Several of his findings conformed to Engel's (1951, 1958, 1959) claims: Patients with pain also had an increased frequency of past illness ($p < .01$) and had significantly more near relations who had had pain. There also was an increased frequency of admission to the hospital in the pain group, but this was not statistically significant, although investigations were vastly more common, as would be expected in those with pain compared with other psychiatric patients. Patients with pain had a tendency to have more operations than did control patients, but this was not statistically significant ($p > .1$) after accounting for age. However, many useless operative procedures had been undertaken specifically for their pain, including laminectomy, stereotactic operation on the thalamus, rhizotomy, trimming of the mylohyoid ridge, uterine curettage, hysterectomy, and laparotomy. Many of these findings might be seen as almost inevitable consequences of the particular complaint rather than as proof of masochistic effort.

Merskey (1965) took note of the occurrence of acts of aggressive behavior by recording all those patients who in adult life had had altercations that had led them to hit other adults or to throw hard objects. The patients with pain did not differ from the others. The women in the groups were as aggressive as the men were— but perhaps they did less damage. Merskey found that resentment was more common in patients with pain, in a ratio of 3:1 ($p < .01$). Resentment was considered present if a patient blamed others for his or her condition or held the view that he or she had been treated badly by others in life. Among 30 such resentful patients with pain, 15 were either markedly resentful before their illness or attributed their condition to the misdeeds of relatives, neighbors, or other nonmedical associates. Three patients mainly blamed doctors for their condition, and 12 blamed doctors and other associates impartially. Those who blamed others tended to blame the alleged miscreant for causing the distress or pain of which complaint was made and only secondarily, if at all, for failing to procure relief.

Resentment and aggressive behavior are thought to be common among patients with chronic pain, and these findings bear them out. Part of the resentment can be attributed to experiences of unsatisfactory treatment, but not a large part, at least from that series. Rather than needing a profound masochistic or unconscious explanation, resentment and aggressive behavior can be explained more simply in patients with chronic pain. Pain is likely to make individuals aggressive for biological reasons. It is part of a fight-or-flight mechanism. When the integrity of the body surface is disrupted it is necessary to respond vigorously if the disruption comes from another living creature. If not, the choice for the individual is to flee or make peace. O'Kelly and Steckley (as cited in Ulrich, 1966; Ulrich, Hutchinson, & Azrin, 1965) reported that, if electric current is run across the bars of the floor of a rat cage, the rats turn around and bite one another. Aggression is one of the main responses to occur in the presence of trauma that gives rise to pain. The evidence for this was reviewed by Ulrich and colleagues (1965, 1966). It is not surprising then that people with chronic pain become irritable and perhaps resentful and difficult. A new, deeper explanation may not be necessary.

This is a banal but practical comment that has received surprisingly little attention. It is probably more important than is the questionable idea that chronic pain causes emotional change rather more than that the emotional change causes the pain. If I have matters right, the consequences of pain will include direct physical distress, unemployment, financial difficulties, marital disharmony, and difficulties in concentration and attention whether due to the pain or to medication, and so on. We should be as wary of personality theories that attribute pain to intangible motives or operant behavior as we are about dynamic postulates.

References

Bardhan, P. N. (1965a). The fathering syndrome. *Armed Forces Medical Journal, 20,* 200–208.

Bardhan, P. N. (1965b). The couvade syndrome. *British Journal of Psychology, 3,* 908–909.

Bostock, J. (1951). The "trap" headache. *Medical Journal of Australia, 1,* 80–82.

Brenner, C., Friedman, A. P., & Carter, S. (1949). Psychological factors in the etiology of chronic headache. *Psychosomatic Medicine, 2,* 53–56.

Breuer, J., & Freud, S. (1974). The psychical mechanisms of hysterical phenomena. In *Studies on hysteria* (pp. 53–69). Harmondsworth, England: Penguin Books. (Original work published 1893.)

Brown, T., Nemiah, J. C., Barr, J. S., & Barry, H. (1954). Psychological factors in low back pain. *New England Journal of Medicine, 251,* 123–128.

Coventry, M. B. (1958). Problem of painful shoulder. *Journal of the American Medical Association, 151,* 177–185.

Crews, F. (1998). *Unauthorised Freud. Doubters confront a legend.* New York: Viking.

Curtis, J. L. (1965). A psychiatric study of 55 expectant fathers. *United States Armed Forces Medical Journal, 6,* 937–950.

Dallenbach, K. M. (1939). Pain: History and present status. *American Journal of Psychology, 52,* 331–347.

Dennis, N., Henriques, F., & Slaughter, C. (1956). *Coal is our life.* London: Eyre & Spottiswoode.

Eisenbud, J. (1937). The psychology of headache. *Psychiatric Quarterly, 2,* 592–619.

Ellman, P., Savage, O. A., Wittkower, E., & Rodger, T. F. (1942). Fibrositis. A biographical study of 50 civilian and military cases. *Annals of Rheumatic Diseases, 3,* 56–76.

Engel, G. L. (1951). Primary atypical facial neuralgia. A hysterical conversion symptom. *Psychosomatic Medicine, 13,* 375–396.

Engel, G. L. (1958). "Psychogenic" pain. *Medical Clinics of North America, 42,* 1481–1496.

Engel, G. L. (1959). "Psychogenic" pain and the pain prone patient. *American Journal of Medicine, 26,* 899–918.

Esterson, A. (1993). *Seductive mirage: An exploration of the work of Sigmund Freud.* Chicago: Open Court.

Flescher, J. (1948). On neurotic disorders of sensibility and body scheme: A bioanalytical approach to pain, fear and repression. *International Journal of Psycho-Analytics, 29,* 156–162.

Forrer, G. R. (1962). Hallucinated headache. *Psychosomatics, 3,* 120–128.

Freud, S. (1955). Beyond the pleasure principle. In *Complete psychological works* (standard ed., Vol. 18). London: Hogarth Press. (Original work published 1920.)

Freud, S. (1957). Mourning and melancholia. In *Complete psychological works* (standard ed., Vol. 14). London: Hogarth Press. (Original work published 1917.)

Freud, S. (1959). Inhibitions, symptoms and anxiety. In *Complete psychological works* (standard ed., Vol. 20). London: Hogarth Press. (Original work published 1926.)

Furmanski, A. R. (1952). Dynamic concepts of migraine. *Archives of Neurological Psychiatry, 67,* 23–31.

Gallinek, A. (1939). The phantom limb, its origin and its relationship to the hallucinations of psychotic states. *American Journal of Psychiatry, 96,* 413–422.

Gidro-Frank, L., & Gordon, T. (1956). Reproductive performance of women with pelvic pain of long duration. *Fertility and Sterility, 7,* 440–447.

Graven, P. S. (1924). A series of clinical notes on headache. *Psychoanalytic Review, 2*, 324–328.

Greenacre, P. (1939). Surgical addiction—A case illustration. *Psychosomatic Medicine, 1*, 325–328.

Grinker, R. R., & Gottschalk, L. (1949). Headaches and muscular pain. *Psychosomatic Medicine, 2*, 46–52.

Halliday, J. L. (1937a). Psychological factors in rheumatism. A preliminary study. *British Medical Journal, 1*, 213–217.

Halliday, J. L. (1937b). Psychological factors in rheumatism. A preliminary study. *British Medical Journal 1*, 264–269.

Hart, H. (1947). Displacement, guilt and pain. *Psychoanalytic Review, 34*, 259–273.

Hirschmuller, A. (1989). *The life and work of Josef Breuer: Physiology and psychoanalysis.* New York: New York University Press.

Holmes, T. H., & Wolff, H. G. (1952). Life situations, emotions and backache. *Psychosomatic Medicine, 14*, 18–33.

Knopf, O. (1935a). Preliminary report on personality studies in thirty migraine patients. *Journal of Nervous and Mental Diseases, 82*, 270–285.

Knopf, O. (1935b). Preliminary report on personality studies in thirty migraine patients. *Journal of Nervous and Mental Diseases, 82*, 400–414.

Kolb, L. C. (1954). *The painful phantom: Psychology, physiology and treatment.* Springfield, IL: Charles C Thomas.

Lancaster, N. P. (1953). Some observations on headaches and personality types. Unpublished MD thesis, University of Manchester, England.

Marcussen, R. M., & Wolff, H. G. (1949). A formulation of the dynamics of the migraine attack. *Psychosomatic Medicine, 2*, 251–256.

Menninger, K. A. (1938). *Man against himself.* New York: Harcourt & Brace.

Merskey, H. (1965). Psychiatric patients with persistent pain. *Journal of Psychosomatic Research, 9*, 299–309.

Merskey, H. (1999). Pain and Psychological Medicine. In P. D. Wall & R. Melzack (Eds.), Textbook of Pain, Fourth Edition (pp. 929–949). Edinburgh: Churchill, Livingston.

Merskey, H., & Spear, F. G. (1967). *Pain: Psychological and psychiatric aspects.* London, UK: Baillière, Tindall & Cassell.

Nemiah, J. C. (1953). Clinic on psychosomatic problems. A case of low-back pain complicated by psychologic factors. *American Journal of Medicine, 15*, 391–398.

O'Kelley, L. E., & Steckley, L. C. (1939). As cited by Ulrich et al., (1965).

Parkes, C. M. (1973). Factors determining the persistence of phantom pain in the amputee. *Journal of Psychosomatic Research 19*, 97–108.

Reik, T. (1914/1934). Couvade and the psychogenesis of the fear of retaliation. In D. Bryan (Trans.), *Ritual psychoanalytic studies* (pp. 27–89). London: Hogarth Press.

Rome, H. P. (1949). Neuromuscular and joint diseases and the psychosomatic approach. *Medical Clinics of North America, 33*, 1061–1069.

Saul, L. J. (1935). A note on the psychogenesis of organic symptoms. *Psychoanalytic Quarterly, 4*, 476–483.

Schilder, P. (1931). Notes on the psychopathology of pain in neuroses and psychoses. *Psychoanalytic Review, 18*, 1–22.

Schilder, P. (1935). The image and appearance of the human body. New York: International Universities Press.

Schilder, P., & Stengel, E. (1928). Schmerzasymbolia. *Zeitschriftfier Neurologie & Psychiatrie, 113*, 143–158.

Schilder, P., & Stengel, E. (1931). Asymbolia for pain. *Archives of Neurology and Psychiatry, 25*, 598–600.

Scott, W. C. M. (1948). Some embryological, neurological, psychiatric and psychoanalytic implications of the body scheme. *International Journal of Psycho-Analytics, 29*, 141–155.

Seidenberg, R. (1947). Psychosexual headache. *Psychiatric Quarterly, 21*, 349–360.

Selinsky, H. (1939). Psychological study of the migrainous syndrome. *Bulletin of New York Academy of Medicine, 15*, 757–763.

Sifneos, P. E. (1956). Clinic on psychosomatic problems: Long-term psychotherapy in a patient with epigastric pain. *American Journal of Medicine, 21*, 275–281.

Simmel, M. L. (1959). Phantoms, phantom pain and "denial." *American Journal of Psychotherapy, 13*, 603–613.

Spear, F. G. (1967). Pain in psychiatric patients. *Journal of Psychosomatic Research, 11*, 187–193.

Sperling, M. (1952). A psychoanalytic study of migraine and psychogenic headache. *Psychoanalytic Review, 39*, 152–163.

Szasz, T. S. (1957). *Pain and pleasure. A study of bodily feelings.* London: Tavistock.

Trethowan, W. H., & Conlon, M. F. (1965). The couvade syndrome. *British Journal of Psychiatry, 3*, 57–66.

Trowbridge, L. S., Cushman, D., Gray, M. G., & Moore, M. (1943). Notes on the personality of patients with migraine. *Journal of Nervous and Mental Diseases, 97*, 509–517.

Ulrich, R. E. (1966). Pain as a cause of aggression. *American Zoologist, 6*, 643–662.

Ulrich, R. E., Hutchinson, P. R., & Azrin, N. H. (1965). Pain-elicited aggression. *Psychology Records, 15*, 111–126.

Weiss, E. (1947). Psychogenic rheumatism. *Annals of Internal Medicine, 26*, 890–900.

Whiskin, F. (1955). A case of persistent ankle pain in spite of adequate orthopaedic treatment. *American Journal of Medicine, 18*, 653–658.

Wittkower, E., Rodger, T. F., & Wilson, A. T. M. (1941). Effort syndrome. *Lancet, 1*, 531–535.

Wright, H. P. (1947). Psychogenic arthralgia. *Annals of Rheumatological Diseases, 6*, 204–207.

Chapter 2
PSYCHOMETRIC TESTING:
THE EARLY YEARS AND THE MMPI

Richard C. Robinson

The Minnesota Multiphasic Personality Inventory (MMPI) was arguably the most widely used objective psychological measure to study chronic pain (Keller & Butcher, 1991; Snyder, 1990). With the introduction of the MMPI-2 and other measures designed specifically for populations with chronic pain, the utility of the MMPI has decreased. However, the extensive research that used this instrument still provides valuable information into the correlates of chronic pain and the personalities of individuals with these conditions.

This chapter highlights the early contributions of the MMPI to the literature on chronic pain. The MMPI has aided in several areas of research, including conceptualizing chronic pain, predicting responses to treatment, and elucidating the possible predisposing factors that could be related to the development of chronic pain conditions. This chapter is limited to the first MMPI; a detailed discussion of the MMPI-2 and pain is found in chapter 5.

MMPI

The MMPI is a 566-item self-report test developed by Starke Hathaway and J. C. McKinley in 1943 to aid in the diagnosis of psychiatric disorders (Graham, 1993). Before that time, most psychological measures were derived through a logical keying approach that had test creators compile questions that intuitively appeared to assess a specific domain of personality or behavior. This approach created tests with relatively high face validities, allowing patients to portray themselves in a manner that might or might not have conformed to their true beliefs of themselves or their actual behavior. Hathaway and McKinley used an empirical keying approach in which test constructors selected an item based on whether it could differentiate between subjects. The authors of the MMPI began from a large pool of questions that had been gathered from various sources, such as textbooks and earlier personality scales. They compared a "normal" group, individuals presumably free of psychopathology, with a "clinical" group, individuals with a psychiatric diagnosis. The normal group contained, but was not limited to, visitors to and relatives of patients at University of Minnesota hospitals. The clinical group consisted of patients in eight psychiatric diagnostic categories: Hypochondriasis; Depression; Hysteria; Psychopathic Deviate; Paranoia; Psychasthenia; Schizophrenia; and Hypomania. Cross-validation was done after analysis identified the items for each clinical group. The Masculinity–Femininity Scale and the Social Introversion Scale were added later (Graham, 1993).

In its final form, the MMPI consists of the 10 clinical scales and 4 validity scales (see Table 2.1): The Cannot Say (?) score, the L Scale, the F Scale, and the K Scale. The Cannot Say (?) score is the number of items that either are omitted or that are answered as both true and false. Graham (1993) posited several reasons a person

Table 2.1—*MMPI Scales*

Validity Scales	Clinical Scales
L Scale	Scale 1 (Hypochondriasis)
F Scale	Scale 2 (Depression)
K Scale	Scale 3 (Hysteria)
	Scale 4 (Psychopathic Deviate)
	Scale 5 (Masculinity-Femininity)
	Scale 6 (Paranoia)
	Scale 7 (Psychasthenia)
	Scale 8 (Schizophrenia)
	Scale 9 (Hypomania)
	Scale 0 (Social Introversion)

could omit an item, including carelessness, confusion, and indecisiveness. Occasionally, items are omitted because individuals are uncomfortable admitting information about themselves. Regardless of the reason, the omission of too many items will invalidate the test (Graham, 1993).

The L Scale was designed to spot individuals who naively present themselves in an overly favorable light (Meehl & Hathaway, 1946, as cited in Graham, 1993). Patients who have a high L score might have difficulty admitting to even minor flaws. For instance, they would have to report that they read every editorial in the newspaper or that they like everyone they meet. Depending on the degree of the elevation, and on other extratest variables, an elevated L Scale suggests a host of situationally based or long-standing characteristics, including denial, defensiveness, or a lack of insight (Graham, 1993).

The F Scale was designed to recognize unusual, deviant, and atypical ways of approaching the MMPI test items (Meehl & Hathaway, 1946, as cited in Graham, 1993). The scale consists of items that fewer than 10% of the adult normal group scored in a specific direction. For example, fewer than 10% of the normal group responded "true" to the statement, "Evil spirits possess me at times." Graham (1993) described three important functions of the F Scale: (a) recognizing abnormal test-taking sets, (b) gauging the severity of psychopathology, and (c) suggesting other clinically relevant information about an individual. An excessively elevated F Scale suggests the possibility of an invalid test, possibly because of a patient's confusion or an attempt to "fake bad." In addition, an elevated score can suggest that a person is seeking the attention of health care providers (Graham, 1993). Generally, the F Scale suggests a person's level of distress or the severity of the psychopathology, with extreme elevations raising the distinct possibility of psychosis.

The K Scale was developed to detect individuals who attempt to portray themselves in either an overly favorable or an overly unfavorable manner, but to detect them in a more sophisticated way than that offered by the L Scale (Meehl & Hathaway, 1946, as cited in Graham, 1993). Elevated scores can suggest defensiveness or the ability to cope with stressors. Conversely, lower scores can suggest a perceived inability to manage difficult circumstances or stressors (Graham, 1993). As with all the validity scales, an excessive elevation suggests the possibility of an invalid test.

Although the MMPI might not have been able to identify and diagnose individuals based on what were believed to be discrete clinical disorders, it has proven useful in developing descriptions and a more thorough understanding of patients (Graham, 1993). Interpretation of the validity scales, followed by an examination of the possible meanings of the elevated clinical scales, lay the necessary groundwork to interpreting a person's MMPI profile. These scales become clinically significant when they exceed a *t* score of 70 (Graham, 1993).

The first three clinical scales (Hypochondriasis, Depression, and Hysteria) intuitively appear the most relevant for patients with chronic pain and, in fact, have repeatedly been investigated with this population. McKinley and Hathaway (1940, as cited in Butcher & Williams, 1993) defined Scale 1 (Hypochondriasis) as an abnormal concern over health. When the MMPI was constructed, participants in the clinical group consisted of individuals who were overly concerned with possible ailments that were believed to have no organic basis. Elevated scores on Scale 1 suggest the possibility of numerous somatic complaints, selfishness, immaturity, and narcissism. Furthermore, people with elevations on Scale 1 tend to voice their complaints aggressively and whiningly (Butcher & Williams, 1993).

The clinical group for Scale 2 (Depression) consisted mostly of bipolar patients during a depressive episode (Butcher & Williams, 1993). Although many individuals with elevations on Scale 2 are depressed, an individual can elevate Scale 2 without meeting the criteria for a Major Depressive Disorder. Rather, Scale 2 may be thought of as an indication of the degree to which patients are satisfied with themselves, their lives, or their current situations. Individuals with an elevated score on Scale 2 tend to be unhappy, pessimistic, self-deprecating, and sluggish, and they can exhibit many of the neurovegetative symptoms consistent with a depressive disorder, including fatigue and mental dullness (Butcher & Williams, 1993).

Scale 3 (Hysteria) was developed to aid in the detection and diagnosis of conversion hysteria. Hathaway and McKinley used 50 patients with a clinical diagnosis of psychoneurosis, most of whom were believed to have a conversion disorder (Butcher & Williams, 1993). Butcher and Williams (1993) described patients with a conversion disorder as exhibiting personalities characterized by "denial and flamboyant social interactions" (p. 68). They are similar to patients with a Histrionic Personality Disorder. These individuals sometimes develop physical problems in reaction to stress (Graham, 1993). Originally, a conversion reaction was believed to be related to a symbolic resolution of an intrapsychic conflict (primary gain) that can be reinforced by attention or special privileges provided by others because of the physical problem (secondary gain). People with an elevated score on Scale 3 tend to react to stress with physical symptoms, they have limited insight into their feelings and motivations, and they can lack anxiety and depression (Butcher & Williams, 1993; Graham, 1993). Moreover, such persons can be immature, childish, and egocentric, and often they require excessive attention and affection from others (Butcher & Williams, 1993; Graham, 1993). Elevations on Scale 3 can reflect difficulty with acknowledging or accepting aggressive or hostile aspects of oneself. Therefore, hostility sometimes is expressed through indirect or passive means or acted out with little insight into the behavior. Although these individuals often demonstrate good interpersonal skills, the quality of their relationships is likely to be superficial (Butcher & Williams, 1993; Graham, 1993).

The first three clinical scales have received most of the attention in the treatment of patients with chronic pain, but the other clinical scales also provide valuable information. Individuals with an elevated score on Scale 4 (Psychopathic Deviate) tend to have difficulty delaying gratification, have trouble with authority, and may engage in antisocial behavior. Scale 5 (Masculinity–Femininity) is interpreted differently for men and women. Men with an elevated Scale 5 score often exhibit creativity, sensitivity, and passivity; women exhibit assertiveness and self-confidence (Snyder, 1990). Individuals who score high on Scale 6 (Paranoia) can exhibit frank psychosis, have a paranoid predisposition, or feel abused or mistreated. An elevation on Scale 7 (Psychasthenia) can suggest that a person is tense, anxious, and nervous. A high score on Scale 8 (Schizophrenia) can be attributed to several reasons, including feelings of alienation and bizarre sensory experiences. Individuals with elevated scores on Scale 9 (Hypomania) tend to throw themselves into excessive and inefficient activity as a way to distract themselves from distressing emotions. Scale 0 (Social Introversion) appears to detect individuals who are painfully shy (Graham, 1993).

The clinical scales can be thought of in several ways. One involves perceiving the scales as reflecting either traits or states. Scales 1, 2, 7, and 8 are typically thought of as state or symptom scales. Scales 3, 4, 5, 6, 9, and 0 are thought of as trait or character scales (Trimboli & Kilgore, 1983). State scales can be more vulnerable and reactive to current psychosocial stressors than trait scales (Trimboli & Kilgore, 1983), and this difference can help clinicians distinguish between Scale 1 and Scale 3. Trimboli and Kilgore (1989) described Scale 1 as a symptom scale in which patients, when stressed, channel emotional distress into somatic complaints. Scale 3 is a character scale, and when elevated, it suggests that a person has difficulty facing conflicting feelings and has a tendency to react to stress with the development of physical symptoms (Butcher & Williams, 1993; Graham, 1993; Trimboli & Kilgore, 1983). It is not surprising to see elevated scores on both scales in the same individual.

Hathaway and McKinley (as cited in Graham, 1993) believed that interpreting the configuration of scores, rather than just the single-scale elevations, provides the best data. Therefore, a description of two of the most common configurations with chronic pain patients involving Scales 1, 2, and 3 is warranted (Keller & Butcher, 1991). First, chronic-pain patients sometimes have high scores on the first three scales, collectively referred to as the *neurotic triad* (see Fig. 2.1). The neurotic triad has been used to refer to the first three clinical scales, but also is a profile configuration in which Scales 1, 2, and 3 are all elevated. Individuals with these elevations tend to have somatic complaints, and the presence of secondary gain is sometimes associated with the symptoms. Depressive feelings and difficulty with sleep are common. These individuals are hypothesized to have conflicted feelings about dependency. However, they often keep other people at a distance or interact with others in unpleasant or demanding ways (Butcher & Williams, 1993; Graham, 1993).

A second common configuration shows scores for Scales 1 and 3 that are significantly higher than that for Scale 2 (see Fig. 2.2). This profile has been called a *Conversion Valley* (Graham, 1993), *Conversion V* (Keller & Butcher, 1991), *Psychosomatic V*, or *Depressive Valley* (Schwartz & Krupp, 1971). An individual produces this profile by endorsing somatic symptoms, denying social anxiety, and denying depressive symptoms (Schwartz & Krupp, 1971). Although these individuals might not meet the criteria for a conversion disorder, they often appear to react to stress with the development of physical symptoms and have limited insight into their feelings. Individuals with this profile tend to be sociable, conforming, and passive-

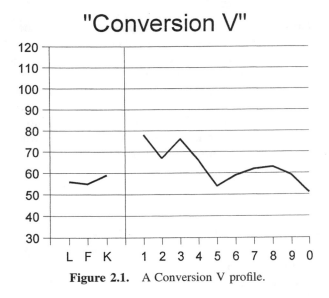

Figure 2.1. A Conversion V profile.

dependent (Graham, 1993). Further, the incidence of the Conversion V profile for patients with chronic pain is 35–60%, but it is 5–15% for general medical patients (Schwartz & Krupp, 1971; Louks, Freeman, & Calsyn, 1978, as cited in Snyder, 1990).

Although the person with the neurotic triad configuration can share some of the symptoms of the Conversion V patient (including somatic complaints), the Conversion V patient is likely to report less psychological distress than is the neurotic triad patient. That is, the Conversion V individual might be able to more effectively distract himself or herself from painful and distressing emotions by focusing on physical symptoms.

The MMPI has provided invaluable data over the years, but as a test instrument it has been replaced. In 1989, the MMPI-2 (Butcher & Williams, 1993) was pub-

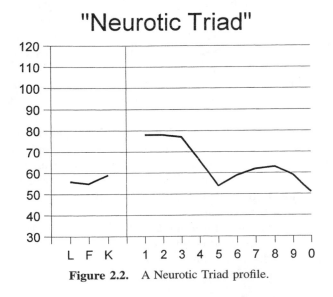

Figure 2.2. A Neurotic Triad profile.

lished, and it addresses several concerns that people had with the original MMPI, which had been criticized for sexist language, poor grammar, and outdated items. For instance, a reference was made to "drop the handkerchief," a game few people remember today. Few items asked about areas that clinicians might find particularly relevant, such as suicide. These criticisms were valid, but the biggest problem had to do with the original standardization sample (Graham, 1993), which was not representative of the U.S. population. It consisted primarily of individuals who were white, married, and living in a rural area or a small town and who had an average of 8 years of education (Dahlstrom, Welsh, & Dahlstrom, 1972).

MMPI and "Functional" versus "Organic" Pain

One early application of the MMPI in medical settings was to help practitioners distinguish *functional* from *organic* pain, a distinction that is today seen as inadequate and overly simplistic. The difference is derived from the biomedical model of pain that postulates a specific complaint should be related to an underlying biological disorder (Turk, 1996). With the introduction of the gate-control theory of pain by Melzack and Wall (1965) and the application of the biopsychosocial model to pain, the distinction between functional and organic appears far less meaningful. Keller and Butcher (1991) succinctly described the difference between the two: "The former implies that the pain problem is caused or maintained by psychosocial factors, whereas the latter assumes a physiologic basis" (p. 33). Love and Peck (1987) described the way the "functional" or "psychogenic" label has been applied to chronic pain conditions, specifically chronic low back pain. Patients often appear to suffer more than would be expected given the equivocal findings of physical examination (Love & Peck, 1987). Unfortunately, clinicians' and researchers' operational definitions of "functional" and "organic" vary according to studies, as does the comprehensiveness of medical evaluations to determine the etiology of a physical complaint. However, although the distinction between "functional" and "organic" might not be entirely useful, empirical investigation of this concept with the MMPI has helped to further our understanding of the patients with chronic pain.

Hanvik (1951) first attempted to differentiate between functional-pain and organic-pain patients. He examined a sample of male inpatients with a primary diagnosis of back pain. Thirty patients were described as "organic," with evidence provided by x-ray. Thirty other cases reportedly had "no clear-cut organic findings" upon physical examination. Hanvik (1951) compared the means of these two groups on the validity and clinical scales (Fig. 2.3).

Figure 2.3 shows that the MMPI profile for functional patients is the conversion V. The first three clinical scales are all elevated, but Scales 1 and 3 are significantly higher than is Scale 2. Hanvik indicated that the patients were, in essence, saying, "I have numerous bodily complaints, but I am relatively unworried, not depressed" (p. 351). The functional group also scored significantly higher on Scales 1, 2, 3, 4, 7, and 8 than did the organic group.

From his work, Hanvik developed the Low Back (Lb) Scale to distinguish functional and organic patients; unfortunately, it lacked substantial psychometric examination for more than 20 years (Freeman, Calsyn, & Louks, 1976; Tsushima & Towne, 1979). French researchers developed the Dorsalles Functionalles (DOR), a

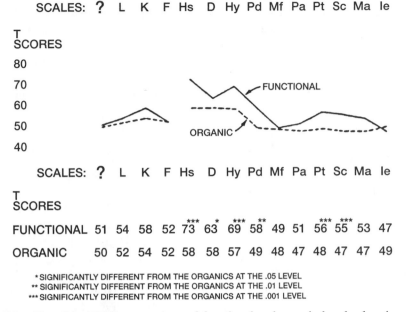

SCALES: **?** L K F Hs D Hy Pd Mf Pa Pt Sc Ma Ie

T
SCORES

	?	L	K	F	Hs	D	Hy	Pd	Mf	Pa	Pt	Sc	Ma	Ie
FUNCTIONAL	51	54	58	52	73***	63*	69***	58**	49	51	56***	55***	53	47
ORGANIC		50	52	54	52	58	58	57	49	48	47	48	47	47	49

* SIGNIFICANTLY DIFFERENT FROM THE ORGANICS AT THE .05 LEVEL
** SIGNIFICANTLY DIFFERENT FROM THE ORGANICS AT THE .01 LEVEL
*** SIGNIFICANTLY DIFFERENT FROM THE ORGANICS AT THE .001 LEVEL

Figure 2.3. Hanvik's (1951) comparison of functional and organic low back pain patients. From "MMPI profiles in patients with low-back pain," by L. J. Hanvik, 1951, *Journal of Consulting Psychology, 15,* p. 351.

63-item MMPI scale also designed to distinguish functional from organic patients (Pichot, Perse, Lebeaux, Dureau, Perez, & Rykewaert, 1972, as cited in Freeman et al., 1976).

The literature is mixed on the utility of the Lb and DOR scales. For instance, Freeman et al. (1976) had some success using these scales to classify patients into one of three groups, "functional," "organic," or "mixed." The mixed group consisted of patients who had an organic basis for their pain that did not fully account for its severity. In a similar study, Calsyn, Louks, and Freeman (1976) concluded that neither the Lb nor the DOR Scale alone was of great use, but when used in an "either/or" fashion, the scales could accurately assign 77.4% of low back pain patients into either a functional or mixed group. Towne and Tsushima (1978) reported that the use of the Lb Scale correctly classified 75% of functional patients, but that once the false-positive rate was included, the rate dropped to 40%. Similar results were obtained by these researchers a year later (Tsushima & Towne, 1979).

Other researchers have found less equivocal results. Sternbach, Wolf, Murphy, and Akeson (1973) reported that patients with positive physical findings compared with patients without positive physical findings did not significantly differ on the Lb Scale. Wilfling, Klonoff, and Kokan (1973) reported that the Lb Scale did not differentiate patients who had been separated into a "good," "fair," or "poor" outcome group after undergoing a spinal fusion. In addition to weak empirical findings, Adams, Heilbronn, Silk, Reider, and Blumer (1981) suggested that the Lb Scale is psychometrically flawed because of its lack of base rates. The Lb Scale therefore might have been a reasonable attempt to make an unreasonable distinction between patients with functional and organic pain.

In addition to his Lb Scale, Hanvik's work was one of the first to suggest the importance of the first three clinical scales and the Conversion V to distinguish functional from organic pain patients (Love & Peck, 1987). However, Lair and Trapp (1962) reported that both organic and functional groups showed the Conversion V profiles. Despite functional pain patients showing higher average elevations on Scales 1, 2, and 3, the overlap appeared too great to discriminate between the two groups. Cox, Chapman, and Black (1978) stated that patients with both chronic pain of unknown etiology and pain related to a surgical event had elevated scores on the first three clinical scales.

Other studies also have raised doubts about the utility of the Conversion V to distinguish patients. Schwartz and Krupp (1971) concluded that the Conversion V does not appear related to the likelihood of receiving a functional diagnosis. Stone and Pepitone-Arreola-Rockwell (1983) found no differences between organic and functional patients, and Leavitt (1985) reported that the Conversion V pattern did not distinguish "organic" from "nonorganic" patients. However, he reported that scores for Scales 1 and 3 were higher in his nonorganic group. It appears that using the Conversion V profile to detect functional from organic pain is unwarranted, because it draws a false distinction between these two groups of patients.

Examination of the Conversion V, or the neurotic triad, is not without merit. Gilberstadt and Jancis (1967) examined individuals seeking admission to a hospital. They found that patients with a Conversion V presented with complaints related to cardiovascular and musculoskeletal problems, and approximately two-thirds of these patients were admitted to the hospital. Several patients had diagnosed heart disease or hypertension. Seven out of 10 of these patients had a history of hypochondriasis or another psychiatric disturbance, suggesting that "hypochondriacs" do become ill. Beals and Hickman (1972) found that patients with back injuries had clinically significant elevations on Scales 1, 2, and 3, with Scales 1 and 2 appearing slightly higher than Scale 3. Rosen, Johnson, and Frymoyer (1983) used Scales 1 and 3, and correctly identified 79% of patients believed to be "inappropriately disabled."

Researchers also have highlighted the importance of other clinical scales. McCreary, Turner, and Dawson (1977) compared 42 organic low back pain patients with 37 functional patients and found that functional patients had significantly higher elevations on Scales 1, 3, 4, 8, 9, and 0. Furthermore, upon examination of means, the functional group approximated a Conversion V. A highly speculative explanation based on these data is that, instead of a single prototypical pain patient, there are subgroups of patients. For instance, there could be one subgroup with a typical Conversion V profile and another with elevated scores on Scale 4 who are manipulative and have difficulty delaying gratification. McCreary et al. (1977) cautioned against making predictions on the basis of personality data alone, because of the high overlap between patients with functional and organic pain. That is, in their study, 25–30% of the functional patients scored below the mean of the organic patients on Scales 1 and 3.

The MMPI has demonstrated difficulty distinguishing between functional and organic patients, an inadequate concept. However, the MMPI might be useful for examining the psychological functioning of chronic pain patients. When studies of such patients present average MMPI profiles, the Conversion V and the neurotic triad appear most common (Adams et al., 1981; Keller & Butcher, 1991). And several studies have found that patients who reported pain and illness had elevated scores on one of the two configurations (e.g., Hansen, Biering-Sorensen, & Schroll, 1995; Leavitt, 1985; McCreary et al., 1977; Schwartz & Krupp, 1971).

Watson (1982) meticulously attempted to unravel the meaning of elevations on the first three clinical scales for chronic pain patients. He compared the item endorsement of a pain group with a sample of general medical patients and a group of college students. Group endorsement differences of 10% or greater were interpreted as significant. From this research, Watson concluded that many of the pain patients endorsed items suggesting vague somatic symptoms that were consistent with hypochondriasis. The pain group also endorsed significant depressive symptomatology. Furthermore, he reported that pain patients appeared to be no more defensive than college students or general medical patients.

Sternbach and colleagues (1973), who coined the term *low-back loser*, were important in shifting the use of the MMPI away from the functional–organic dichotomy while highlighting the importance of psychological factors. They defined the *low-back loser* as a person "whose complaint of back pain has persisted for six months or more; who is unable to work and is supported by social security, welfare, or disability payments; and who despite previous surgery, continues to seek medical or surgical relief" (p. 226). This group was subdivided in several ways, and the researchers initially examined the MMPI scores for 117 consecutive patients admitted to a pain clinic who had complained of low back pain, many of whom did not fit the description of the low-back loser. The sample included patients with acute and chronic pain, patients with and without physical findings, patients with and without litigation involvement, and patients with and without disability. Patients with physical findings, compared with those without physical findings, were significantly different on Scale 9, and the mean profile of this group showed elevations on Scales 1, 2, and 3. The researchers noted the absence of a Conversion V. They interpreted the combined profile as indicating a "psychophysiological reaction with depression" (p. 227). Their work highlights the importance of understanding the psychosocial components of individuals in pain by reframing the argument away from the dichotomy of real versus imaginary pain.

Perhaps, from the data, one might hypothesize that some patients would react to physical discomfort in a similar manner regardless of the physical findings. For instance, a patient who has chronic low back pain but only vague physical findings and a cancer patient with numerous tumors could similarly direct most of their attention and energy toward their physical symptoms. A cancer patient's attention to the undeniable physical disease, at times, can serve to impede the ability to think about, or to acknowledge, more painful and distressing emotions. Many cancer pain patients, or medically ill patients, might endorse concerns with their physical well-being, a sense of dissatisfaction, and *unusual bodily experiences*, such as tingling (Swenson, Pearson, & Osborne, 1973). However, one can imagine a Conversion V subgroup of cancer pain patients who are able to talk at length about numerous uncomfortable physical symptoms but who have difficulty acknowledging the fear, anxiety, and sadness they feel. One also can imagine a neurotic triad subgroup whose numerous physical complaints and psychological distress are voiced aggressively enough to challenge even the most understanding of health care professionals. Although more cancer patients might fall into the first category and more patients with chronic low back pain might fall into the second two categories, the overlap is evident, and it underlines the importance of psychological factors.

Snyder (1990) accurately and succinctly commented on the vast literature on this topic in his chapter on the MMPI and pain:

> Overall, findings from these studies suggest that high scores on the MMPI, and particularly on those scales comprising the neurotic triad, confirm a significant psychological component to the patient's pain complaints and functional limitations, but do not rule out underlying physical pathology. The higher the profile, the more likely that psychological factors play a significant and disproportionately greater role in the patient's pain syndrome. (p. 243)

When pain complaints are viewed through a biopsychosocial model, the functional–organic dichotomy becomes more of a continuum, and the MMPI helps to clarify the psychological components of a person's pain experience. Therefore, the difficulty distinguishing between functional and organic pain could represent less of a shortcoming with the MMPI and more of a problem with the functional–organic concept.

MMPI and Treatment Outcomes

The MMPI also has been studied to help predict who will respond to treatment and who will have difficulty. The treatments studied have ranged from spinal fusion to comprehensive pain treatment or functional restoration programs. Initially, the studies focused attention on scale elevations as a predictor. Wilfling et al. (1973) studied 26 male patients from a population of veterans who had received lumbar intervertebral fusions for relief from low back pain. The patients were assigned to three groups— "good," "poor," or "fair"—based on the success or failure of the fusion in restoring them to normal functioning. The orthopedist based the decision on employment, pain, motor signs, and patient self-reports. As expected, the good group produced a relatively normal MMPI profile. However, the poor group had clinically significant elevations on Scales 1 and 2, with a near clinically significant elevation on Scale 3. The fair group had clinically significant elevations on Scales 1 and 3, with a near clinically significant elevation on Scale 2. The poor and fair groups also showed lower scores on the Ego Strength Scale (Wilfling et al., 1973), a subscale of the MMPI that, when elevated, reflects an ability to cope with daily stressors and difficult life situations (Graham, 1993).

Whereas Wilfling et al. (1973) examined MMPI profiles after treatment, Wiltse and Rocchio (1975) examined the MMPI profiles of low back pain patients before chemonucleolysis. In addition to the MMPI, the researchers used surgeon ratings, patient biographical data, and scores from other tests. The patients' outcomes were rated 1 year after the injection based on organic and symptomatic aspects of success. Scales 1 and 3 of the MMPI were found to be the best predictors of treatment outcome. In addition, reviewing data from 274 patients who had been hospitalized for persistent back pain symptoms, these researchers concluded that scores on Scales 1 and 3 tended to increase with the number of back operations a patient had undergone (Wiltse & Rocchio, 1975).

The list of studies that have found the first three scales relevant to surgical outcomes is relatively large. Herron and Pheasant (1982) studied 69 patients who had diskogenic disease. Scales 1 and 3 were modestly related to outcomes preoperatively, but were strongly related to treatment outcomes postoperatively. Long

(1981) administered the MMPI preoperatively to low back pain patients and found a significant difference between surgery success and failure on Scale 1. Blumetti and Modesti (1976) found similar results when they studied patients who had one of several surgical interventions, such as dorsal column stimulator, rhizotomy, cordotomy, or stereotaxic thalamotomy. At 6 months, subjects were rated as falling into one of four categories ranging from "unchanged" to "abolished" pain. Nineteen improved cases were then compared with 23 unimproved cases. The unimproved cases scored significantly higher on Scales 1 and 3. In addition, Gentry, Newman, Goldner, and VonBaeyer (1977) concluded from their study that the MMPI predicted future activity level and reported pain.

There are several interesting points raised by this research. First, scales other than the first three do not regularly and consistently appear to differentiate treatment successes from failures. The amount of anxiety an individual experiences (Scale 7), ability to delay gratification (Scale 4), and ability to receive support from others (Scale 0) do not seem as relevant as is an excessive preoccupation with physical functioning. One might argue that the general presence of any psychopathology is less important than an individual's characteristic ways of handling distress and the meaning that physical symptoms develop. That is, elevations on Scales 1 and 3 could suggest that a person's physical discomfort has begun to serve a psychological purpose (such as providing a distraction from painful emotions related to a failed relationship).

Second, Scale 3 has been described as a character scale, and, as such, it is believed to measure a relatively stable trait (Trimboli & Kilgore, 1983). Little can be reliably and conclusively drawn from this fact, but it supports the thesis that a person's characteristic ways of handling negative emotions and general psychological distress is important. A person with an elevated Scale 3 has limited insight into psychological functioning and often reacts to stress with physical symptoms. Such patients tend to rely heavily on other people and have difficulty directly expressing negative emotions. Rather, negative feelings can occur as passive–aggressive or indirect behavior. For instance, a patient who has chronic low back pain and who has an elevated score on Scale 3 might deny any dissatisfaction with a spouse who has been critical of the patient's absence from work. Rather than expressing anger at the spouse for a less-than-supportive stance, the patient might stop performing minor household chores previously performed, complaining instead of a decrease in physical functioning. As one can see, there are more factors involved in the above example aside from the characteristics associated with Scale 3, although those characteristics certainly deserve attention.

Along similar lines, Herron, Turner, and Weiner (1986) did a study that explored and compared the meaning of elevations on the Millon Clinical Multiaxial Inventory (MCMI; Millon, 1982), another type of personality test, and the MMPI in an attempt to predict treatment response to lumbar laminectomy. The investigators administered the MCMI and MMPI preoperatively to 129 patients, who were later divided into "good," "fair," or "poor" surgical outcome groups. Consistent with previous findings, patients in the fair and poor groups scored higher on the first three clinical scales of the MMPI, as well as on Scale 7 (Psychasthenia). Furthermore, these patients showed higher scores on the asocial, gregarious, and neurotic depression scales of the MCMI. The researchers commented that these are not the scales of the MCMI that one would intuitively assume to be elevated. Rather, the alcohol misuse, drug misuse, hysterical, submissive, and aggressive scales appear to be more relevant, but did not show a statistically significant difference among the groups. Obviously, a discrepancy exists between the MCMI Hysterical Scale and the MMPI Scale 3. However, the Gregarious Scale of the MCMI differentiated between the groups, and gregariousness, albeit a superficial gregariousness, is associated with an elevation on Scale 3 (Herron et al., 1986).

Not all researchers have found a strong relationship between elevations on Scales 1 and 3 and poor treatment outcomes. Brandwin and Kewman (1982) attempted to use the MMPI to predict responses to electrical spinal epidural stimulation. The researchers reported that scores on Scales 1 and 3 were lower for patients who responded poorly to treatment, but that higher scores on Scale 2 were associated with poor response. Kuperman, Golden, and Blume (1979) compared organic and functional pain patients. They reported that Scale 1 was positively associated with poor treatment outcome for organic patients; Scale K was positively associated with poor outcomes for functional patients. Watkins, O'Brien, Draugelis, and Jones (1986) concluded that preoperative MMPI scores proved unreliable indicators of surgical success. However, they reported that when men were examined, improved functioning was associated with a decrease in Scales 1 and 3. The data are mixed for invasive procedures, but examination of Scales 1 and 3 could prove beneficial as one aspect of a screening procedure.

The MMPI has been used to predict response to comprehensive pain management programs. For instance, Barnes, Smith, Gatchel, and Mayer (1989) investigated patients with chronic low back pain who attended a functional restoration program. Patients were examined 1 and 2 years after completing the program and placed into "success," "failure," or "drop-out" groups based on completion of the program and returning to work. The success group had significantly lower scores on Scales 1, 2, and 3 (Barnes et al., 1989). Roberts and Reinhardt (1980) examined a comprehensive treatment program and divided patients into those who received treatment, those who refused treatment, and those rejected for treatment by the program. There were no differences between groups on the MMPI scales, but the treatment group's scores on Scales 1 and 3 decreased and ego strength increased with treatment. A decrease in Scale 3 suggests that it might not be a true character scale or that character traits can be altered with treatment that is not specifically targeted toward those traits. Whichever the case, the issue is truly complex.

Again, the importance of the first three clinical scales is highlighted, but they are by no means as strong an indicator as one would want to predict who will respond to treatment. The MMPI is useful as a part of a screening process in which other relevant pieces of biographical and background data are integrated with its findings. It might be difficult to tailor treatment based solely on elevations of the first three clinical scales, and more sophisticated ways of examining MMPI profiles have developed that are discussed later in this chapter.

MMPI and the Development of Chronic Pain

As early as 1959, Engel hypothesized that, although pain might originally develop from an external source, it often becomes a psychological phenomenon. He described the characteristics that he believed predispose individuals to chronic pain. Engel's risk factors include a history of defeat, significant guilt, unsatisfied aggressive impulses, and a propensity to develop pain in response to a real or imagined loss. Merskey (1965) hypothesized that chronic pain patients are likely to be semi-skilled workers who had difficult lives and were hypochondriacal or depressed. Blumer and Heilbronn (1982) described individuals with a pain prone disorder as having several features in common, including a hypochondriacal preoccupation, a history of "workaholism," symptoms consistent with depression, and a family history of depression and alcoholism. As can be seen, many of these characteristics are consistent with elevations on the neurotic triad scales.

The MMPI has been used to help elucidate the relationship between chronic pain and personality factors. Large-scale prospective studies are the gold standard for investigating personality factors and chronic pain, but examination of acute and chronic pain conditions, as well as the effects of treatment on MMPI scales, can provide useful initial results. A more thorough review of this topic is provided in Chapter 5 of this volume.

Sternbach and colleagues (1973) compared the MMPI profiles of patients with acute and chronic pain and examined the profiles for predictive signs. It was immediately apparent that chronic pain patients scored significantly higher on Scales 1, 2, and 3. However, acute pain patients had a more pronounced Conversion V and higher scores on Scales 6 (Paranoia) and 9 (Hypomania). The researchers hypothesized that patients with acute pain were binding their depressive affect with somatic preoccupation, the result of which was increased agitation. They also hypothesized that as time went on the patients with chronic pain were no longer able to as effectively bind their depressive affect, resulting in more depression and physical concern.

Studies have raised questions about the interactions among pain, chronicity, personality, and treatment. Barnes, Gatchel, Mayer, and Barnett (1990) examined the effects of treatment. The researchers administered the MMPI both before and 6 months after an intensive, 3-week rehabilitation program for patients with chronic low back pain. Before treatment, patients had elevated Scales 1, 2, and 3. However, 6 months after successfully completing the program—when most of the patients had returned to work—all three scales were at normal levels. Garron and Leavitt (1983) reported that increasing chronicity was associated with increases on MMPI Scales 1, 2, 3, 7, and 9. The researchers concluded that chronic pain leads to somatic preoccupation and vegetative symptoms of depression without a necessary increase in depressive mood.

Hendler (1982) described a 4-stage model of pain that includes the progression of pain from acute to subacute to chronic to subchronic. He also described what one might find on the MMPI, as well as on other psychological measures, during each period. For his discussion of the model, the patients were assumed to begin as well-adjusted, so that abnormal responses could be better understood. The acute phase occurs in the first 2 months after acquiring pain. During this stage, the patient expects the pain to subside, and the individual's MMPI profile is normal. During the subacute phase, from 2 to 6 months, the patient begins to become distressed. The MMPI reflects this with elevations on Scales 1 and 3, suggesting an increased somatic focus. Hendler compared this with the denial stage described by Kübler-Ross, because the patient is attempting to deny the potential for chronic pain and disability. Patients in the chronic phase—6 months to 8 years—experience an increase in depression, and thus an increase in Scale 2 is expected. Subsequently, the chronic pain patient also may experience anger. During the subchronic phase—between 3 and 12 years—the patient develops ways to live with the pain. The MMPI shows an elevation in Scale 1, but Scales 2 and 3 are expected to be lower than in the previous stage.

Gatchel (1996) presented a similar model, but one that allows for a possible predisposition to react to the stress of chronic pain with the development of psychopathology. He referred to the psychological changes that occur as a person progresses from acute to chronic pain as a "layering of behavioral/psychological problems over the original nociception of the pain experience itself" (p. 34). His model is based on a 3-stage progression from acute to subacute to chronic disability, after the experience of pain as a result of an identifiable injury. Stage 1 encompasses the resulting emotional reactions (fear, anxiety, worry) that arise as a consequence of perceived pain. Stage 2 begins when the pain persists beyond a reasonable acute period. In this stage, the development or exacerbation of psychological and behavioral problems occurs. Gatchel (1996) noted that the form of the difficulties depends primarily on the premorbid personality and psychological characteristics of the individual (a diathesis), as well as on the patient's current socioeconomic and environmental conditions. For instance, an individual with a tendency to become depressed might develop a depressive disorder in response to the economic and social stress of being unable to work as a result of pain (Gatchel, 1996).

This complex interaction of physical and psychosocioeconomic factors leads to Stage 3. As the patient's life begins to revolve completely around the pain, the patient begins to accept the "sick role." By doing so, the patient is excused from normal responsibilities and social obligations, which can serve to reinforce the maintenance of the role. Gatchel (1996) emphasized that the model does not assume there is a "pain personality." Rather, it assumes that "there is a general nonspecificity in terms of the relationship between personality/psychological problems and pain" (p. 35). The MMPI has provided support for this conceptualization of the pain process. Gatchel, Polatin, and Kinney (1995) studied 324 patients with acute back pain by means of several instruments, including the MMPI. Logistic regression analyses could correctly classify 88% of the patients as working or unemployed based on patient reports of pain and disability, presence of an Axis II personality disorder, and scores on MMPI Scale 3.

Bigos et al. (1991) published a longitudinal, prospective study on 3020 aerospace company employees, in an attempt to identify risk factors for back pain. After 4 years, 279 employees reported back problems. In addition to current or recent back problems and work perception, the authors concluded that Scale 3 was a primary predictor variable. Hansen et al. (1995) reported that low back pain was associated with elevations on Scales 1, 2, and 3. The researchers examined the MMPI prospectively and found that scale elevations were not predictive of future low back pain, but that they were associated with pain at the time of evaluation.

Although the MMPI does not conclusively prove the importance of personality factors in the development of chronic pain, the literature strongly suggests that personality factors are not irrelevant. The MMPI provides useful information about the psychological overlay of chronic pain conditions, and it points to the possibility of predisposing personality factors that are yet to be fully understood.

MMPI and Configurational Subgrouping

In addition to examining group elevations, the MMPI has been used for classifying profiles into subgroups. (For a more thorough explanation of the literature on this topic, see Keller and Butcher's, 1991, comprehensive review of MMPI typologies and pain.) Sternbach (1974) described several profiles that he believed might be relevant for predicting response to treatment. Patients in the first group have what is called a depressive reaction, in which Scales 1, 2, and 3 are all clinically elevated, but Scale 2 is the highest. Sternbach hypothesized that persons in this group respond well to treatment. They are aware of, distressed by, and dissatisfied with their condition and their situation. The next group has a hypochondriacal reaction in which elevations on Scales 1, 2, and 3 produce the neurotic triad. These patients, consumed with somatic concerns, are possible treatment failures. A third group, those with somatization reactions, was characterized by the familiar Conversion V, but neither success nor failure was predicted for them. The "manipulative reactions" group was the last profile and was characterized by an elevation on Scale 4. These patients tend to be "game-players and manipulators" (p. 330) and are thought to use the services of health care professionals for secondary gains.

Naliboff, Cohen, and Yellen (1983) applied more explicit rules to divide patients into six profiles. The researchers examined 157 patients with chronic low back pain, migraine headaches, hypertension, or diabetes. They found an association between configurations and self-reported limitations. Specifically, the hypochondriacal code-type appeared related to severe limitations.

Other researchers have divided patients into groups based on MMPI profiles. Louks, Freeman, and Calsyn (1978) expanded their work with low back pain patients, previously categorized as "functional," "mixed," or "organic." They divided patients into the profile groups originally described by Pichot and colleagues (1972, as cited by Louks et al., 1978): denial, Conversion V without defensiveness, Conversion V with defensiveness, depressed–anxious, psychotic, and normal. Pichot's group reported that pathological MMPI profiles, and thus psychopathology, are associated with functional pain. Bradley, Prieto, Hopson, and Prokop (1978) criticized the Pichot study for several flaws in methodology. Bradley's group argued that the functional–organic distinction should not be the focus of attention. Rather, they stated the importance of studying the pain-related behaviors of subgroups and matching treatments to effectively address the needs of the various subgroups.

McCreary, Turner, and Dawson (1979) used MMPI codetypes to help predict responses to standard medical treatment. MMPI profiles were divided into neurotic profiles (1/2, 2/3, 1/3, and 1/2/3), with severe and mild subcategories; psychotic profiles (elevation on Scale 8); and good risk profiles (any that did not fit into the above categories). The investigators reported that patients with poor outcomes had elevated scores on Scale 3 and pathological MMPI profiles. However, the pathological codetypes produced a large number of false-positives. Other studies also report useful information from configural profiles (Adams, Heilbronn, & Blumer, 1986; Heaton, Getto, Lehman, Fordyce, Brauer, & Groban, 1982; Long, 1981).

Initially, many investigators identified profiles based on clinical experience, but others have used more empirical means, specifically cluster analysis, to categorize patient profiles. Bradley, Prokop, Margolis, and Gentry (1978) examined 3 independent cohorts of 233 male and 315 female patients with low back pain. The goal was to identify replicable subgroups. The researchers examined men and women separately and found 3 subgroups for men and 4 subgroups for women. The women demonstrated a "neurotic triad" group, a "Conversion V" group, a "within normal limits" group, and a "general elevation" group. The men demonstrated a "neurotic triad" group; a "within normal limits" group; and a group with elevations on Scale F, the neurotic triad, and Scale 8 (Schizophrenia).

Prokop, Bradley, Margolis, and Gentry (1980) replicated the Bradley, Prokop, et al. (1978) study with patients who had multiple pain complaints. Three cohorts were used for women, and there was not a complete replication across the cohorts. However, the researchers found a "within normal limits" profile, a "Conversion V" profile, and a "neurotic triad" profile. The male sample consisted of a "neurotic triad" profile, a "within normal limits" profile, an elevated Scale 2 profile, and a "general elevation" profile.

Other investigators found results similar to those of Bradley, Prokop, et al. (1978) (e.g., Bernstein & Garbin, 1983; Hart, 1984), and some began to investigate relevant extratest correlates (Leavitt & Garron, 1982). For instance, Armentrout, Moore, Parker, Hewett, and Feltz (1982) studied 240 male pain patients using a hierarchical clustering procedure. They found 3 groups: a "normal" group with no significant elevations, a "hypochondriacal" group with significant elevations on the neurotic triad scales, and a "psychopathological" group with elevations on multiple clinical scales. The researchers found no significant differences among the groups with regard to age, education, income, IQ, assertiveness, type of pain, or duration of pain, but they reported that the groups differed in self-reports of pain severity and in the effects of pain on their lives.

McGill, Lawlis, Selby, Mooney, and McCoy (1983) examined 92 patients in an inpatient program for treatment of low back pain. The investigators reported that they replicated the cluster solution that Bradley, Prokop, et al. (1978) found for men and women alike. The profile groups appeared to differ with regard to the duration of pain, the presence of a clear precipitant, the number of hospitalizations, the number of back surgeries, and pretreatment pain estimate. Moreover, a significant difference was found after treatment with regard to pain estimate. However, no differences were found with regard to drug use, hours in bed, and range of motion. The estimate of pain for each group was the same before treatment as it was after treatment (McGill et al., 1983).

Bradley and Van der Heide (1984) studied 314 patients from a back pain clinic. When hierarchical clustering procedures were used, 4 male and 4 female subgroups were found. Patients in the subgroups with elevated profiles showed greater interference with daily activities. Patients with elevations primarily on Scales 1, 2, and 3 demonstrated greater affective distress and disruption of activities than did a second group of patients who had elevated scores for the first 3 clinical scales along with Scales 4 (Psychopathic Deviate) and 8 (Schizophrenia).

Rosen, Grubman, Bevins, and Frymoyer (1987) examined 362 patients with acute or chronic low back pain. The investigators used cluster analysis, and found 2 normal and 3 clinically elevated MMPI profile typologies. The normal subgroups contained patients who were less disabled than were patients in the clinically elevated subgroups. Patients in the neurotic triad group had the greatest duration of symptoms, the most abnormal physical findings, and the lowest number of functional activities. Patients in another neurotic triad group, with subclinical elevations on some of the other clinical scales, showed less physical impairment but more vocational disability, financial compensation, and past surgeries. The general elevation group in this study consisted primarily of acute pain patients and, in many respects, was similar to the normal subgroups with regard to functioning. Other researchers have found a relationship between profile type and depression (Atkinson, Ingram, Kremer, & Saccuzzo, 1986).

Unfortunately, the use of profile types to study treatment outcomes has produced mixed results (McCreary, 1985; Moore, Armentrout, Parker, & Kivlahan, 1986). For instance, Guck, Meilman, Skultety, and Poloni (1988) examined 635 chronic pain patients who received multidisciplinary treatment. The researchers reported no real relationship between cluster membership and self-reported treatment outcome. However, Bombardier, Divine, Jordan, Brooks, and Neelon (1993) examined two independent samples of more than 500 chronically ill patients using a 4-cluster solution similar to those mentioned above. The clusters were found in both samples, and MMPI profiles were associated with differences in psychiatric diagnoses, depression, psychosomatic symptoms, and functional impairment after treatment.

Costello, Hulsey, Schoenfeld, and Ramamurthy (1987) summarized most of the literature involving MMPI cluster types. They examined the various MMPI profile categorizations or cluster solutions from 10 studies and used the acronym P-A-I-N to describe the different typologies (Fig. 2.4), which were based on the categorizations or cluster solutions of previous research. Type P involved elevations on most of the clinical scales and appeared to be the most disturbed profile. The profile was associated with difficulty in the realms of psychological, educational, and vocational functioning. Type A was the familiar Conversion V profile. Type I appeared to be a hypochondriacal profile associated with physical impairment, multiple procedures,

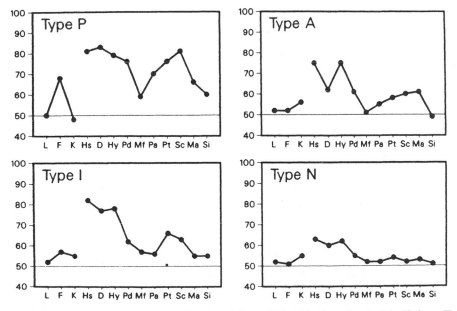

Figure 2.4. The P-A-I-N typology. Reprinted from *Pain, 30,* Costello, R. M., Hulsey, T. L., Schoenfeld, L. S., and Ramamurthy, S. (1987). P-A-I-N: A four-cluster MMPI typology for chronic pain, p. 203. Copyright 1987, with permission from Elsevier Science.

and multiple hospitalizations. Type N patients were described as relatively normal. When patients in this group had an elevated score for a scale, it was Scale K. The within normal limits group appears to be a relative description. An elevated K score can be produced by individuals who are successfully managing difficulties or it can suggest a defensive response style.

Conclusion

The use of the MMPI has contributed to the study of patients with chronic pain. Although the utility of this instrument has decreased with the introduction of the MMPI-2 and other instruments designed for chronic pain patients, the value of the vast research remains. Specifically, the importance of the psychological overlay with chronic pain patients is repeatedly demonstrated in the literature. The MMPI highlights how patients react to their pain, and how patients might be predisposed to reacting to pain in particular ways.

Clearly, the first three clinical scales have significant relevance to pain patients. The scales do not consistently differentiate functional from organic patients, but they do suggest that physical symptoms can be used to distract from painful emotions or to produce distressful affect. Furthermore, scales 1 and 3 demonstrate utility in predicting who will respond to invasive procedures, although they do a poorer job if they are used to predict a response to more comprehensive results.

Cluster analysis has been useful for describing MMPI profile types, and the method has been extended to the MMPI-2 (Keller & Butcher, 1991). Although the research has produced mixed results with regard to treatment outcomes, it seems repeatedly to find characteristic profile types for chronic pain patients. The literature does not support a single pain-prone personality, but the work with the MMPI suggests the possibility of several types of personalities that might be prone to develop chronic pain. Much more prospective research and complex conceptualizations are required to unravel this enigma. However, the research with the MMPI prevents the casual dismissal of possible predisposing personality factors.

References

Adams, K. M., Heilbronn, M., & Blumer, D. P. (1986). A multimethod evaluation of the MMPI in a chronic pain patient sample. *Journal of Clinical Psychology, 42*(6), 878–886.

Adams, K. M., Heilbronn, M., Silk, S. D., Reider, E., & Blumer, D. P. (1981). Use of the MMPI with patients who report chronic back pain. *Psychological Reports, 48*(3), 855–866.

Armentrout, D. P., Moore, J. E., Parker, J. C., Hewett, J. E., & Feltz, C. (1982). Pain-patient MMPI subgroups: The psychological dimensions of pain. *Journal of Behavioral Medicine, 5*(2), 201–211.

Atkinson, J. H., Jr., Ingram, R. E., Kremer, E. F., & Saccuzzo, D. P. (1986). MMPI subgroups and affective disorder in chronic pain patients. *Journal of Nervous and Mental Disease, 174*(7), 408–413.

Barnes, D., Gatchel, R. J., Mayer, T. G., & Barnett, J. (1990). Changes in MMPI profile levels of chronic low back pain patients following successful treatment. *Journal of Spinal Disorders, 3*(4), 353–355.

Barnes, D., Smith, D., Gatchel, R. J., & Mayer, T. G. (1989). Psychosocioeconomic predictors of treatment success/failure in chronic low-back pain patients. *Spine, 14*(4), 427–430.

Beals, R. K., & Hickman, N. W. (1972). Industrial injuries of the back and extremities. Comprehensive evaluation—An aid in prognosis and management: A study of one hundred and eighty patients. *Journal of Bone and Joint Surgery—American Volume, 54*(8), 1593–1611.

Bernstein, I. H., & Garbin, C. P. (1983). Hierarchical clustering of pain patients' MMPI profiles: A replication note. *Journal of Personality Assessment, 47*(2), 171–172.

Bigos, S. J., Battie, M. C., Spengler, D. M., Fisher, L. D., Fordyce, W. E., Hansson, T. H., Nachemson, A. L., & Wortley, M. D. (1991). A prospective study of work perceptions and psychosocial factors affecting the report of back injury [published erratum appears in *Spine* (1991) June; *16*(6): 688]. *Spine, 16*(1), 1–6.

Blumer, D., & Heilbronn, M. (1982). Chronic pain as a variant of depressive disease: The pain-prone disorder. *Journal of Nervous and Mental Disease, 170*(7), 381–406.

Blumetti, A. E., & Modesti, L. M. (1976). Psychological predictors of success or failure of surgical intervention for intractable back pain. In J. J. Bonica & D. Albe-Fessard (Eds.), *Advances in pain research and therapy* (Vol. 1, pp. 323–325). New York: Raven.

Bombardier, C. H., Divine, G. W., Jordan, J. S., Brooks, W. B., & Neelon, F. A. (1993). Minnesota Multiphasic Personality Inventory (MMPI) cluster groups among chronically ill patients: Relationship to illness adjustment and treatment outcome. *Journal of Behavioral Medicine, 16*(5), 467–484.

Bradley, L. A., Prieto, E. J., Hopson, L., & Prokop, C. K. (1978). Comment on "Personality Organization as an Aspect of Back Pain in a Medical Setting." *Journal of Personality Assessment, 42*(6), 573–578.

Bradley, L. A., Prokop, C. K., Margolis, R., & Gentry, W. D. (1978). Multivariate analyses of the MMPI profiles of low back pain patients. *Journal of Behavioral Medicine, 1*(3), 253–272.

Bradley, L. A., & Van der Heide, L. H. (1984). Pain-related correlates of MMPI profile subgroups among back pain patients. *Health Psychology, 3*(2), 157–274.

Brandwin, M. A., & Kewman, D. G. (1982). MMPI indicators of treatment response to spinal epidural stimulation in patients with chronic pain and patients with movement disorders. *Psychological Reports, 51*(3, pt. 2), 1059–1064.

Butcher, J. N., & Williams, C. L. (1993). *Essentials of MMPI-2 and MMPI-A interpretation.* Minneapolis: University of Minnesota Press.

Calsyn, D. A., Louks, J., & Freeman, C. W. (1976). The use of the MMPI with chronic low back pain patients with a mixed diagnosis. *Journal of Clinical Psychology, 32*(3), 532–536.

Costello, R. M., Hulsey, T. L., Schoenfeld, L. S., & Ramamurthy, S. (1987). P-A-I-N: A four-cluster MMPI typology for chronic pain. *Pain, 30*(2), 199–209.

Cox, G. B., Chapman, C. R., & Black, R. G. (1978). The MMPI and chronic pain: The diagnosis of psychogenic pain. *Journal of Behavioral Medicine, 1*(4), 437–443.

Dahlstrom, W. G., Welsh, G. S., & Dahlstrom, L. E. (1972). *An MMPI handbook: Vol.1. Clinical interpretation* (rev. ed.). Minneapolis: University of Minnesota Press.

Engel, G. L. (1959). "Psychogenic" pain and the pain prone patient. *American Journal of Medicine, 26*, 899–918.

Freeman, C., Calsyn, D., & Louks, J. (1976). The use of the Minnesota Multiphasic Personality Inventory with low back pain patients. *Journal of Clinical Psychology, 32*(2), 294–298.

Garron, D. C., & Leavitt, F. (1983). Chronic low back pain and depression. *Journal of Clinical Psychology, 39*(4), 486–493.

Gatchel, R. J. (1991). Early development of physical and mental deconditioning in painful spinal disorders. In T. G. Mayer, V. Mooney, & R. J. Gatchel (Eds.), *Contemporary conservative care for painful spinal disorders* (pp. 278–279). Philadelphia: Lea & Febiger.

Gatchel, R. J. (1996). Psychological disorders and chronic pain: Cause-and-effect relation-ships. In R. J. Gatchel & D. C. Turk (Eds.), *Psychological approaches to pain manage-ment: A practitioner's handbook* (pp. 33–52). New York: Guilford Press.

Gatchel, R. J., Polatin, P. B., & Kinney, R. K. (1995). Predicting outcome of chronic back pain using clinical predictors of psychopathology: A prospective analysis. *Health Psy-chology, 14*(5), 415–420.

Gentry, W. D., Newman, M. C., Goldner, J. L., & VonBaeyer, C. (1977). Relation between graduated spinal block technique and MMPI for diagnosis and prognosis of chronic low-back pain. *Spine, 2,* 210–213.

Gilberstadt, H., & Jancis, M. (1967). "Organic" vs. "functional" diagnoses from 1–3 MMPI profiles. *Journal of Clinical Psychology, 23*(4), 480–483.

Graham, J. R. (1993). *MMPI-2: Assessing personality and psychopathology* (2nd ed.). New York: Oxford University Press.

Guck, T. P., Meilman, P. W., Skultety, F. M., & Poloni, L. D. (1988). Pain-patient Minnesota Multiphasic Personality Inventory (MMPI) subgroups: Evaluation of long-term treatment outcome. *Journal of Behavioral Medicine, 11*(2), 159–169.

Hansen, F. R., Biering-Sorensen, F., & Schroll, M. (1995). Minnesota Multiphasic Personality Inventory profiles in persons with or without low back pain. A 20-year follow-up study. *Spine, 20*(24), 2716–2720.

Hanvik, L. J. (1951). MMPI profiles in patients with low-back pain. *Journal of Consulting Psychology, 15,* 350–353.

Hart, R. R. (1984). Chronic pain: Replicated multivariate clustering of personality profiles. *Journal of Clinical Psychology, 40*(1), 129–133.

Heaton, R. K., Getto, C. J., Lehman, R. A., Fordyce, W. E., Brauer, E., & Groban, S. E. (1982). A standardized evaluation of psychosocial factors in chronic pain. *Pain, 12*(2), 165–174.

Hendler, N. H. (1982). The four stages of pain. In N. H. Hendler, D. M. Long, & T. N. Wise (Eds.), *Diagnosis and treatment of chronic pain* (pp. 1–8). Littleton, MA: John Wright.

Herron, L. D., & Pheasant, H. C. (1982). Changes in MMPI profiles after low-back surgery. *Spine, 7*(6), 591–597.

Herron, L., Turner, J., & Weiner, P. (1986). A comparison of the Millon Clinical Multiaxial Inventory and the Minnesota Multiphasic Personality Inventory as predictors of success-ful treatment by lumbar laminectomy. *Clinical Orthopaedics and Related Research,* 232–238.

Keller, L. S., & Butcher, J. N. (1991). *Assessment of chronic pain patients with the MMPI-2.* Minneapolis: University of Minnesota Press.

Kuperman, S. K., Golden C. J., & Blume, H. G. (1979). Predicting pain treatment results by personality variables in organic and functional patients. *Journal of Clinical Psychology, 35,* 832–837.

Lair, C. V., & Trapp, E. P. (1962). The differential diagnostic value of MMPI with somatically disturbed patients. *Journal of Clinical Psychology, 18,* 146–147.

Leavitt, F. (1985). The value of the MMPI conversion "V" in the assessment of psychogenic pain. *Journal of Psychosomatic Research, 29*(2), 125–131.

Leavitt, F., & Garron, D. C. (1982). Patterns of psychological disturbance and pain report in patients with low back pain. *Journal of Psychosomatic Research, 26*(3), 301–307.

Long, C. J. (1981). The relationship between surgical outcome and MMPI profiles in chronic pain patients. *Journal of Clinical Psychology, 37*(4), 744–749.

Louks, J. L., Freeman, C. W., & Calsyn, D. A. (1978). Personality organization as an aspect of back pain in a medical setting. *Journal of Personality Assessment, 42*(2), 152–158.

Love, A. W., & Peck, C. L. (1987). The MMPI and psychological factors in chronic low back pain: A review. *Pain, 28*(1), 1–12.

McCreary, C. (1985). Empirically derived MMPI profile clusters and characteristics of low back pain patients. *Journal of Consulting & Clinical Psychology, 53*(4), 558–560.

McCreary, C., Turner, J., & Dawson, E. (1977). Differences between functional versus organic low back pain patients. *Pain, 4*(1), 73–78.

McCreary, C., Turner, J., & Dawson, E. (1979). The MMPI as a predictor of response to conservative treatment for low back pain. *Journal of Clinical Psychology, 35*(2), 278–284.

McGill, J. C., Lawlis, G. F., Selby, D., Mooney, V., & McCoy, C. E. (1983). The relationship of Minnesota Multiphasic Personality Inventory (MMPI) profile clusters to pain behaviors. *Journal of Behavioral Medicine, 6*(1), 77–92.

McKinley, J. C., & Hathaway, S. R. (1940). A multiphasic personality schedule (Minnesota): II. A differential study of hypochondriasis. *Journal of Psychology, 10*, 255–268.

Melzack R., & Wall, P. (1965). Pain mechanisms: A new theory. *Science, 150*, 971–979.

Merskey, H. (1965). The characteristics of persistent pain in psychological illness. *Journal of Psychosomatic Research, 9*, 291–298.

Millon, T. (1982). *Millon Clinical Multiaxial Inventory manual* (3rd ed.). Minneapolis, MN: National Computer Systems.

Moore, J. E., Armentrout, D. P., Parker, J. C., & Kivlahan, D. R. (1986). Empirically derived pain-patient MMPI subgroups: Prediction of treatment outcome. *Journal of Behavioral Medicine, 9*(1), 51–63.

Naliboff, B. D., Cohen, M. J., & Yellen, A. N. (1983). Frequency of MMPI profile types in three chronic illness populations. *Journal of Clinical Psychology, 39*(6), 843–847.

Prokop, C. K., Bradley, L. A., Margolis, R., & Gentry, W. D. (1980). Multivariate analysis of the MMPI profiles of patients with multiple pain complaints. *Journal of Personality Assessment, 44*(3), 246–252.

Roberts, A. H., & Reinhardt, L. (1980). The behavioral management of chronic pain: Long-term follow-up with comparison groups. *Pain, 8*(2), 151–162.

Rosen, J. C., Grubman, J. A., Bevins, T., & Frymoyer, J. W. (1987). Musculoskeletal status and disability of MMPI profile subgroups among patients with low back pain. *Health Psychology, 6*(6), 581–598.

Rosen, J. C., Johnson, C., & Frymoyer, J. W. (1983). Identification of excessive back disability with the Faschingbauer Abbreviated MMPI. *Journal of Clinical Psychology, 39*(1), 71–74.

Schwartz, M. S., & Krupp, N. E. (1971). The MMPI "conversion V" among 50,000 medical patients: A study of incidence, criteria, and profile elevation. *Journal of Clinical Psychology, 27*, 89–95.

Snyder, D. K. (1990). Assessing chronic pain with the Minnesota Multiphasic Personality Inventory (MMPI). In T. W. Miller (Ed.), *Chronic pain: Clinical issues in health care management* (pp. 215–257). Madison, CT: International Universities Press.

Sternbach, R. A. (1974). Psychological aspects of pain and the selection of patients. *Clinical Neurosurgery, 21*, 323–333.

Sternbach, R. A., Wolf, S. R., Murphy, R. W., & Akeson, W. H. (1973). Traits of pain patients: The low-back "loser." *Psychosomatics, 14*(4), 226–229.

Stone, R. K., Jr., & Pepitone-Arreola-Rockwell, F. (1983). Diagnosis of organic and functional pain patients with the MMPI. *Psychological Reports, 52*(2), 539–548.

Swenson, W. M., Pearson, J. S., & Osborne, D. (1973). *An MMPI source book: Basic item, scale, and pattern data on 50,000 medical patients*. Minneapolis: University of Minnesota Press.

Towne, W. S., & Tsushima, W. T. (1978). The use of the Low Back and the Dorsal scales in the identification of functional low back pain patients. *Journal of Clinical Psychology, 34*, 88–91.

Trimboli, F., & Kilgore, R. B. (1983). A psychodynamic approach to MMPI interpretation. *Journal of Personality Assessment, 47*(6), 614–626.

Tsushima, W. T., & Towne, W. S. (1979). Clinical limitations of the Low Back Scale. *Journal of Clinical Psychology, 35*(2), 306–308.

Turk, D. C. (1996). Biopsychosocial perspectives on chronic pain. In R. J. Gatchel & D. C. Turk (Eds.), *Psychological approaches to pain management: A practitioner's handbook* (pp. 33–52). New York: Guilford Press.

Watkins, R. G., O'Brien, J. P., Draugelis, R., & Jones, D. (1986). Comparisons of preoperative and postoperative MMPI data in chronic back patients. *Spine, 11*(4), 385–390.

Watson, D. (1982). Neurotic tendencies among chronic pain patients: An MMPI item analysis. *Pain, 14*, 365–385.

Wilfling, F. J., Klonoff, H., & Kokan, P. (1973). Psychological, demographic and orthopaedic factors associated with prediction of outcome of spinal fusion. *Clinical Orthopaedics and Related Research, 90*, 153–160.

Wiltse, L. L., & Rocchio, P. D. (1975). Preoperative psychological tests as predictors of success of chemonucleolysis in the treatment of the low-back syndrome. *Journal of Bone and Joint Surgery—American Volume, 57*(4), 478–483.

Part II

Advances in Personality Testing in Patients With Chronic Pain

Chapter 3
ASSESSING PERSONALITY WITH THE MILLON BEHAVIORAL HEALTH INVENTORY, THE MILLON BEHAVIORAL MEDICINE DIAGNOSTIC, AND THE MILLON CLINICAL MULTIAXIAL INVENTORY

Neil Bockian, Sarah Meager, and Theodore Millon

The goal of clinical diagnosis in traditional medicine is identification of the disease process and formulation of a plan to treat the disease. When psychosocial factors are added to the medical symptomatology, the patient cannot be seen simply as a vessel who carries a group of predictable or constant symptoms available for evaluation. Rather, psychosocial events and the patient's premorbid personality co-vary to create a changing constellation. Under these circumstances, clinical analysis must not only systematically evaluate these varied elements, but it must also elucidate their interrelationships and dynamic flow. Current behaviors and attitudes should be interpreted in conjunction with the physical aspects of the presenting problem. The premorbid background of the patient must be delineated in an effort to clarify the historical context or pattern of the syndrome. Moreover, personality and environmental circumstances must be appraised to optimize therapeutic recommendations. Ultimately, the goal of psychological assessment is the development of a preventive or remedial plan.

It is now well established that pain, along with most medical conditions, is profoundly influenced by psychological factors. Descartes' dualism—that mind and body are separate—is increasingly seen as an untenable philosophical underpinning for understanding and treating medical problems. Clinical psychological analysis with medical patients is both an abbreviated and a more extensive evaluation than for the psychiatric patient, as characterized by Millon (1969). The first task is the description of the clinical picture. The presenting medical problem is often the most obvious aspect, but it often serves as a precipitant of difficulties of a more extensive or long-lasting nature. The physical problem must be evaluated for its effects on the physiology of the individual and for its influence on the emotions of the patient and those who surround the patient. Thus, it is important to evaluate the individual's overt behaviors, stated reports of feelings along with the inferred intrapsychic processes, and biophysical processes.

This chapter introduces two scales that have been used to assess personality: the Millon Clinical Multiaxial Inventory (MCMI[1]; Millon, 1977, 1987; Millon, Millon, & Davis, 1994, 1997) and the Millon Behavioral Health Inventory (MBHI[1]; Millon, Green, & Meagher, 1982). A brief description of the development of these scales and their underlying personality theory is provided. A new scale, the Millon Behavioral Medicine Diagnostic (MBMD; Millon, Antoni, Millon, & Davis, in press), is described, although its development is in its "adolescence." The MBHI and MBMD were developed with patients undergoing evaluation or treatment in medical settings

---

for physical disorders, including those associated with pain. Their major intent is to provide information relevant to behavioral assessment and treatment decisions about patients.

General Personality and Coping Patterns

Based on psychopathological models (that pain is a somatization of underlying psychological problems), it was natural to search for a "pain-prone personality." Some consider pain proneness a useful concept (Large, 1986; Sivik, 1991). On the other hand, Sadigh (1998) noted that, "since the advent of psychoanalysis, nearly a hundred years ago, a number of studies have attempted to predict the connection between personality traits and a tendency for developing chronic muscle pain. . . . The evidence, however, remains inconclusive" (p. 4). In a prospective study of whiplash patients, for example, Borchgrevink, Stiles, Borchgrevink, and Lereim (1997) found that mean MCMI–I profiles at intake were in the average range on all scales, and they interpreted this as evidence against personality playing a causal role in the development of chronic pain. Elliott, Jackson, Layfield, and Kendall (1996) noted that, rather than playing an important causal role, personality problems most likely precede pain problems and complicate treatment. Others have concluded that many of the findings with medical populations are a result of coping with difficult, long-term conditions (Naber, Weinberger, Bullinger, Polsby, & Chase, 1988). It is reasonable to theorize that individuals with personality disorders have reduced social and intrapsychic resources and are therefore more vulnerable to the difficulties imposed by a chronic pain condition; they would thus tend to populate pain centers with greater-than-average frequency.

Three of the Millon inventories are presented in this chapter. Although many clinicians associate the diagnosis of personality disorders with the MCMI, most research conducted with pain patients has been done using the MBHI. Therefore, a large part of this chapter will be devoted to presenting the MBHI and reviewing the empirical evidence that has been generated involving pain patients since the measure was introduced in 1982. A description of the new scales on the soon to be released MBMD will then be reviewed. Finally, the MCMI will be covered briefly, and the limited empirical evidence that involves assessment of patients with pain will be presented.

Personality Styles and Health-Related Attitudes: The MBHI

The MBHI was developed specifically with medical–behavioral decision-making issues in mind (Millon et al., 1982). A major goal in its construction was to keep the total number of items small enough to encourage its use in all types of diagnostic and treatment settings, yet large enough to permit the assessment of a wide range of clinically relevant behaviors. It is geared to an 8th-grade reading level, and it contains 150 items.

Diagnostic instruments such as the MBHI have increased utility if they are linked systematically to a comprehensive clinical theory or are anchored to empirical validation data gathered in their construction (Loevinger, 1957). The eight basic *coping styles* that constitute the first scales of the MBHI are derived from Millon's (1969) theory of personality. The theory is based on a biosocial learning model that sets forth basic principles of personality and the combinations of these principles that led to deducing the coping styles that are included on the MBHI. The six Psychogenic Attitude scales were developed to reflect psychosocial stressors found in the research literature to be significant precipitators or exacerbators of physical illness. The final six scales in the current form were derived empirically for the MBHI, either to appraise the extent to which emotional factors complicate particular psychosomatic ailments or to predict psychological complications associated with several diseases.

Self-administered and suitable either for group or for individual administration, the inventory can be completed by most patients in 20–25 minutes. Because the MBHI has multiple scales, it is also multiple-keyed, and the test authors and manufacturer suggest that it is best machine scored. This method automatically converts the raw scores on the 20 scales into base-ratio (BR) scores and can provide the clinician with a narrative report that interprets the results. The conversions to BR scores were determined by known or estimated prevalence data to maximize correct classifications, as argued by Meehl and Rosen (1955).

Norms for the MBHI are based on several groups of nonclinical and numerous samples of medical patients involved in diagnosis, treatment, or follow-up. The nonclinical group included in the construction phase of test development consisted of participants drawn from several settings (colleges, health maintenance organizations, nursing schools, medical schools, and factories, among others) and consisted of 212 men and 240 women. The test construction patient group, drawn from a diverse clinical population (surgical clinics, pain centers, dialysis units, cancer programs), consisted of 1194 persons, of which 130 men and 170 women were selected as a representative cross-section for purposes of developing norms. An additional series of patient populations, consisting of 437 men and 482 women, was involved in development and cross-validation of the six empirically derived scales. In all, 443 patients and 452 nonclinical individuals were used to validate the instrument. Interpretation is based on single-scale elevations and profile configurations.

Basic Coping Styles

The following descriptions of the personality style scales are drawn from the MBHI manual (Millon et al., 1982)[2]. These characteristics usually blend with other features when an interpretive paragraph is generated from a configural profile of several scales. The highest two or three scales form a configuration, which then combines and synthesizes the various coping dimensions exhibited by the patient.

Scale 1: The Introversive Style

High scorers are rather colorless and emotionally flat, tending to be quiet and restrained in their speech. They often appear unconcerned about their problems and are lacking in energy, just plodding along through life in a dull way. They are usually vague when reporting symptoms, and it is often difficult to get them to take an active role in their own health care. Physicians should give clear and explicit directions and not expect these patients to take the initiative in following a treatment plan. Simple concrete steps delivered through a highly structured treatment plan will be most helpful in patients who score highest on this coping scale.

Scale 2: The Inhibited Style

High scorers tend to be fearful of others and are often shy and ill at ease. Health care providers must be careful how they phrase comments, inasmuch as these patients are highly anxious and easily hurt. Because these patients are distrustful of what others might do to them, the health care provider must devote extra effort to establishing rapport. These patients also have low opinions of themselves, which they fear others will exploit. Hence, they often keep their problems to themselves. However, they do want understanding and attention. With a sympathetic attitude, it should be possible to gain their cooperation. A patient and sympathetic approach is likely to work best in earning this type of person's trust and adherence to required treatment regimens.

Scale 3: The Cooperative Style

High scorers tend to be good-natured, gentle, and generous with others. They are eager to attach themselves to a supportive health care provider and will follow advice closely. These patients rarely take the initiative in treatment, and will expect to be told exactly what to do. They tend to belittle themselves and are inclined to deny the existence of real problems. Thus, it will be necessary to probe carefully and ask questions explicitly. A sense of security is derived for these patients from specific and clear-cut directives. These patients become dependent and may resist when suggestions are made for referral to other doctors or clinics. Providing high scorers on this scale with too many treatment alternatives may be contraindicated in that it will increase their anxiety. They generally prefer that they be told the "best" alternative for their specific circumstances.

Scale 4: The Sociable Style

High scorers are superficially very sociable, talkative, and charming. However, these patients are rather changeable in their likes and dislikes. They may appear to be very cooperative with the physician in following the treatment plan, but this alliance and cooperation is often short-lived. These patients frequently are more concerned with "appearing nice and attractive" than they are with solving their problem. They tend to be more vocal than other patients in their reporting of symptoms, and their dependability in meeting appointments and taking medications is likely to be low.

Scale 5: The Confident Style

High scorers act in a calm and confident manner. However, they have a great fear of bodily injury and will thus be motivated to follow any treatment plan that will ensure their well-being. They expect to be given special treatment and will tend to take advantage of everyone on staff. Although the physician may find this abrasive, it is important that he or she manage these patients fairly and explain the course of treatment fully. If these patients are impressed with the critical importance to their health of following the medical regimen, they will do it carefully. Although these patients are typically demanding, the extra time and energy required of health care personnel is likely to result in increased compliance on the part of the patient.

Scale 6: The Forceful Style

High scorers tend to be domineering and tough-minded, and they are often hostile and angry. Health care professionals should be careful not to let themselves feel intimidated or provoked, because these patients behave bluntly with everyone. A straightforward approach in which the clinician "pulls no punches" and makes no apologies is best in increasing chances for patient compliance. Given their tendency to distrust others, these patients may not follow the planned treatment program, doing instead what they want. These patients react to frightening situations with anger and hostility. When feeling uncertain of their bearings, high scorers instinctively respond with challenge. In dealing with these patients, the clinician needs to maintain a fine balance between being either overly authoritative or overly indecisive.

Scale 7: The Respectful Style

High scorers are very prompt, efficient, and disciplined. They hold their feelings inside and will try to impress the health care professional as being well-controlled, serious-minded, and responsible. Illness represents weakness or laziness for these patients, and they might have denied symptoms and delayed seeking treatment for long periods. Nonetheless, they tend to be responsible about taking prescribed medications and following professional advice. They will seek detailed answers to well-considered questions regarding their illness. It is essential that they feel a part of the treatment planning. Their perceived self-efficacy through the management of their illness mitigates their tendency to deny and allows them a sense of self-control. These patients usually take medications and follow therapeutic recommendations carefully. They do not like being sick because it signifies weakness and inefficiency. Whatever measures can be taken to enhance their sense of control will enhance treatment compliance.

Scale 8: The Sensitive Style

High scorers tend to be unpredictable, moody, and troublesome. They are often erratic in following a treatment plan (overmedicating or undermedicating without telling the physician). These patients often seem displeased and dissatisfied with their physical and psychological state. At times, they will complain profusely about treatment but then quickly switch to expressing guilt. Mood changes seem to occur for no clear reason. Rapport may be established easily on some days but be excruciatingly difficult on others. These patients are critical and demanding, and they are often unforgiving of perceived mistakes or inadequacies in others. Typically, these patients are "over utilizers" of the system and will require much attention and coddling from the professional staff.

Psychogenic Attitudes Scales

The Psychogenic Attitudes scales represent the personal feelings and perceptions of the patient regarding different aspects of psychological stress, which are presumed to increase psychosomatic susceptibility or aggravate the course of a current disease. The first two of these scales pertain to relatively objective events that have been experienced either as chronically or as recently stressful. The next two scales relate to attitudes that intensify the subjective impact of past or future stressful events. The third set of two scales attempts to gauge the status of two significant sources of potential stress—interpersonal relationships and bodily functioning.

Scores are gauged by comparing the attitudes of the test respondent to those expressed by a cross-section of healthy and physically ill adults of the same gender. Each of these scales is to be first analyzed on an individual basis. Scores lower than BR = 35 are indicative of lower-than-average levels of concern regarding the construct measured by that scale and a projected better-than-average management of an illness, should one exist or occur. Scores falling between 35 and 74 are considered average and have neither positive nor negative consequences. Scale elevations in the "presence" range of BR 75–84 indicate that they could pose serious difficulties both for patients' health status and for their capacity to manage disease, if present. Score elevations of BR > 85 signify a major area of concern for the patient that will likely affect health.

Scale A: Chronic Tension

The Chronic Tension Scale gauges level of stress, a factor that has repeatedly been found to relate to the incidence of a variety of diseases. More specifically, qualitative studies of chronic stress, such as persistent job tensions or marital problems, have been carried out with particular reference to their consequences for heart disease, often addressed as the Type A–Type B behavior pattern (Friedman & Rosenman, 1974; Jenkins, 1976; Rahe, 1977). Constantly on the go, Type A individuals live under considerable self-imposed pressure and have trouble relaxing. Some research has suggested that it is not necessarily a global Type A behavior that contributes to coronary artery disease but the more specific qualities of anger and hostility that are part of the Type A constellation (Dembroski & Costa, 1987). Frequently endorsed for some aspects of this behavior, such individuals are often found in positions of responsibility and are well-targeted for preventive intervention.

Scale B: Recent Stress

The Recent Stress Scale addresses patients' perceptions of events in the recent past that were experienced as stressful. This is a phenomenological assessment similar to the Social Readjustment Rating Scale (Holmes & Rahe, 1967) and the Life Experience Survey (Sarason, Johnson, & Siegal, 1978). High scorers on this scale are assumed to have an increased susceptibility to serious illness for the year following test administration. Recent marked changes in their lives predict a significantly higher incidence of poor physical and psychological health than that found in the population at large (Andrew, 1970; Rahe & Arthur, 1968; Yunik, 1979). Identifying patterns of susceptibility is particularly important in health settings, where preventive interventions often prove both beneficial and cost-effective. Therefore, regular and frequent contact with these patients would be advisable during this period to anticipate and avert the possibility of illness.

Scale C: Premorbid Pessimism

The Premorbid Pessimism Scale represents a dispositional attitude of helplessness–hopelessness that has been implicated in the appearance or exacerbation of such diseases as multiple sclerosis, ulcerative colitis, and cancer (Mei-Tal, Meyerowitz, & Engel, 1970; Paull & Hislop, 1974; Schmale, 1972; Stavraky, Buch, Lott, & Wonklin, 1968). It differs from other "depression" indices by noting characterological tendencies toward a negative view of the world. High scorers on this scale are disposed to interpret life as a series of troubles and misfortunes and are likely to intensify the discomforts they experience with real physical and psychological difficulties (Levine, 1980; Yunik, 1979). Again, this scale is particularly salient for identifying individuals whose personal life and health could suffer as a consequence of their feelings.

Scale D: Future Despair

The Future Despair Scale focuses on the patient's willingness to plan and look forward to the future (Engel, 1968; Wright, 1960). This scale is more likely than the Premorbid Pessimism Scale to tap the person's response to current difficulties and circumstances than it is to detect a general or lifelong tendency to view things negatively. High scorers do not look forward to a productive future life, and they view medical difficulties as seriously distressing and potentially life threatening. This scale assesses a respondent's willingness to plan and look forward to the future. High scorers have a poor prognostic outlook and a consequently poor prognosis that characterize them as needing considerable support and encouragement from health personnel.

Scale E: Social Alienation

Social Alienation assesses familial and friendship support, both real and perceived, that appears to relate to the influence of various life stressors (Cobb, 1977; Rabkin

& Streuning, 1976). The sense of aloneness has been detailed in sociological literature (Comstock & Partridge, 1972; Moss, 1977; Parkes, Benjamin, & Fitzgerald,
1969). High scorers are prone to physical and psychological ailments. A poor adjustment to hospitalization is also common. These patients perceive low levels of
family and social support and might not seek medical assistance until illness is
extremely discomforting. By using this scale on the MBHI to identify these patients,
special efforts can be made to aid them in developing alternative support systems.

Scale F: Somatic Anxiety

All the above stressors seem to be significantly modulated upward or downward by
the preoccupations and fear that individuals may express about their physical state,
a characteristic addressed in the Somatic Anxiety Scale. Studies of what may be
called somatic anxiety reflect the general concerns that people have about their bodies
(Lipsitt, 1970; Lowy, 1977; Lucente & Fleck, 1972; Mechanic & Volkart, 1960).
High scorers on this scale tend to be hypochondriacal and susceptible to various
minor illnesses. They experience an abnormal amount of fear concerning bodily
functioning and are likely to overreact to the discomforts of surgery and hospitalization (Green, Meagher, & Millon, 1980). Such preoccupations often lead patients
to excessive searches for medical treatment.

Psychosomatic Correlates Scales

The scales in this section are relevant only to patients who have been medically
diagnosed as exhibiting one of several specific disease syndromes (allergy, gastrointestinal problems, cardiovascular difficulties). These scales were derived empirically. The scores for each scale gauge the extent to which a patient's responses are
similar to comparably diagnosed patients whose illnesses have been judged by the
health care provider to be substantially psychosomatic or whose course has been
complicated by emotional or social factors. Scores of BR < 60 indicate little likelihood that psychosomatic components are contributory to disease processes. Scores
between 61 and 74 provide only a weak basis for concluding that the disorder is
partially somatic in nature. Scores of 75–84 indicate that psychosomatic factors have
contributed to or have prolonged a disease process. BR scores above 85 presume
that psychological precipitants are likely to have been a major source of the disorder
and greatly contribute to the severity and persistence of illness.

Scale MM: Allergic Inclination

High scorers among patients with allergic disorders (e.g., dermatitis, asthma) experience emotional factors as significant precipitants of their disease process. The role
of these influences among low scorers is likely to be minimal.

Scale NN: Gastrointestinal Susceptibility

High scores among patients with gastrointestinal disorders—ulcer, colitis, dyspepsia
—are likely to react to psychological stress with an increase in the frequency and

severity of symptomatology. Stress is not a significant precipitant among low scorers with these ailments.

Scale OO: Cardiovascular Tendency

High scorers among patients with cardiovascular symptoms, such as hypertension or angina pectoris, are susceptible to a significant increase in complaint symptomatology under conditions of tension. Emotional factors are not likely to contribute significantly to such symptomatology among low scorers.

Prognostic Indices Scales

The Prognostic Indices scales assist clinicians in determining whether psychosocial or emotional factors are likely to complicate the usual prognostic course of patients with specific chronic or life-threatening illnesses. These scales also can identify future treatment problems or difficulties that could arise in the course of an illness.

Scale PP: Pain Treatment Responsivity Scale

High scorers among patients with an intermittent or persistent pain syndrome (low back pain, tension headache, temporomandibular joint dysfunction) are prone to respond to isolated medical or surgical treatments with a less-than-optimal outcome. Pain-related behavior, such as excessive symptom report or withdrawal, can be maintained by psychological factors in these patients. Low scorers often report a reasonably good response to physically oriented treatment programs. Obviously, this is an important scale to scrutinize carefully when treating patients with pain.

Scale QQ: Life-Threat Reactivity

High scorers who currently have a chronic or progressive life-threatening illness (metastatic carcinoma, renal failure, congestive heart disease) are likely to deteriorate more rapidly than is typical among patients with a comparable physical illness. Psychological and social support is highly recommended for those scoring high on this scale. Low scorers are judged as likely to progress through a more benign and favorable course.

Scale RR: Emotional Vulnerability

High scorers facing major surgery or other life-dependent treatment programs, such as open-heart surgical procedures, hemodialysis, or chemotherapy, are more vulnerable to severe psychological complications, such as disorientation, depression, or frank psychotic episodes. Intensive pre- and postoperative support can decrease such developments. Severe reactions of this nature are not probable among low scorers.

Validation of the MBHI

The MBHI was developed following procedures recommended by Loevinger (1957) and Jackson (1970), in that validation was continuous throughout all phases of test construction rather than a procedure for assessing or corroborating the instrument's accuracy at the end. The three aspects of this validation procedure are called theoretical–substantive, internal–structural, and external-criterion stages.

Theoretical–Substantive Validation Stage

More than 1000 items were gathered from numerous sources, including other psychological measures of normal and abnormal personality; some were written specifically for item pool purposes. Items were developed to cover the full range of characteristics to be tapped by the personality and the psychogenic scales. At this stage, the number of items in the personality style scales ranged from 60 to 135. The Psychogenic Attitude scale items ranged from 37 to 57. The item set for the 6 empirically derived scales was drawn entirely from the final pool based on the 14 Coping Style and Psychogenic Attitude scales; they were not subjected to initial theoretical–substantive analysis. Items were balanced at this stage so that approximately half of them could be answered "true" to signify the style or attitude, and half could be answered "false." The balance was built in to correct for "acquiescence" bias (Jackson & Messick, 1961).

Items were deleted according to the following general criteria: (a) too complicated for patient understanding, (b) obvious social desirability bias, (c) lack of clarity in phrasing, and (d) probable extreme endorsement frequency. Items were retained if they exemplified the traits of the scale for which they were written, and efforts were made to cover the full range of behaviors and attitudes typified by a given scale. To achieve this, researchers asked 10 health professionals knowledgeable of personality theory and experienced with psychological traits in medically ill individuals to independently sort these items into their theoretically appropriate personality and psychogenic categories. Inclusion required that the item be sorted into the "correct" (or same) scale by at least 7 of the 10 reviewers.

Internal–Structural Validation Stage

In accordance with the theoretical model, items should give evidence not only of substantial within-scale homogeneity, but also of selective overlap with theoretically related scales. Item and scale overlap within the MBHI was both expected and constructed, in line with theoretical considerations. This contrasts with other instruments, such as the Minnesota Multiphasic Personality Inventory (MMPI), where overlap among items on different scales is solely a function of empirically obtained covariations. A detailed explanation of this rationale may be found in the MCMI—III revised manual (Millon, Millon, & Davis, 1997). According to the theory underlying both the MCMI (Millon, 1969; Millon & Davis, 1996) and the MBHI, no personality style or psychogenic attitude is likely to consist of entirely homogeneous and discrete psychological dimensions. Rather, these styles and attitudes comprise complex characteristics, as well as having distinctive features that share many traits. Items are expected to exhibit their strongest, but not their only, association with the specific scale for which they were developed. The ultimate test of an item's or scale's efficiency is not statistical but discriminatory or predictive; procedures that enhance high item–scale homogeneity through studies of internal consistency are the best methods for optimizing rather than maximizing discriminations among scales.

The initial items were chosen in accord with theoretical–substantive validation data and were reduced on grounds of preliminary internal consistency and structural validation to the 289 best items. This form was administered to more than 2500 persons in a variety of settings; half of the test participants were students at urban universities. Medical populations were not included in this evaluation phase. Several procedures were followed after this form had been administered to these participants. Most important, item–scale homogeneities were calculated using measures of internal consistency; additionally, true-and-false endorsement frequencies were obtained. Point-biserial correlations (corrected for overlap) were calculated between each personality scale. To maximize scale homogeneity, investigators retained for further evaluation only items that showed their highest correlation with the scale to which they were originally assigned. With few exceptions, items showing a correlation below .30 were eliminated. The median biserial correlation for all items for all personality scales was .47. Sixty-four items were retained for inclusion in the MBHI from the provisional 289-item inventory; these comprise the core group of Coping-Style items for the final 150-item inventory.

Items for the Psychogenic Attitude scales were developed on theoretical–substantive grounds after the development of the 64 core personality items. Lists of 35–60 items were developed for each scale on the basis of previous research by other investigators into the characteristics to be measured. These item lists were then rated by clinicians with experience in assessing the effects of psychological influences on physical illness. Only items "correctly" placed by more than 75% of the raters were considered for inclusion in the inventory. Efforts were made to include some representation of the several diverse traits comprising each scale. By this procedure, 83 items were added to the core group of 64 personality items; an additional 3 "correction" items were included, resulting in a final form of 150 items.

External–Criterion Stage

The final 150-item form of the inventory was administered in a large number of medical settings to develop a series of empirically derived scales. The idea, both as a construction approach and as a method of validation, was that items on a test scale should be selected because of an empirically verified association with a significant and relevant criterion measure. The procedure by which this association was gauged also was direct. Preliminary items were administered to two groups of participants who differed on the criterion measure. The "criterion" group exhibited the trait with which the item was to be associated; the "comparison" group did not. In the case of the MBHI, all participants were patients with a given diagnosis, but they varied according to clinical judgments regarding the degree to which various psychological or social complications were involved. After administration, true–false endorsement frequencies obtained with each group were calculated for each item. Items that differentiated the criterion group statistically from the comparison group were judged "externally valid." This was the approach followed in attempting to develop empirical scales that either would identify (correlate) or would predict (prognose) specific clinically relevant criteria. Point-biserial correlations between each of the 150 items and between each of the scales were recalculated and reexamined. Items that showed high correlations (usually .30 or greater) with any scale other than those theoretically incompatible were added as items to that scale.

A central factor in evaluating any psychological instrument is whether the results it obtains are reliable. It is particularly difficult to address this question with instruments designed to measure personality traits; it is even more difficult when attitudes that can reflect transient or situational states are being appraised. Change is inevitable in these states. Thus, low test–retest reliabilities can be a function of changing circumstances rather than intrinsic measurement errors. At $4\frac{1}{2}$ months, the Coping Style scales showed reasonably high test–retest reliabilities ($x = .82$, range = $.77-.88$). The Psychogenic Attitude scales also displayed high reliabilities, averaging about .85, as did the empirically derived scales, at about .80, with the single exception of Emotional Vulnerability. Kuder–Richardson Formula 20 (KR20; 1937) coefficients were calculated to assess internal consistency. The KR20 coefficients for all scales ranged from .66 to .90, with a median of .83. Correlational data have been obtained using a variety of different and often homogeneous patient and nonpatient samples. Among the inventories used were the MMPI, the SCL-90, the I-E Scale, the Beck Depression Inventory, the Personal Orientation Inventory, the Life Events Survey, the Webber–Johansson Temperament Survey, and the California Personality Inventory, which are discussed at length in the MBHI manual (Millon et al., 1982).

The MBHI addresses interpersonal style and attitudes shown to be significant to the management of health concerns, likelihood of psychological components of medical problems, and specific prognostic issues. It uses this information to make probabilistic statements about the patient's behavior in relation to illness and its management and toward health care personnel. Directly addressing specified disease processes and their management, the manual provides the basis for making recommendations across a variety of medical problems regarding the likelihood of illness occurring and probable progress, as well as optimal management of the disease process.

Research and Clinical Uses of the MBHI

The MBHI can be used both for research and for purposes of individual clinical prediction. For example, the effect of coping styles on outcome and patient management is readily studied with the MBHI. It can predict behaviors such as isolation, hostility toward health personnel, and excessive complaining and emotionality. It also shows significant value as a clinical tool. Detailing patients' styles of relating to the world, attitudes toward their specific medical problems, and health care personnel, the MBHI provides a framework in which to establish treatment plans. Information obtained from scores on the Psychogenic Attitude scales allows the clinician to evaluate patients' level of concern across a wide range of issues.

Numerous studies have shown that the MBHI is extremely effective for a variety of purposes in the general medical setting (Antoni & Goodkin, 1988, 1989; Byrnes, Antoni, Goodkin, Efantis-Potter, Simon, & Munaij, 1996; Goodkin, Antoni, & Blaney, 1986; Kolitz, Antoni, & Green, 1988; Lutgendorf et al., 1996). The MBHI has been used to examine how personality style relates to behavioral and cognitive responses immediately after the onset of acute coronary symptoms in patients experiencing a first myocardial infarction, which could potentially facilitate life-saving or disability-reducing early interventions (Kolitz et al., 1988).

At least four studies have related MBHI-indexed personality coping styles and other psychosocial factors to the subclinical promotion of cervical neoplasia, the cellular changes that precede the development of invasive cervical carcinoma (Antoni & Goodkin, 1988, 1989; Byrnes et al., 1996; Goodkin et al., 1986). These findings suggest that the MBHI is useful in identifying psychosocial characteristics (such as MBHI Premorbid Pessimism, Future Despair, Social Alienation, Somatic Anxiety, and Respectful personality styles) that combine with lifestyle and behavioral risk factors and pathophysiological risk factors—which are incrementally predictive of the development of neoplastic disease—as well as changes in underlying immune system mechanisms that control the growth of the primary pathogenic process.

The MBHI also has been used to examine associations between personality–coping styles and the progression of breast cancer. Cancer patients with poorer outcomes were significantly more likely to display an emotionally nonexpressive coping style (higher MBHI Respectful, Introversive, or Cooperative scores). Follow-up analyses revealed that higher scores for the nonexpressive coping style were correlated with a greater tumor size in these women (Goldstein & Antoni, 1989). Another study used the MBHI to examine the association between personality coping styles and immune system functioning in men ultimately diagnosed with HIV infection (Lutgendorf et al., 1996). As in the case of the cervical neoplasia study, an emotional nonexpressive coping style (as measured on the MBHI Respectful and Introversive Style scales) was associated with greater impairments in indices of immune system functioning.

The MBHI also has been used to predict how individuals react to a new medical diagnosis such as HIV-positive status (Ironson et al., 1990). HIV+ men who were randomized to a stress management intervention showed significantly lower pre-to-post notification increases in distress (Antoni et al., 1991; LaPerriere et al., 1990) than did those randomized to the assessment-only control. Higher MBHI Respectful Scale scores predicted decreased positive outlook and increased denial as a coping strategy over the course of the study. Subsequent analyses revealed that greater increases in denial coping over the postnotification period predicted greater decrements in immune system functioning 1 year later (Antoni, Esterling, Lutgendorf, Fletcher, & Schneiderman, 1995) and a greater likelihood of progression to AIDS over a 2-year follow-up period (Ironson et al., 1994). A study by Starr et al. (1996) demonstrated that HIV-infected gay men who had elevations on the Inhibited, Forceful, and Sensitive scales coped more poorly (e.g., were more depressed, had lower social support, and had more frequent unprotected sex), and those with elevations on the Social and Confident scales coped relatively well (e.g., had lower depression, higher self-efficacy, more social support). These findings indicate that the MBHI has predicted help-seeking in response to symptoms, efficacy of secondary prevention interventions, and adjustment to disease and the course of disease. All of these factors are also potentially relevant to the assessment of patients with chronic pain.

MBHI and Chronic Pain Populations

Descriptive Studies

In a primarily descriptive study, Labbe, Goldberg, Fishbain, Rosomoff, and Steele-Rosomoff (1989) compared MBHI profiles of 247 patients with chronic pain with a nonmedical control sample. The purpose was to establish normative data for the former group. Female patients were statistically more likely than were male patients to have elevations on the Future Despair and Somatic Anxiety scales and less likely to have elevations on the Cooperative Scale. Male patients scored higher than did female patients on Introversive, Premorbid Pessimism, Future Despair, and Somatic Anxiety, and they scored lower on the Cooperative and Sociable scales. The authors conclude that patients with pain are "not that much different on the MBHI Coping Styles and Psychogenic Attitude Scales than a non-medical population" (p. 387). They noted that their results are consistent with findings in other studies with patients with chronic pain (the patients are more depressed and anxious), and differences in cooperativeness and sociability were often positively correlated to long and difficult relationships with the medical system.

In a descriptive study that used multivariate techniques to analyze the MBHI, Murphy and Tosi (1995) assessed a sample of 67 patients with chronic low back pain. They list 4 subtypes of chronic pain patients, labeled (a) "introversive," (b) "denial–minimizer," (c) "conformers," and (d) "severe psychophysiological reaction." The parallel to previous MMPI studies is apparent (with a healthy or denial profile, as well as an overwhelmed profile). The MBHI is better suited than the MMPI to detect a conforming type, as that construct is closely related to MBHI Scales 7 (Respectful) and 3 (Cooperative). Although the introversive dimension did not appear in the MMPI studies, it could be related to dimensions of depression, or it might relate to other studies that have found mean elevations on MMPI Scale 0 (Social Introversion; Harper & Richman, 1978).

Predictive Studies

In addition to its use for describing pain patients, the MBHI can facilitate predictions for important outcome variables. In studies that use both the MMPI and the MBHI, the MBHI has generally been found to be at least as effective as the MMPI for purposes of predicting outcomes. In general, the MBHI has been well-received, and it has been recommended for use with pain patients (Capra, Mayer, & Gatchel, 1985; Murphy, Sperr, & Sperr, 1986). For example, Gatchel, Deckel, Weinberg, and Smith (1985) found that numerous MBHI scales were useful for predicting outcome among outpatient pain patients. They examined a total of 70 patients: 25 with headaches, 24 age-matched pain patients (nonheadache), and 21 "normal" (nonpain) control patients. All patients completed the MBHI prior to receiving 16 one-hour weekly treatment sessions. They used daily logs to measure the number of headaches, hours of headaches, average intensity of headaches, and number of medications. Treatment response was assessed by comparing the 2-week pretreatment variables with the 2-week posttreatment variables entered in the daily logs. Pearson product moment correlations were used to assess the relationships between the MBHI and the outcome measures. Numerous MBHI scales predicted the number and duration of headaches. Higher scores on the Inhibited and Sensitive scales were associated with greater frequency of headaches, and higher scores on the Sensitive Scale were associated with greater duration of headaches (less improvement). Average headache intensity was not predictable statistically, and only one variable—Emotional Vulnerability—predicted the number of medications used. Pain Treatment Responsivity also predicted both the frequency and the duration of headaches. Emotional Vulnerability was the single best predictor ($r = .71$) of the number of headaches, and it was the only variable associated with three of the four outcome measures. Gatchel and associates (1985) also found that four scales were able to differentiate those with headaches from those with other forms of chronic pain (Inhibited, Sensitive, Chronic Tension, and Allergic Inclination).

Wilcoxson, Zook, and Zarski (1988) reported that a composite score based on several MBHI scales (Chronic Tension, Recent Stress, Allergic Inclination, Inhibited Style, Respectful Style, Pain Treatment Responsivity, Life-Threat Reactivity, and Premorbid Pessimism) successfully predicted gains in time sitting, time standing, number of stairs climbed, time on a treadmill, treadmill speed, and hand-grip strength among male and female pain patients completing a 20-day outpatient pain rehabilitation program. Using a composite score reflecting success across all of these areas of treatment improvement, a discriminant function analysis revealed that these MBHI scales, in combination with demographic information on age, gender, marital status, and educational level, correctly classified 97% (29/30) of patient outcomes. This compared favorably to the MMPI, which correctly classified 80% (28/35) of the cases. Similarly, the MBHI has predicted recovery of physical function in patients with low back pain, such that decreases in the Introversive and Emotional Vulnerability scales predicted functional restoration; further, the Sensitive Style, Recent Stress, Emotional Vulnerability, and Gastrointestinal Susceptibility scales discriminated patients who dropped out of a functional restoration program from those who completed it (Gatchel, Mayer, Capra, Diamond, & Barnett, 1986).

Sweet, Breuer, Hazlewood, Toye, and Pawl (1985) used the MBHI and the MMPI to predict treatment outcome for 52 patients in a multidisciplinary chronic pain and headache treatment center. Each patient received an individual treatment plan, which often included multiple modalities (including physical therapy and biofeedback). A psychologist assigned a global outcome on a 5-point Likert scale, with anchors at 2 (worse after treatment) and 6 (significant improvement). A patient received a score of 2 if he or she felt worse, regardless of other indicators. Scores of 3–6, however, were based on a comprehensive evaluation that included self-reports and observations of emotional status, return to employment or similar activities, decreased pain, decreased pain medication, and increased physical activity. Forty-four of the 52 patients had outcome data in categories 2–6. The researchers found that the MBHI Pain Treatment Response Scale accurately predicted outcome approximately 70% of the time. Although clinically useful, Sweet et al. expressed concerns regarding the scale's high overlap with other MBHI scales and with its lack of unique variance. In a forward stepwise multiple-regression analysis, this scale did not have enough unique variance to be retained as a predictor variable. Regression analyses showed that combinations of scales on the MMPI and the MBHI had similar predictive validity, with a slight advantage to the MMPI.

In another study, the MBHI was used to predict the ability to tolerate physical discomfort as part of a medical procedure (Rozensky, Honor, Tovian, Herz, & Holland, 1985). The study evaluated 30 cancer patients who were receiving hyperthermia treatments to enhance the effectiveness of their chemotherapy and radiation treatments. Patients with scores above 74 on the Sensitive, Cooperative, and Forceful scales tolerated higher average wattage than did others in the sample. Patients who scored below the median on Pain Treatment Response and Future Despair also had better tolerance than did others. Scores below the median on Somatic Anxiety, Inhibited, and Emotional Reactivity approached significance in predicting improved outcome. The authors' conclusions were somewhat tentative because of the small number of patients who exceeded the cutoff score, but they suggest that patients who were "more hopeful about the future, less sensitive, more cooperative, more forceful, less responsive to pain, and less emotionally reactive were more tolerant of the hyperthermia treatment" (p. 75).

Although most studies have found the MBHI to be predictive of outcome, there is at least one exception. Murphy et al. (1986) found that both the MMPI and the MBHI were ineffective in predicting important outcomes (such as clinic visits for pain, narcotic prescriptions, or general pain status) for 20 consecutive admissions to a pain program. The MBHI approached significance for predicting pain-related hospitalizations; no other findings were significant for the MBHI or the MMPI. The psychologist ratings, based on an interview and personal interpretation of the MMPI, were able to make reasonably accurate predictions, especially with regard to general pain status. Although the relatively small sample size probably played a role in the difference between this and other studies, it is still true that there could be specific aspects of the sample or the type of variable under evaluation that account for the relatively weak findings.

With chronic pain patients, then, as with other medical patients, the MBHI has been found to be related to outcome in important ways. Scores on the scales for Pessimism, Emotional Vulnerability, Somatic Anxiety, and Despair are relatively elevated among patients with chronic pain. Lower scores on some MBHI variables (such as Introversive Style, Sensitive Style, Emotional Vulnerability) have been shown to be associated with a variety of improved outcomes (Gatchel et al., 1985; Murphy, Tosi, & Pariser, 1989; Sweet et al., 1985; Wilcoxson et al., 1988). This is consistent with several well-known clinical patterns associated with chronic pain. Pain patients are often referred to mental health clinicians after medical treatments have "failed," leading to feelings of hopelessness, helplessness, and being unheard. By the time they see a psychologist or psychiatrist, patients with chronic pain often are irritable and prone to making numerous complaints (related to the Sensitive Style). Those who are lower on this dimension might be relatively resilient. Some variables measured by the MBHI—such as Somatic Anxiety, Emotional Vulnerability, Sensitive Style, and Inhibited Style—may be seen as targets of treatment; in such instances, the MBHI would be a useful outcome measure.

Future Directions: The MBMD

Despite the impressive results generated by studies using the MBHI to assess psychosocial characteristics relevant to a variety of primary and secondary prevention domains in different patient populations, there are several important psychosocial characteristics the MBHI does not evaluate. These include (a) information on the presence of psychiatric indicators, such as anxiety and emotional lability, that can influence patients' adjustments to their medical conditions; (b) information on coping styles that reflect recently derived personality disorders (Millon & Davis, 1996); (c) information on other psychological factors related to cognitive appraisals (self-esteem, functional efficacy), resources (spiritual and religious), and contextual factors (functional abilities); (d) information on specific lifestyle behaviors (alcohol and substance abuse, smoking, eating patterns, exercise routine); (e) information on patients' communication styles (tendencies toward disclosure, social desirability, devaluation when communicating, preference for more or fewer details when receiving medical information); and (f) more detailed information useful for predicting patient adherence to a recommended regimen, medication abuses, and emotional responses to stressful medical procedures, which, in turn, can be useful in health care management decision making and triage for mental health treatment. Awareness of the potential usefulness of this information for maximizing health maintenance and minimizing health care costs has provided the impetus for our work toward the forthcoming expanded health-oriented instrument: the MBMD.

The space here does not permit a presentation of the recent empirical evidence that has driven the development of this new instrument, but information is available in an article by Antoni, Millon, and Millon (1997) that reviews the literature extensively. What follows is a brief description of the individual scales that represent the domains covered in the MBMD.

Modifying Indices

The Modifying Indices Domain characterizes components of a patient's communication style. As in the MCMI, the scales are Disclosure, Desirability, Debasement, and Validity. The Disclosure Scale captures the tendency of patients to be open about sharing personal information. The Desirability Scale characterizes patients' inclinations to present themselves in an overly positive light, even at the expense of concealing symptoms. The Debasement Scale reveals the inclination of patients to present a problematic image of themselves. The Validity Scale identifies patient inattention, random response patterns, or marked confusion while responding to items. The ability of the health care provider to identify systematic distortions, biases, and preferences in patient self-reports can improve the precision of history-taking and symptom monitoring, and it can facilitate patient–provider rapport, resulting in improved help-seeking upon emergence of new symptoms, as well as better adherence to prescribed pharmacologic and self-care regimens.

Psychiatric Indicators

The five scales of the Psychiatric Indicators Domain cover major areas of psychopathology that can influence health maintenance and health care delivery. These scales correspond to the *Diagnostic and Statistical Manual of Mental Disorder's* (DSM; American Psychiatric Association, 1987, 1994) Axis I–related phenomena that are most prevalent and relevant to medical populations. They are Anxiety, Depression, Cognitive Dysfunction, Emotional Lability, and Guardedness. These features can affect medical outcomes in a variety of ways. For instance, Anxiety might place patients at heightened risk for adverse reactions to particularly stressful medical procedures; Depression might be associated with adherence problems, inadequate self-care, and severe emotional reactions to changes in the medical diagnosis or prognosis. Cognitive Dysfunction can indicate that patients are unable to accurately communicate aspects of their physical condition to the health care provider, or it might reflect a side effect of a medication or an underlying organic pathology that should be followed up with a comprehensive neuropsychological and neurological assessment. Patients with high levels of Emotional Lability could be at heightened risk for extreme affective reactions to stressful medical protocols, medication abuse, and poor adherence to medical regimens. Finally, the Guardedness Scale assesses the presence of psychiatric problems characterized by suspicious thinking and pervasive mistrust that could affect a patient's ability to relinquish control to the health care team when necessary and that could lead to significant difficulties in patient–physician communications. Although elevations on these scales do not provide precise Axis I diagnoses, they do provide supporting evidence for such a diagnosis that can be corroborated with a reliable and valid measure of Axis I pathology, such as the Schedule for Affective Disorders and Schizophrenia (Spitzer & Endicott, 1979) or the Structured Clinical Interview (SCID; Spitzer, Williams, Gibbon, & First, 1988) for the *DSM*.

Personality/Coping Style

As with the Coping Style scales of the MBHI, the Personality/Coping Style scales of the MBMD assess patient characteristics that reflect the cognitive, behavioral, and interpersonal strategies people use to acquire positive reinforcers and to avoid pain and discomfort in medical settings as well as in other areas of their lives. These styles of coping are derived directly from Millon's personality theory (Millon & Davis, 1996) and are described here specifically as they relate to medical patients' transactions with health care personnel and the medical environment. The scales that represent the Personality/Coping Style domain expand on the MBHI Coping Style scales in two ways. First, three new scales have been added, corresponding to the three personality styles (Depressive, Sadistic, Masochistic) that have been added to Millon's classification system since the development of the MBHI (Millon & Davis, 1996). A second way the MBMD Personality/Coping Style scales differ involves the naming of scales. In the MBMD, there is a greater effort to use adjectives that reflect how the patient is likely to be viewed by the health care provider, thus emphasizing the interpersonal qualities of the coping style. The 11 MBMD Personality/Coping Style scales are (a) Introversive, (b) Inhibited, (c) Dejected, (d) Cooperative, (e) Sociable, (f) Confident, (g) Nonconforming, (h) Aggressive, (i) Respectful, (j) Oppositional, and (k) Denigrated. Although these scales are designed to measure characteristics that *qualitatively* reflect components of *DSM* personality disorders, scores that reach the cut-off for "presence" (BR > 74) and "prevalence" (BR > 84) on these scales are more likely to *quantitatively* reflect a style of coping that is not in the range of an overt or diagnosable disorder.

Health Moderators

The scales in the Health Moderators Domain of the MBMD were designed to represent the intra- and interpersonal characteristics of patients that directly influence or moderate the effects of patients' psychiatric and personality features for several medical outcomes, such as use of medical services, treatment success, recovery–rehabilitation rate, and adherence to a medical regimen. The scales in the domain pertain to three major areas shown consistently in empirical studies (see Antoni, Millon, & Millon, 1997, for a literature review) to be associated with such medical outcome measures: (a) cognitive appraisals, (b) resources, and (c) contextual factors.

There are four MBMD scales that reflect psychosocial issues subsumed under the cognitive appraisal characteristics that can influence health maintenance and health care delivery: (a) Illness Concerns, (b) Functional Efficacy, (c) Pain Reactivity, and (d) Future Outlook. The Illness Concerns Scale reflects the patient's focus on and awareness of changes in bodily states, such as tension–relaxation and arousal–fatigue. This characteristic can either influence an individual's ability to monitor and report changes in sensations and symptoms in a beneficial manner (hyperglycemic states, subtle signs of ischemia), or it can cause a patient to ruminate about less important sensations or physical states. It also can prompt overuse of medical services. The Functional Efficacy Scale measures perceived control over current and future health-related phenomena and perceived control over other events in life. Pain Reactivity assesses the presence and intensity of physical pain. The Future Outlook Scale assesses outlook toward future health status; high scores characterize an attitude of pessimism and hopelessness. Based on prior research, this characteristic was hypothesized to influence several medical outcomes, including adherence to and confidence in medical regimens, emotional reactions to diagnostic test results, and possibly the actual physical course of disease.

Two scales on the MBMD characterize patient resources that can act directly on medical outcomes through behavioral channels or can work indirectly by buffering the influence of different sources of stress: Social Support and Spiritual Faith. The Social Support Scale reveals patients' perceptions of the adequacy of current sources of social support in their lives—family members, friends, and other significant people. The Spiritual Faith Scale assesses the degree to which patients rely on religious or spiritual resources to deal with the stressors, fears, and uncertainties of their medical condition. Information on these two important aspects of patient resources can be useful in providing the patient with more individualized care based on significant supports and philosophies. This should facilitate the treatment plan (self-care, adherence to medications, making and maintaining lifestyle changes) and provide buffers in stressful periods

Treatment Prognostics

The Treatment Prognostics Domain of the MBMD synthesizes all of the information from the other domains to make predictions about the patient's probable reactions to diagnosis and treatment as a way to optimize management of the patient's care. The Treatment Prognostics Domain scales are (a) Interventional Fragility, (b) Medication Abuse, (c) Information Discomfort, (d) Service Utilization, (e) Problematic

Compliance, (f) Psychiatric Referral, and (g) Management Risk. The Interventional Fragility Scale predicts the likelihood that the patient will have a decompensatory reaction to treatment. The Medication Abuse Scale predicts difficulties with or misuse of prescribed medications. This might take the form of changing dosages, combining medications inappropriately, or using expired prescriptions. The Information Discomfort Scale anticipates willingness to share and to be receptive to personal health data. The Service Utilization Scale anticipates excessive desire to use medical resources beyond those warranted by the diagnosis. The Problematic Compliance Scale predicts the likelihood of compliance with medical regimens, ranging from taking oral medications to adopting dietary and other lifestyle changes. The Psychiatric Referral Scale identifies which patients are at psychological risk and should be referred for psychiatric or psychological help. The Management Risk Scale predicts the risks of treatment complications due to coping style, the current psychological issues, available resources for managing stress, and probability of the resumption of risk behaviors.

Lifestyle Behaviors

As supported by empirical evidence reviewed in Antoni et al. (1997), several aspects of patient lifestyles can affect many facets of health maintenance and health care delivery. Some behaviors have health-compromising effects (substance use); others can promote good health (physical exercise). The Lifestyle Behaviors (Alcohol, Drug, Eating, Caffeine, Exercise, and Smoking) Domain of the MBMD provides information that gives the health care provider a comprehensive picture of factors that could influence health outcomes by acting as obstacles to the patient's ability to adhere to medication regimens and to make necessary lifestyle changes.

Personality Disorders and Acute Distress: The MCMI

We now discuss an instrument that was not developed to be specifically used with a medical patient population, although its utility for evaluating personality characteristics is plain to see when treating patients with pain. The MCMI (Millon, 1977) has undergone two revisions since its introduction (Millon, 1987; Millon, Millon, & Davis, 1994) and is now the MCMI–III. The instrument has 175 items geared to an 8th-grade reading level, and it takes approximately 25 minutes to complete. The same three-step validation process described for the MBHI was used for the MCMI. It yields 27 scales (Table 3.1). The first three are modifying indices; the other 24 scales correspond to the *DSM*'s Axis I and Axis II. The clinician who is familiar with the standard diagnostic system is therefore already generally familiar with the interpretation of the MCMI scales. A detailed examination of the MCMI is not provided in this chapter, but interested readers are directed to the manual (Millon et al., 1994) and to several excellent texts (Choca, Shanely, & Van Denberg, 1992; Craig, 1993; Millon, 1997).

Although the MCMI was designed primarily for psychiatric settings, individuals with moderate to severe psychopathology do, of course, receive treatment in medical facilities, and it is often helpful for clinicians to undertake a formal assessment in

Table 3.1—*MCMI–III Scales*

Type	Letter/Number and Name
Modifying Indices	X Disclosure
	Y Desirability
	Z Debasement
Clinical Personality Patterns	1 Schizoid
	2A Avoidant
	2B Depressive
	3 Dependent
	4 Histrionic
	5 Narcissistic
	6A Antisocial
	6B Aggressive (Sadistic)
	7 Compulsive
	8A Passive–Aggressive
	8B Self-Defeating
Severe Personality Pathology	S Schizotypal
	C Borderline
	P Paranoid
Clinical Syndromes	A Anxiety Disorder
	H Somatoform Disorder
	N Bipolar: Manic Disorder
	D Dysthymic Disorder
	B Alcohol Dependence
	T Drug Dependence
	R Post Traumatic Stress
Severe Syndromes	SS Thought Disorder
	CC Major Depression
	PP Delusional Disorder

Note. Copyright © 1997 DICANDRIEN, Inc. Published and distributed exclusively by National Computer Systems, Inc., Box 1416, Minneapolis, MN 55440. Reproduced with permission.

that context. Individuals with borderline and antisocial personality disorders, for example, can be extremely disruptive in a medical treatment setting, and effective intervention often hinges on understanding the relevant personality variables (Bockian, 1994). One concern of using the MCMI in a medical setting, however, is that psychopathology will be overestimated. As with the MBHI, the MCMI uses population base rates to determine cutting lines. For example, assume that the prevalence of borderline personality disorder was 20% in the psychiatric normative sample used in developing the MCMI. A score of BR = 75 would be set to correspond to a particular raw score that was achieved by 20% of the sample, so that 20% of the sample would be considered borderline. However, in a medical sample (with, for example, a 10% prevalence of borderline personality disorder), the same raw score would overestimate the presence of a personality disorder—by about double. By increasing the threshold score from which one assumes the presence of a personality disorder, one can compensate for the lower prevalence of personality disorders in a particular population. In medical settings, Hsu and Maruish (1992, as cited in Elliot et al., 1996) recommended a BR > 84, which in most medical settings would be an appropriate adjustment.

In the chronic pain setting, however, a sufficiently high prevalence of personality disorders has been found such that a much smaller adjustment than usual, if any, might be necessary. The prevalence of personality disorders in patients with chronic pain has been found to range from 40% to 60%. If this prevalence rate is replicated with broader, larger samples, it is high enough to warrant the use of the MCMI without interpretive modification. Until and unless such studies are conducted, however, we recommend the continued use of a cutoff of BR > 84.

MCMI Studies of Personality Disorders in Patients With Pain

Descriptive Studies, Prevalence

A limited number of studies have used the MCMI to describe various populations with chronic pain. In a study comparing 42 individuals with chronic temporomandibular joint pain with a matched nonclinical control group on the MCMI–II, there were differences between the two groups on the Obsessive–Compulsive, Dependent, and Schizoid Personality Disorder scales (Baggi, Rubino, Zanna, & Martignoni, 1995). It should be noted, however, that none of these scales was clinically elevated, and all three had scores of BR = 52 to BR = 64. The highest elevations for the pain group were on the Histrionic (74.9), Passive–Aggressive (68.7), and Narcissistic (68.9) scales.

In another study, Snibbe, Peterson, and Sosner (1980) used the MCMI–I with a workers' compensation sample of patients, 6 of whom had low back pain. Anxiety was found to be substantially elevated (mean score above 85), and depression was moderately elevated (mean score above 75). The highest personality scale was Negativistic/Passive–Aggressive, which approached 75. Thus, for this sample of patients, unlike the patients in the study of Baggi et al. (1995), some of the scales approached clinical significance. Obviously, more research is needed to develop a more accurate determination of prevalence rates in various pain populations when using the MCMI.

Predictive Studies

Another area of interest for pragmatic and theoretical purposes is predicting pain treatment outcomes. To date, studies that have investigated the utility of the MCMI with pain patients have focused mostly on the prediction of treatment outcome. The findings generally have been encouraging. For example, Jay, Grove, and Grove (1987) studied the MCMI as a predictor of treatment outcome in a pain clinic. They explicitly set out to replicate and extend the study by Gatchel et al. (1985), which used the MBHI to predict outcome. Jay's group hypothesized that, because a scale derived from the MCMI—Emotional Vulnerability—was the best predictor of outcome, then perhaps the MCMI would capture more of the variance than would the MBHI. As with the Gatchel et al. (1985) study, three groups were used: headache ($n = 25$); pain–nonheadache ($n = 26$); and "normal" (in this case, graduate students, $n = 20$) control. As with the study by Gatchel et al. (1985), four variables separated headache from nonheadache pain patients: Passive–Aggressive, Anxiety, Dysthymia, and Alcohol Abuse (headache patients were higher on all four scales). Numerous scales differentiated the combined pain groups (i.e., headache plus nonheadache pain) from the normal control group. The best discriminator was anxiety. The Axis II scales that significantly differentiated between the groups were Schizoid, Avoidant, Passive–Aggressive, Schizotypal, and Borderline Personality Disorder.

In another investigation, Elliott and associates (1996) evaluated 101 individuals in an outpatient chronic treatment program. Personality disorders were found to be predictive of length of treatment, with *DSM-IV* Cluster A (odd-eccentric) and Cluster B (dramatic-emotional) personality disorder groups' treatment significantly shorter than Cluster C (anxious–fearful) and groups with no personality disorder. Personality disorder scales, especially the Passive–Aggressive Scale, also were found to be positively associated with improvement in depression. Personality disorders were associated with changes in pain scores. Individuals with Cluster B personality disorders had the least improvement (and, in fact, worsened), those with Cluster C disorders had an intermediate level of improvement, and those with Cluster A or with no personality disorders had the most improvement.

A prospective study by Uomoto, Turner, and Herron (1988) used the MCMI and MMPI to predict outcome in 129 patients undergoing spinal surgery (laminectomy). Using discriminant analysis to predict good versus fair–poor outcome, both instruments, separately, were able to make correct predictions approximately 70% of the time, which could be increased to 75.8% by combining the instruments. Moreover, a correct identification rate of 78.6% was achieved by a regression equation, using the MCMI Dependent, Avoidant, Anxiety, Psychotic Thinking, Alcohol Abuse, and Histrionic scales, in addition to a combination of demographic variables.

Finally, Borchgrevink et al. (1997) attempted to predict long-term pain in patients versus those who would recover within 6 months (neck sprain). Eighty-nine patients were divided into subtypes at 6 months: (a) previously symptomatic (those with pain before the accident that caused the sprain, $n = 14$), (b) symptomatic (those with continued problems who were previously symptom free, $n = 34$), and (c) recovered (those who had symptoms immediately after their accident but recovered, $n = 41$). The MCMI did not differentiate between the groups, which, in conjunction with other research findings, led the authors to conclude that prolonged disability is unrelated to premorbid personality.

The limited research to date suggests that self-report measures, such as the MBHI and MCMI, can provide predictors of pain outcomes with some degree of accuracy. The preliminary studies suggest that these two instruments could predict a dichotomous (good vs. fair–poor) outcome with 70–80% accuracy. Depending on the frequency of good outcomes, this can be a solid improvement over chance. Of course, a great deal of additional clinical research is needed to further substantiate how robust such measures will be as predictor variables.

Summary and Conclusions

Despite the substantial amount of work done in the area of personality assessment in chronic pain, there are numerous areas that require further exploration. A fair amount of work has been done using the MCMI and MBHI to predict treatment outcomes and, although prediction is useful in its own right, in this instance it serves the more important purpose of providing opportunities to further develop theoretical understanding of the connection between psychological factors and pain. We would argue that a theory-driven model, tailored to specific outcome criteria, would yield more satisfactory results. For example, elevations on one personality scale could predict return to work; elevations on another could predict more effective pain control. Multiscale prototypes (Choca et al., 1992; Romm, Bockian, & Harvey, 1999) could be derived for individuals, comparing groups with poor outcomes to those with good outcomes. Starting with theory, models of patients with pain likely to have good (or poor) outcomes could be tested using structural equation modeling or similar techniques. Larger studies and meta-analyses would provide greater clarity as well. It could be that, in selected instances, medical prognosis or other physical measures could prove useful. Finally, it might be that variables other than personality *type* are essential in predicting outcome. *Severity* of disorder (rather than type) could make a substantial contribution. For example, having *any* MCMI scale >85, or >100, could be a good predictor of problematic outcome, regardless of which scale is elevated. Various specific domains of thought and behavior (Millon & Davis, 1996, p. 139) also could be useful constructs for clarifying the pain–personality relationship. By comparing the efficacy of different predictive models, the theoretical understanding of important factors underlying treatment should become more apparent.

In terms of practical clinical utility, the three instruments reviewed in this chapter, especially the MBHI and the MBMD, can be quite helpful to health care professionals dealing with patients experiencing pain. Information is provided about such factors as the patient's style of relating to health care personnel and major psychosocial stressors, as well as probable response to pain treatment interventions. Traditional personality assessment methods designed for psychiatric populations (such as the MMPI) might not be completely valid for a medical pain population because the statistical norms and clinical signs can differ significantly.

References

American Psychiatric Association. (1987). *Diagnostic and statistical manual of mental disorders* (3rd ed., rev.). Washington, DC: Author.

American Psychiatric Association. (1994). *Diagnostic and statistical manual of mental disorders* (4th ed.). Washington, DC: Author.

Andrew, J. M. (1970). Recovery from surgery, with and without preparatory instruction, for three coping styles. *Journal of Personality and Social Psychology, 15*, 223–226.

Antoni, M. H., Baggett, L., Ironson, G., August, S., LaPerriere, A., Klimas, N., Schneiderman, N., & Fletcher, M. A. (1991). Cognitive–behavioral stress management intervention buffers distress responses and immunologic changes following notification of HIV-1 seropositivity. *Journal of Consulting and Clinical Psychology, 59*(6), 906–915.

Antoni, M. H., Esterling, B. A., Lutgendorf, S., Fletcher, M. A., & Schneiderman, N. (1995). Psychosocial stressors, herpes virus reactivation and HIV-1 infection. In M. Stein & A. Baum (Eds.), *Chronic diseases: Perspectives in behavioral medicine* (pp. 135–168). Mahwah, NJ: Erlbaum.

Antoni, M. H., & Goodkin, K. (1988). Life stress and moderator variables in the promotion of cervical neoplasia. I: Personality facets. *Journal of Psychosomatic Research, 32*(3), 327–338.

Antoni, M. H., & Goodkin, K. (1989). Life stress and moderator variables in the promotion of cervical neoplasia. II: Life event dimensions. *Journal of Psychosomatic Research, 33*(4), 457–467.

Antoni, M. H., Millon, C., & Millon, T. (1997). The role of psychological assessment in health care: The MBHI, MBMC, and beyond. In T. Millon (Ed.), *The Millon inventories: Clinical and personality assessment* (pp. 409–448). New York: Guilford.

Baggi, L., Rubino, I. A., Zanna, V., & Martignoni, M. (1995). Personality disorders and regulative styles of patients with temporo-mandibular joint pain dysfunction syndrome. *Perceptual and Motor Skills, 80*, 267–273.

Bockian, N. R. (1994). Systemic–behavioral treatment of a personality disorder and abusive behavior on a spinal cord injury unit: A case illustration. *SCI Psychosocial Process, 7*(4), 153–160.

Borchgrevink, G. E., Stiles, T. C., Borchgrevink, P. C., & Lereim, I. (1997). Personality profile among symptomatic and recovered patients with neck sprain injury, measured by MCMI–I acutely and 6 months after car accidents. *Journal of Psychosomatic Research, 42*(4), 357–367.

Byrnes, D., Antoni, M. H., Goodkin, K., Efantis-Potter, J., Simon, T., & Munaij, J. (1996, March). *Life stress, HPV infection, immunity, and cervical intraepithelial neoplasia in HIV-1 seropositive minority women.* Paper presented at the annual meeting of the Society of Behavioral Medicine, Washington, DC.

Capra, P., Mayer, T. G., & Gatchel, R. (1985). Adding psychological scales to your back pain assessment. *Journal of Musculoskeletal Medicine, 2*, 41–52.

Choca, J., Shanely, L. A., & Van Denburg, E. (1992). *Interpretive guide to the Millon Clinical Multiaxial Inventory.* Washington, DC: American Psychological Association.

Cobb, S. (1977). An epilogue: Mediation on psychosomatic medicine. In Z. J. Lipowski, D. R. Lipsett, & P. C. Whybrow (Eds.), *Psychosomatic medicine: Current trends and clinical applications* (pp. 612–617). New York: Oxford University Press.

Comstock, G. W., & Partridge, K. B. (1972). Church attendance and health. *Journal of Chronic Diseases, 25*, 665–672.

Craig, R. J. (1993). *The Millon Clinical Multiaxial Inventory: A clinical research synthesis.* Hillsdale, NJ: Erlbaum.

Dembroski, T. M., & Costa, P. R., Jr. (1987). Coronary prone behavior. Components of the Type A pattern and hostility. *Journal of Personality, 55*, 211–235.

Elliott, T. R., Jackson, W. T., Layfield, M., & Kendall, D. (1996). Personality disorders and response to outpatient treatment of chronic pain. *Journal of Clinical Psychology in Medical Settings, 3*(3), 219–234.

Engel, G. L. (1968). A life setting conducive to illness: The giving up–given up complex. *Bulletin of the Menninger Clinic, 32*, 355–365.

Friedman, M., & Rosenman, R. H. (1974). *Type A behavior and your heart.* New York: Knopf.

Gatchel, R. J., Deckel, A. W., Weinberg, N., & Smith, J. E. (1985). The utility of the Millon Behavioral Health Inventory in the study of chronic headaches. *Headache, 25*, 49–54.

Gatchel, R. J., Mayer, T. G., Capra, P., Diamond, P., & Barnett, P. (1986). Millon Behavioral Health Inventory: Its utility in predicting physical function in patients with low back pain. *Archives of Physical Medicine and Rehabilitation, 57*, 878–882.

Goldstein, D., & Antoni, M. H. (1989). The distribution of repressive coping styles among non-metastatic and metastatic breast cancer patients as compared to non-cancer patients. *Psychology and Health: An International Journal, 3*, 245–258.

Goodkin, K., Antoni, M., & Blaney, P. (1986). Stress and hopelessness in the promotion of cervical intraepithelial neoplasia to invasive squamous cell carcinoma of the cervix. *Journal of Psychosomatic Research, 30*, 67–76.

Green, C., Meagher, R., & Millon, T. (1980, November). *The management of the "problem" patient in the medical setting.* Paper presented at the meetings of the Society of Behavioral Medicine, New York.

Harper, D. C., & Richman, L. C. (1978). Personality profiles of physically impaired adolescents. *Journal of Clinical Psychology, 34*(3), 636–642.

Holmes, T. H., & Rahe, R. H. (1967). The social readjustment rating scale. *Journal of Psychosomatic Research, 11*, 213–218.

Ironson, G., Friedman, A., Klimas, N., Antoni, M. H., Fletcher, M. A., LaPerriere, A., Simoneau, J., & Schneiderman, N. (1994). Distress, denial and low adherence to behavioral intervention predict faster disease progression in gay men infected with human immunodeficiency virus. *International Journal of Behavior Medicine, 1*, 90–105.

Ironson, G., LaPerriere, A., Antoni, M. H., O'Hearn, P., Schneiderman, N., Klimas, N., & Fletcher, M. A. (1990). Changes in immune and psychological measures as a function of anticipation and reaction to news of HIV-1 antibody status. *Psychosomatic Medicine, 52*, 247–270.

Jackson, D. N. (1970). A sequential system for personality scale development. In C. D. Spielberger (Ed.), *Current topics in clinical and community psychology* (Vol. 2, pp. 61–92). New York: Academic Press.

Jackson, D. N., & Messick, S. (1961). Acquiescence and desirability as response determinants in the MMPI. *Educational and Psychological Measurement, 21*, 771–790.

Jay, G. W., Grove, R. N., & Grove, K. S. (1987). Differentiation of chronic headache from non-headache pain patients using the Millon Clinical Multiaxial Inventory (MCMI). *Headache, 27*, 124–129.

Jenkins, C. D. (1976). Psychologic and social precursors of coronary disease. *New England Journal of Medicine, 284*, 307–317.

Kolitz, S., Antoni, M. H., & Green, C. (1988). Personality style and immediate help-seeking responses following the onset of myocardial infarction. *Psychology and Health, 2*, 259–289.

Labbe, E. E., Goldberg, M., Fishbain, D., Rosomoff, H., & Steele-Rosomoff, R. (1989). Millon Behavioral Health Inventory norms for chronic pain patients. *Journal of Clinical Psychology, 45*(3), 383–390.

LaPerriere, A., Antoni, M. H., Ironson, G., Klimas, N., Ingram, F., Fletcher, M. A., & Schneiderman, N. (1990). Exercise training buffers emotional distress and immune decrements in gay males learning of their HIV-1 antibody status. *Biofeedback and Self-Regulation, 15*(3), 229–242.

Large, R. G. (1986). DSM-III diagnoses in chronic pain: Confusion or clarity? *Journal of Nervous and Mental Disease, 174*(5), 295–303.

Levine, R. (1980). *The impact of personality style upon emotional distress, morale, and return to work in two groups of coronary bypass surgery patients.* Unpublished master's thesis, University of Miami, Florida.

Lipsitt, D. R. (1970). Medical and psychological characteristics of "crocks." *The International Journal of Psychiatry in Medicine, 1*, 15–25.

Loevinger, J. (1957). Objective tests as instruments of psychotherapy. *Psychological Reports, 3*, 635–694.

Lowy, F. H. (1977). Management of the persistent somatizer. In Z. J. Lipowski, D. R. Lipsett, & P. C. Whybrow (Eds.), *Psychosomatic medicine: Current trends and clinical applications* (pp. 227–229). New York: Oxford University Press.

Lucente, F. E., & Fleck, S. (1972). A study of hospitalization anxiety in 408 medical and surgical patients. *Psychosomatic Medicine, 34*, 304–312.

Lutgendorf, S., Antoni, M. H., Ironson, G., Klimas, N., Starr, K., Schneiderman, N., & Fletcher, M. A. (1996, March). *Coping and social support predict distress changes in symptomatic HIV-seropositive gay men following a cognitive behavioral stress management intervention.* Paper presented at the annual meeting of the Society of Behavioral Medicine, Washington, DC.

Mechanic, D., & Volkart, E. H. (1960). Stress, illness behavior, and the sick role. *American Sociological Review, 26*, 51.

Meehl, P. E., & Rosen, A. (1955). Antecedent probability and the efficiency of psychometric signs, patterns or cutting scores. *Psychological Bulletin, 52*, 194–216.

Mei-Tal, V., Meyerowitz, S., & Engel, G. L. (1970). The role of psychological process in a somatic disorder: Multiple sclerosis. 1. The emotions of illness onset and exacerbation. *Psychosomatic Medicine, 32*, 67–86.

Millon, T. (1969). *Modern psychopathology: A biosocial approach to maladaptive learning and functioning.* Philadelphia: Saunders.

Millon, T. (1977). *Millon Clinical Multiaxial Inventory manual.* Minneapolis: National Computer Systems.

Millon, T. (1987). *Millon Clinical Multiaxial Inventory manual II.* Minneapolis: National Computer Systems.

Millon, T. (Ed.) (1997). *The Millon inventories: Clinical and personality assessment.* New York: Guilford Press.

Millon, T., Antoni, M., Millon, C., & Davis, R. (in press). *Millon Behavioral Medicine Diagnostic.* Minneapolis: National Computer Systems.

Millon, T., & Davis, R. D. (1996). *Disorders of personality: DSM-IV and beyond.* New York: Wiley.

Millon, T., Green, C., & Meagher, R. (1982). *The Millon Behavioral Health Inventory Manual.* Minneapolis: National Computer Systems.

Millon, T., Millon, C., & Davis, R. D. (1994). *Millon Clinical Multiaxial Inventory manual —III.* Minneapolis: National Computer Systems.

Millon, T, Millon, C., & Davis, R. D. (1997). *Millon Clinical Multiaxial Inventory—III manual* (2nd ed.) Minneapolis: National Computer Systems.

Moss, E. (1977). Biosocial resonation: A conceptual model of the links between social behavior and physical illness. In Z. J. Lipowski, D. R. Lipsett, & P. C. Whybrow (Eds.), *Psychosomatic medicine: Current trends and clinical applications* (pp. 90–99). New York: Oxford University Press.

Murphy, J. K., Sperr, E. V., & Sperr, S. J. (1986). Chronic pain: An investigation of assessment instruments. *Journal of Psychosomatic Research, 30*(3), 289–296.

Murphy, M. A., & Tosi, D. J. (1995). Typological description of the chronic low back pain syndrome using the Millon Behavioral Health Inventory. *Psychological Reports, 76*, 1227–1234.

Murphy, M. A., Tosi, D. J., & Pariser, R. F. (1989). Psychological coping and the management of pain with cognitive restructuring and biofeedback: A case study and variation of cognitive experiential therapy. *Psychological Reports, 64*(3, part 2), 1343–1350.

Naber, D., Weinberger, D. R., Bullinger, M., Polsby, M., & Chase, T. N. (1988). Personality variables, neurological and psychopathological symptoms in patients suffering from spasmodic torticollis. *Comprehensive Psychiatry, 29*(2), 182–187.

Parkes, M., Benjamin, B., & Fitzgerald, R. G. (1969). Broken heart: A statistical study of increased mortality among widowers. *British Medical Journal, 1*, 740–743.

Paull, A., & Hislop, I. G. (1974). Etiologic factors in ulcerative colitis: Birth, death, and symbolic equivalence. *International Journal of Psychiatry in Medicine, 5*, 57–64.

Rabkin, J. G., & Streuning, E. L. (1976). Life events, stress, and illness. *Science, 194*, 1013–1020.

Rahe, R. H. (1977). Subjects' recent life changes and their near future illness susceptibility. *Advances in Psychosomatic Medicine, 8,* 2–19.

Rahe, R. H., & Arthur, R. J. (1968). Life-change patterns surrounding illness experience. *Journal of Psychosomatic Research, 11,* 341–345.

Rozensky, R. H., Honor, L. F., Tovian, S. M., Herz, G., & Holland, M. A. (1985). Tolerance of pain by cancer patients in hyperthermia treatment. *Journal of Psychosocial Oncology, 3*(2), 75–82.

Sadigh, M. R. (1998). Chronic pain and personality disorders: Implications for rehabilitation practice. *Journal of Rehabilitation, Oct.–Dec.,* 4–8.

Sarason, I. G., Johnson, J. H., & Siegal, J. M. (1978). Assessing the impact of life changes: Development of the life experiences survey. *Journal of Consulting and Clinical Psychology, 46,* 932–946.

Schmale, A. H. (1972). Giving up as a final common pathway to changes in health. In Z. J. Lipowski (Ed.), *Psychological aspects of physical illness.* Basel, Switzerland: Karger.

Sivik, T. M. (1991). Personality traits in patients with acute low-back pain: A comparison with chronic low-back pain patients. *Psychotherapy and Psychosomatics, 56*(3), 135–140.

Snibbe, J. R., Peterson, P. J., & Sosner, B. (1980). Study of psychological characteristics of a workers' compensation sample using the MMPI and Millon Clinical Multiaxial Inventory. *Psychological Reports, 47,* 959–966.

Spitzer, R., & Endicott, J. (1979). *Schedule for affective disorders and schizophrenia—lifetime version.* New York: New York State Institute, Biometrics Research.

Spitzer, R. L., Williams, J. B., Gibbon, M., & First, M. B. (1988). *Structured clinical interview for DSM-III-R.* New York: New York State Psychiatric Institute.

Starr, K., Antoni, M. H., Penedo, F., Costello, N., Lutgendorf, S., Ironson, G., & Schneiderman, N. (1996, March). *Cognitive and affective correlates of emotional expression in symptomatic HIV-infected gay men.* Paper presented at the annual meeting of the Society of Behavioral Medicine, Washington, DC.

Stavraky, K. M., Buch, C. N., Lott, J. S., & Wonklin, J. M. (1968). Psychological factors in the outcome of human cancer. *Journal of Psychosomatic Research, 12,* 251–259.

Sweet, J. J., Breuer, S. R., Hazlewood, L. A., Toye, R., & Pawl, R. P. (1985). The Millon Behavioral Health Inventory: Concurrent and predictive validity in a pain treatment center. *Journal of Behavioral Medicine, 8*(3), 215–226.

Uomoto, J. M., Turner, J. A., & Herron, L. D. (1988). The use of the MMPI and MCMI in predicting outcome of lumbar laminectomy. *Journal of Clinical Psychology, 44*(2), 191–197.

Wilcoxson, M. A., Zook, A., & Zarski, J. J. (1988). Predicting behavioral outcomes with two psychological assessment methods in an outpatient pain management program. *Psychology and Health, 2,* 319–333.

Wright, B. A. (1960). *Physical disability: A psychological approach.* New York: Harper.

Yunik, S. (1979). *The relationship of personality variables and stressful life events to the onset of physical illness.* Unpublished doctoral dissertation, University of Miami, Florida.

Chapter 4
NONPATHOLOGICAL FACTORS IN CHRONIC PAIN: IMPLICATIONS FOR ASSESSMENT AND TREATMENT

James B. Wade and Donald D. Price

This chapter focuses on assessments of the influence of nonpathological factors on pain. Accomplishing this aim requires an explicit recognition that pain consists of sensory, cognitive–evaluative, and affective motivational dimensions (Gracely, 1979; Melzack, 1975; Price, Harkins, & Baker, 1987). These dimensions have been reconceptualized as having different subcomponents and as representing different stages of pain processing (Harkins, Price, & Braith, 1989; Price, 1988; Wade, Doughtery, Archer, & Price, 1996; Wade, Dougherty, Hart, Rafii, & Price, 1992; Wade, Price, & Hamer, 1990). A model of pain processing has been proposed that consists of 4 stages (See Figure 4.1, p. 91) (Price 1988; Wade et al., 1996; Wade, Dougherty, Hart, Rafii, & Price, 1992).

The first stage of pain processing is the sensory-discriminative dimension, which consists of spatial, temporal, and intensive features. Probably its most important component is the perceived intensity of the painful sensation. Pain sensation intensity can be measured with visual analogue scaling (VAS) and verbal descriptor scaling and by cross-modality matching methods (Price & Harkins, 1992). The second stage reflects immediate unpleasantness (the first stage of affective processing), and it consists of the perceived degree of distress, annoyance, intrusion, or threat intimately associated with the pain sensation. This dimension involves only limited cognitive processing and, similar to the unpleasantness associated with fatigue, dizziness, and nausea, is usually closely associated with the intensities of the physical sensation (Price et al., 1987). Like pain sensation intensity, immediate unpleasantness can be measured with VAS (Price et al., 1987; Price, McGrath, Rafii, & Buckingham, 1983; Wade et al., 1990).

Evidence that VAS can measure these first 2 stages of pain processing separately comes from several sources. First, sensory and affective VAS ratings of experimental heat pain have been shown to be reliably different. When patients use the same length sensory and affective VAS to rate different nociceptive temperatures (41–51°C) applied to the skin of the forearm, the mean unpleasantness ratings are consistently and significantly lower than are the mean sensory ratings (Price, 1988; Price et al., 1983, 1987). This result could reflect the relatively low concern about enduring physical harm or other long-term deleterious consequences associated with experimental as compared with clinical pain. A second line of evidence for the separateness between the first 2 stages of pain processing has been demonstrated by the fact that psychological factors can selectively amplify or reduce VAS unpleasantness ratings in different pain conditions. For example, patients with cancer pain have been shown to have higher unpleasantness VAS ratings than sensory VAS ratings, whereas the reverse was true for patients with labor pain. In addition, psychological set was found to alter unpleasantness but not sensory VAS ratings in labor pain (Price et al., 1987).

Two recent studies (Rainville, Duncan, Price, Carrier, & Bushnell, 1997; Rainville, Carrier, Hofbauer, Bushnell, & Duncan, in press) provide a neurophysiological basis for the distinction between the first 2 stages of pain processing. In the first study of experimentally induced heat, participants were given two types of hypnotic suggestion, designed either to enhance or to attenuate the immediate unpleasantness (Stage 1 affect) but not the pain sensation intensity associated with a noxious heat stimulus. Positron emission tomography scan imaging permitted the identification of specific brain regions associated with the processing of both the pain sensation intensity (Stage 1) and the immediate unpleasantness associated with the painful sensation (Stage 1 affect). This selective modulation of pain unpleasantness resulted in a parallel modulation of neural activity within the anterior cingulate cortex but not within the somatosensory S-1 cortex. The fact that separate higher cortical brain regions are involved in the experience of these two pain stages provides additional support for their uniqueness.

The second study (Rainville et al., in press) extended this approach by comparing two experimental conditions. Hypnotic suggestions were targeted specifically toward altering pain unpleasantness in the first condition and toward altering pain sensation intensity in the second. Similar to the first study by Rainville et al. (1997), pain unpleasantness ratings but not pain sensation intensity ratings were changed in the first condition. However, both pain sensation intensity and pain unpleasantness ratings changed in parallel in the second condition. This experiment helps to establish the direction of causation—pain sensation is the cause of pain unpleasantness and not vice-versa.

The third stage of pain processing represents a second stage of pain-related affect that can be conceptualized generally as "suffering." It is closely related to the meanings and implications that pain holds for one's life (Price, 1988). Thus, an individual's attitudes, beliefs, and memories about real or imagined long-term consequences of having pain bear on the individual's adaptation to this stage. It is composed of evaluations and beliefs (such as the perceived ability to endure pain, perceived interference, control in reducing pain intensity, hope for cure) and consequently of negative emotions related to these evaluative components (such as depression, fear, anxiety, anger, frustration). Attempts have been made to validate measures of this stage of pain processing by developing and administering VAS for each of these pain-related negative emotions (Harkins, Price, & Martelli, 1986; Wade et al., 1996; Wade, Doughtery, Hart, Rafii, & Price, 1992; Wade et al., 1990). The combined ratings of five emotions and illness beliefs were shown to represent a psychological stage that was unique and separate from that of the immediate pain-related unpleasantness (Wade et al., 1996; Wade, Doughtery, Hart, Rafii, & Price, 1992; Wade et al., 1990). Two studies (Harkins et al., 1989; Wade, Doughtery, Hart, & Cook, 1992) showed that neuroticism selectively and potently enhanced this stage of pain processing.

The fourth and final stage of pain processing is that of the overt behavioral expression of pain. This stage reflects the activities of daily living that are influenced by pain (such as the number of hours spent in bed during the day because of pain). This stage can be evaluated by self-report inventories and by structured observation methods. Figure 4.1 depicts this 4-stage model of pain processing.

In addition to psychophysical, psychological, and neurophysiological data, a fourth line of evidence for this 4-stage model of pain processing comes from multivariate (LISREL; Joreskeg, & Sorbom, 1976) analysis (Wade et al., 1996). Path analyses with 506 patients with chronic pain demonstrated that VAS could be used to assess pain sensation intensity, pain-related unpleasantness (Stage 1 affect), and pain-related suffering (Stage 2 affect) and that a structured interview (Getto & Heaton, 1985) could assess pain-related behavior. The authors divided suffering into subcomponents of illness beliefs and negative emotions. Consistent with our previous theory and several other empirical studies (Rainville et al., 1997, in press) the linear stage sequence shown in Figure 4.1 best fits the relationship between the 4 stages. Successive stages did not have recursive effects on earlier pain stages.

Confirmatory LISREL analysis, with an additional 502 pain patients, supported the integrity of these findings. These data provide important converging lines of

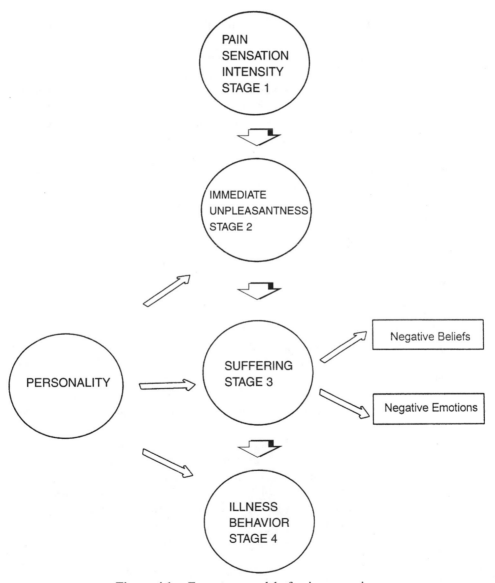

Figure 4.1. Four-stage model of pain-processing.

evidence for the validity and cogency of the model, which we believe generalizes to chronic illness conditions other than chronic pain. For example, similar to considering pain sensation intensity as Stage 1 of the 4-stage model, one could easily substitute other intense physical sensations, such as chronic fatigue. By inference, the subsequent 3 components of the pain-staging model (immediate sensation-related unpleasantness, suffering, illness behavior) would similarly characterize stages of illness processing. Although the rest of this chapter focuses on available evidence examining the influence of nonpathological factors on the 4 stages of chronic pain, it is quite possible that the factors also could affect similar stages within other chronic, debilitating medical conditions.

Demographic Factors and Pain Processing

Since the writings of the ancient Greek scholars (Aurelius, trans. 1980; Greene, Sophocles, trans. 1957), investigators have considered the influence of nonpathological factors on pain processing. Several studies addressing the association between ethnicity and pain have led to contradictory conclusions. Modern investigations (Garron & Leavitt, 1979; Greenwald, Bonica, & Bergner, 1987; Weisenberg, Kreindler, Schachat, & Werboff, 1975; Woodrow, Friedman, Siegelaub, & Collen, 1972) have noted that White people, African Americans, and Puerto Ricans differ in response to a variety of painful conditions. In one study, (Sternbach & Tursky, 1965) Italian American individuals were noted to differ from individuals of Irish descent on autonomic and psychophysical measures. Similarly, Woodrow et al. (1972) reported that White individuals endured more pain than did Asian Americans, and African Americans occupied an intermediate position. These findings contrast those of Lipton and Marbach (1984) who reported that Irish American, Italian American, Jewish, African American, and Puerto Rican patients with facial pain were similar on measures of attitude, pain response, and description. Finally, Zatzick and Dimsdale (1990), in a review of the literature, concluded that there is little evidence to suggest cultural differences in response to pain.

Studies that examine the relationship between age and pain are similar to those in the pain-and-ethnicity literature for two reasons. First, the studies have focused primarily on the first stage of pain processing, pain sensation intensity. Second, they have resulted in contradictory findings (Harkins, Price, & Martelli, 1986; McMillan, 1989; Sorkin, Rudy, Hanlon, Turk, & Stieg, 1990; Woodrow et al., 1972). The earlier studies using a variety of experimental pain stimuli and threshold or tolerance measures point to an increase in pain threshold with advancing age (Chapman & Jones, 1944; McMillan, 1989; Procacci, Bozza, Buzzelli, & Della Corte, 1970; Sherman & Robillard, 1964). Other studies (e.g., Mumford, 1965) have found no age effects for pain tolerance or threshold. More recent studies (Harkins et al., 1986) using direct scaling techniques to evaluate threshold and suprathreshold levels of experimental pain sensitivity demonstrate much stronger similarities than differences across the lifespan.

For the most part, pain-and-gender studies suggest that women have a lower pain threshold (Ellermeier & Westphal, 1995; Leon, 1974) and tolerance (Dubreuil & Kohn, 1986; Woodrow et al., 1972) than do men. These studies used a variety of experimentally induced pain techniques such as heat, cold, pressure application, and electric shock. As for the literature concerning ethnicity and age, most of the pain-and-gender studies focus on the sensory-discriminative dimension (Stage 1 of the pain-processing model). Little regard is given to the next three stages. Of the studies that did include an assessment of unpleasantness, suffering (Bush, Harkins, Harrington, & Price, 1993), or pain threshold (Lander, Fowler-Kerry, & Hargreaves, 1989) using either experimentally induced or clinical pain, no gender-related differences were detected.

A final nonpathological variable of interest concerns that of the medical diagnosis itself. Clinicians have speculated that, in complex regional pain syndrome (CRPS), the pain sensation intensity seems more severe than expected based on the degree of tissue damage alone (Blumberg, Griesser, & Hornyak, 1990). These observations, along with the presence of significant psychiatric comorbidity in CRPS patients (Haddox, 1990; Lynch, 1992), suggest that suffering and illness behavior are disproportionately higher in such patients. Indeed, there has been speculation that an underlying personality defect could predispose an individual to develop this painful condition (De Vilder, 1980). Despite these assertions, there is a scarcity of literature comparing this pain disorder with other pain conditions, such as failed back surgery and myofascial dysfunction.

In a large population of chronic pain patients ($n = 1434$), we examined the extent to which the demographic factors, such as medical diagnosis (failed back surgery syndrome, CRPS, myofascial pain dysfunction), gender, age, and ethnicity (African American, White) influenced the magnitude of the four stages of pain processing (Wade, 1999). We used methodology similar to that of Wade et al. (1996) who used LISREL to assess the causal interrelationships between the four pain stages. Only age had large and selective effects on later stages of pain (Stage 2 affect and illness behavior), with older adults manifesting less emotional suffering and lifestyle disruption as a result of their pain. One explanation for this result could be that the older participants would not be dealing with other concerns, such as how to pay their children's college tuition or other midlife problems. Pain could be viewed by older adults as less "threatening," resulting in less suffering. Like the Wade et al. (1996) study, a linear sequence best fit the relationship between the four stages of pain processing. This study, (Wade, 1999) provided additional support for the conceptual strength of the four-stage model and for the validity of the measures used to assess the stages. Although the scarcity of studies conceptualizing pain as a multidimensional experience raised several questions about the influence of demographic factors on pain processing, it appeared that at least the general manner in which the stages of pain were processed was similar. With the exception of differences associated with age, at least the general dimensions and stages of pain processing appear to be universal across pain conditions, gender, and ethnicity.

Normal Personality Structure and Pain Processing

This section reviews the impact of normal personality factors on medical illness and pain processing. The first part traces the development of the Big-Five factor model of personality, whose acceptance by personality researchers led to the development of objective personality measures such as the NEO PI-R (Costa & McCrae, 1992). The second part discusses application of normal personality structure to chronic pain and illness.

Big-Five Factor Model of Personality

It is important first to draw a distinction between *normal personality structure* and *psychopathology*. Both terms describe aspects of personality, but psychopathology has its roots in a disease-based model. For the individual, an assessment is made regarding the presence or absence of psychopathology. Its presence is always problematic and implies maladaptation. The Minnesota Multiphasic Personality Inventory-2 (MMPI-2) is a widely used measure of psychopathology (Piotrowski & Lubin, 1990). Psychopathology can remit in entirety with or without treatment. In contrast, normal personality has its derivation in personality trait theory. It represents a comprehensive framework for the description of individual differences. The fundamental underpinning of this personality theory is that an individual's interpersonal, experiential, and enduring emotional world consists of a set of basic dimensions. These dimensions represent universal and enduring factors in all individuals, regardless of demographic or cultural difference. An individual's loading on them is not affected by stressful life events, changes in developmental life stage, or prior experience (McCrae, 1993).

Sir Francis Galton (1884) might have been the first to note that important differences in individual human interaction could be described using single terms. Influenced by Thurstone's use of factor analysis assessing temperament differences (Thurstone, 1934, 1953), Cattell, Eber, and Tatsuoka (1970) began their exploration of personality by analyzing some 4500 trait-descriptive terms included in the Allport and Odbert (1936) compendium. Other analyses (Borgatta, 1964a, 1964b; Digman & Takemoto-Chock, 1981; Norman, 1963; Smith, 1967, 1969; Tupes & Christal, 1958, 1961) of Cattell's variables consistently yielded only 5 factors. Similarly, factor analytic studies using other data sets have produced a 5-factor solution (Digman & Inouye, 1986; Goldberg, 1990, 1992; McCrae & Costa, 1985b, 1987). The Big-Five factors typically are numbered and labeled as follows: Factor I, Surgency (or Extraversion); Factor II, Agreeableness; Factor III, Conscientiousness; Factor IV, Emotional Stability (vs. Neuroticism); and Factor V, Culture. Within the recent past, others have renamed Factor V as Openness to Experience (McCrae & Costa, 1987) or Intellect (Peabody & Goldberg, 1989). Despite this seeming agreement, there are those today who do not accept the Big-Five factor model of normal personality. Two of the most prominent critics are Cattell and colleagues (1970) and Eysenck (1967). Whereas Cattell has argued that more than 5 factors are necessary to describe normal personality, Eysenck has asserted that 5 is too many. He claims that Agreeableness and Conscientiousness are subcomponents of the construct Psychoticism. He offers a 3-factor model composed of Psychoticism, Extraversion, and Neuroticism (Eysenck 1991, 1992).

Two popular instruments for assessing the 5-factor model are the NEO PI-R and the Hogan Personality Inventory (HPI; Hogan, 1986). The HPI has its conceptual origins in Hogan's (1983) socioanalytic theory. Therefore, although it is grounded in the 5-factor model, its focus is conceptually broader. The HPI consists of 310 items organized into 6 scales: Intellectance (Openness), Adjustment (Neuroticism), Prudence (Conscientiousness), Ambition (Extraversion), Sociability (Extraversion), and Likeability (Agreeableness). Hogan divided Extraversion into 2 major components, Ambition and Sociability. He emphasized the need to make a distinction between status seeking (Ambition) and the enjoyment of social interaction (Sociability). The six scales of the HPI are currently organized into 43 subscales called HICs (Homogeneous Item Clusters). The HICs vary in length from 3 to 7 items, and the scales consist of from 5 to 10 HICs.

The NEO acronym reflects the fact that the original version of the NEO PI was designed to assess only 3 of the Big-Five personality factors. Influenced by the work of Digman and Takemoto-Chock (1981) and Goldberg (1981, 1982), Costa and McCrae (1985) maintained that 5 orthogonal factors comprehensively account for phenotypic personality differences. Two factors, II (Agreeableness) and III (Conscientiousness), were added to the original 3 test scales to form the current version of the NEO PI-R, which now consists of 181 items, answered on a 5-point scale from *strongly disagree* to *strongly agree*. The NEO PI-R comes in two forms: Form S, which is an instrument that reflects self-ratings, and Form R, which represents ratings of others. Form R is reported to have comparable reliability and validity when completed by knowledgeable raters, such as spouses or long-time friends. These two versions contain the same items except that the pronouns are changed from "I" to "he" or "she." Each domain is measured by 48 items grouped into 6 sets of 8 items each. The sets are the domain facets and can be used to clarify information about the overall domain score.

The NEO PI was developed using a rational and factor analytic method on large samples of normal adult volunteers. Test items were evaluated and selected to produce maximally discriminant facet scales. Principal component analysis was the primary statistical tool used for test construction. The test was devised with an emphasis on external criteria (discriminant and convergent validity), rather than internal checks (simple structure). A factor approach, called validimax (McCrae & Costa, 1989a), involves maximizing the loadings of items on one factor while minimizing their loadings on others. This methodology underscores the fundamental goal of capturing, in their purest form, the Big-Five factors, while maximizing the test's convergent and discriminative validity. The validimax approach lent itself to developing an abbreviated version of the NEO PI-R, the Five Factor Inventory (FFI; Costa & McCrae, 1992). This short-form version consists of 60 items and provides an assessment of each factor. No information is available about facet scores. The FFI was constructed by selecting the highest loading items and is reported to account for about 75% of the variance in convergent criteria as the original NEO PI-R (Costa & McCrae, 1992). NEO PI-R scales are balanced to control for the effects of acquiescent responding, and a series of studies has suggested that the scales are not overly sensitive to social desirability effects. Internal consistency reliabilities for the 5 domain scales range from .76 to .93 (McCrae & Costa, 1983).

Hogan (1986) used the 5-factor model as a starting point but grafted socioanalytic theory onto it. This philosophical emphasis led Hogan to separate the Extraversion domain into separate factors, Ambition and Sociability. His test did not adhere to the belief that the HICs on the HPI produce maximally discriminant facet scales, which was a requirement of the NEO PI-R. In contrast, the overriding goal of the HPI was to develop a tool that would prove useful in predicting behavior. Specifically, Hogan attempted to show that the HPI was a valuable predictor of work-related performance.

In contrast, Costa and McCrae (1985) relied on factor analysis to produce a tool that measured the 5 factors without redundancy among domains. Their measure is a precise representation of the 5-factor model, with uniquely defined facets within each of the major domains. They intentionally excluded a facet for assessing bodily symptoms, because they did not want to confound the NEO PI-R with a construct they intended to predict (health complaints). Nevertheless, there is limited empirical support for the NEO PI-R subfacets' differential validity. In support of the test's usefulness, several studies have shown that the NEO PI-R domain scales replicate across different raters (self or significant other). During the 1980s, Costa and McCrae published an impressive number of studies demonstrating an association between information captured by the NEO PI-R and other adjective-based personality rating measures questionnaires, such as those developed by Jackson (Costa & McCrae, 1988), Speilberger (Costa & McCrae, 1987), Wiggins (McCrae & Costa, 1989b), and Eysenck (McCrae & Costa, 1985a). These and other works highlighted the universality of the 5-factor model by demonstrating that the NEO PI-R captures important information described by other popular personality tests, such as the Meyer–Briggs Type Indicator (McCrae & Costa, 1989a) and the MMPI (Costa, Busch, Zonderman, & McCrae, 1986).

Application of Normal Personality Structure to Chronic Pain and Illness

Several measures of normal personality have been studied in medical populations. Popular personality assessment tools include the Eysenck Personality Questionnaire (Eysenck & Eysenck, 1975), which has been used in several versions with a variety of clinical disorders (e.g., Boyce & Parker, 1985; Roy, Custer, Lorenz, & Linnoila, 1989). Several studies have used the California Psychological Inventory (Gough, 1957) and the 16 Personality Factor Test (Cattell & Eber, 1964) (e.g., Nagelberg, Hale, & Ware, 1984; Reuter, Wallbrown, & Wallbrown, 1985). Most of the studies that evaluate the association between medical illness and normal personality focus on 2 of the Big-Five factors, Neuroticism and Extraversion. In explaining the association between neuroticism and pain, a few studies have offered the explanation that neuroticism might be causally related to pain disorders (Breslau, Chilcoat, & Andreski, 1996; Philips & Jahanshahi, 1985). The logic stems from the fact that neuroticism is a chronic condition of proneness to distress. Chronic irritability and distress can contribute to physical changes associated with disease progression. An alternative view is that the lifestyle habits of individuals with high neuroticism predispose them to develop physical illness.

Pietri-Taleb, Riihimäki, Viikari-Juntura, and Lindström (1994) administered measures of normal personality to a group of 1015 machine operators, carpenters, and office workers. Participants were followed for 3 years. Machine operators with higher neuroticism scores subsequently developed severe neck pain. In another 3-year longitudinal study, Breslau et al. (1996) prospectively followed a randomly selected group of young adult members of a health maintenance organization. High neuroticism scores were associated with individuals who reported new onset of migraine headache. The authors concluded that neuroticism could be causally related to the development of migraine.

Whereas previously mentioned studies consider neuroticism a risk factor for medical illness, a second thrust of this literature suggests neuroticism either directly or indirectly influences illness-related suffering (the second stage of affective processing). Neuroticism reflects a tendency to experience chronic, negative, distressing emotions and to engage in a ruminative style that leads to fearfulness, low self-esteem, and feeling helpless. Therefore, individuals high in neuroticism could engage in a pattern of thinking that leads them to catastrophize or magnify the negative aspects of their situations.

In one study, (Larsen, 1992) neuroticism led patients to recall physical symptoms as being worse than they actually were. High-neuroticism patients retrospectively recalled having more physical symptoms than were shown in their actual daily symptom recordings. Similarly, Affleck, Tennen, Urrows, and Higgins (1992), using a sample of patients with rheumatoid arthritis, found that higher neuroticism scores were associated with more distress—regardless of the pain intensity and extent of depressive symptomology. In a large community-based sample of elderly adults, Gertrudis, Kempen, and Ormel (1997) found that personality characteristics, such as neuroticism, influence perceptions regarding medical-related quality of life. After controlling for the extent of lifestyle disruption due to medical illness, high neuroticism scores were associated with less satisfactory quality of life. The authors posited that the relationship between chronic pain and neuroticism reflects the fact that individuals with high neuroticism catastrophize their situation. This ineffective coping strategy involves a preoccupation with the worst possible outcomes and an excessive reliance on negative self-statements (Keefe, Brown, Wallson, & Caldwell, 1989; Rosenstiel & Keefe, 1983). In a series of chest pain studies (Costa 1987; Costa et al., 1985; Roll & Theorell, 1987) neuroticism was associated with somatic complaints but was not etiologically related to objective signs of pathophysiological disease. Thus, neuroticism is believed to result in a distress-prone style independent of objective physical signs.

Although several studies have explored the relationship between normal personality traits and pain, most have focused largely on 1 or 2 of the 4 pain stages. For example, BenDebba, Torgerson, and Long (1997) followed patients with low back pain for up to 2 years posttreatment and evaluated the relationship between psychological distress due to the chronic pain condition, neuroticism, and extraversion. They found patients who scored high on a neuroticism scale had higher levels of psychological distress than did individuals who scored lower on the same scale. This relationship remained, although substantially weakened, at both the 1- and 2-year posttreatment interval. In contrast, greater extraversion scores were negatively related to psychological distress, although the correlations were consistently small. The authors did not systematically examine the influence of neuroticism and extraversion on pain sensation intensity (Stage 1 of the pain-processing model), immediate unpleasantness (Stage 2), negative illness beliefs or chronic pain–related emotions (Stage 3), or illness behavior (Stage 4).

Lauver and Johnson (1997) specifically assessed the relationship between neuroticism and illness behavior in an older group of patients with chronic pain (mean age 65 years). Using multiple regression, they controlled for the amount of social support the patients received. Neuroticism was a significant predictor of observable pain behavior. High neuroticism scores were associated with a quantitative increase in maladaptive illness behavior.

In this chapter, we have emphasized that it is critical to characterize pain as being represented by 4 separate stages. Doing so allows the clinician to clarify at which point in the pain-processing schema personality factors and therapeutic interventions exert their influence. Unfortunately, few studies have systematically characterized the influence of personality on each pain-processing stage. One of the few studies to do so (Harkins et al., 1989) found that neuroticism was unrelated to the sensory-intensive dimension (Stage 1) for both experimental pain and myofascial pain dysfunction related to orofacial pain. Neuroticism exerted small but statistically reliable enhancement of pain unpleasantness (Stage 2) of both experimental and clinical pain. In contrast to small or negligible effects on Stages 1 and 2, neuroticism exerted a large enhancement of emotional suffering (Stage 3) and illness behavior (Stage 4) in the same patients. Individuals at both extremes of extraversion reported similar levels of emotional disturbance as a result of pain.

In a study of patients with chronic pain, Wade, Dougherty, Hart, Rafii, and Price (1992) examined the relationship between neuroticism and extraversion on the 4 stages of pain processing. The Pain Experience Analog Scales (VAS) (Price et al., 1983), the Psychosocial Pain Inventory (Getto & Heaton, 1985), and the NEO PI-R (Costa & McCrae, 1985) were administered to 205 pain patients. Canonical correlation was used to control for pain sensation intensity in evaluating affective dimensions of pain and to control for neuroticism and extraversion in assessing effects of the other personality variables on stages of pain processing. Consistent with the findings of Harkins et al. (1989), neither neuroticism nor extraversion were related to pain sensation intensity. Neuroticism alone was related to immediate pain-related unpleasantness. This finding is consistent with previous reports (Gracely, 1989; Gracely, McGrath, & Dubner, 1978). Both neuroticism and extraversion demonstrated a strong facilitative role with regard to the latter stages of pain processing (Stage 3, Suffering; Stage 4, Illness Behavior).

In the Wade, Dougherty, Hart, Rafii, and Price (1992) study, multiple-regression analyses indicated that lifelong vulnerability to anxiety and, to a lesser extent, to depression are the most important contributors to the relationship between personality and pain processing. The importance of anxiety in the development of emotional suffering has been emphasized previously in studies examining the genesis of psychopathology (Cattell et al., 1970; Costa & McCrae, 1976). In the Wade, Dougherty, Hart, Rafii, and Price (1992) study, anxiety emerged as the most important factor in predicting the degree of illness behavior associated with pain. These data suggest that lifelong vulnerability to anxiety and depression, prominent aspects of neuroticism, are the best predictors of chronic unhappiness (Costa & McCrae, 1985).

Although several studies (BenDebba et al., 1997; Harkins et al., 1989; Wade, Dougherty, Hart, Rafii, & Price, 1992) have suggested that extraversion is related to suffering, its relationship is weaker than that of neuroticism. In the Wade, Dougherty, Hart, Rafii, and Price (1992) study, assertiveness, a facet score of extraversion, was the most important predictor of pain suffering. Both assertiveness and activity level were the only extraversion facet scores associated with illness behavior. The relationship between extraversion and behavior is complicated. It appears that highly assertive patients manifest more pain behavior at home and during clinical interviews when they are unobtrusively observed. In contrast, they also report less lifestyle disruption (i.e., sickness impact) and fewer incidents of solicitous behavior (e.g., received less secondary gain from family members). Several reports (Eysenck, 1967; Gordon & Hitchcock, 1983; Harkins et al., 1989) provide support for the finding that extraverts express their suffering more frequently than do introverts.

Several epidemiological studies suggest that psychological factors are important in the aftermath of major medical events (Gertrudis et al., 1997). Personality traits have been related to long-term physical health (Friedman et al., 1993; Smith & Williams, 1992). Brickman, Young, Blaney, Rothberg, and De-Nour (1996) evaluated whether personality traits influence diabetic patients' ability and willingness to follow prescribed treatment regimens for achieving glycemic control. They found neuroticism and conscientiousness were related to long-term survival. Persons moderate in neuroticism and high in conscientiousness had renal deterioration times that were 12 years longer than did others in the sample. Russo, Katon, Lin, Von Korff, Bush, Simon, and Walker (1997) assessed whether personality characteristics predicted health outcome in a depressed primary-care population, independent of disease status, demographics, depression, and psychiatric diagnosis. Their outcome factors were disability (days missed from work), somatization (unexplained medical symptoms), and pain severity. Neuroticism was significantly related to all three. Extraversion also was associated with health outcomes, independent of demographics; disease status; and psychiatric diagnosis, although its relationship to outcome was weaker than that of neuroticism. As had Wade, Dougherty, Hart, Rafii, and Price (1992), Russo's group found the relationship between extraversion and disability status complicated. Extraversion was a significant predictor of disability status, but increasing extroversion scores were associated with less reported disability. Extraversion could serve to attenuate the influence of neuroticism on later stages of pain processing. Similarly, as had other researchers (Harkins et al., 1989; Wade, Dougherty, Hart, Rafii, & Price, 1992), Russo et al. found no relationship between extraversion and pain sensation intensity in primary care patients. The fact that several studies have attained similar findings across heterogeneous populations using different personality measures of extraversion and neuroticism supports the generalizability of these findings.

The literature finds that personality factors have their greatest influence on Stage 3 (suffering) and Stage 4 (illness behavior) of pain processing. This reinforces the uniqueness of these later-stage pain components. Similarly, in the Wade, Dougherty, Hart, Rafii, and Price (1992) study, with the exception of anxiety, different NEO PI-R facet scores were associated with suffering (depression, positive emotions, assertiveness, and activity level) and immediate pain-related unpleasantness. These data highlight the separateness of these earlier pain dimensions. Although the literature demonstrates an association between measures of normal personality (mainly neuroticism and extroversion) and pain-related suffering, it does not clearly assign a causal relationship between these variables. One possibility is that enduring anxiety and lifelong depression contribute to a pattern of catastrophizing, which exacerbates emotional disturbance in chronic pain patients. An alternative hypothesis is that an increase in lifestyle disruption resulting from pain leads to an intensification of catastrophizing and subsequent suffering.

Treatment Implications of the Big-Five Factors

This section concerns the domains that constitute the 5-factor model of normal personality and their implications for treatment. Administering a measure of normal personality structure to a patient helps to elucidate the patient's emotional state, to facilitate treatment plan development, and to clarify obstacles that would interfere with treatment. In comparison with normative samples, the NEO PI-R profiles of patients seeking psychotherapy are a standard deviation higher in neuroticism, and one-half standard deviation lower in agreeableness and conscientiousness (Fagan et al., 1991; Miller, 1991; Muten, 1991). These study group comparisons did not result in extraversion or openness domain score differences. Neuroticism is thought to reflect an individual's vulnerability to emotional distress or a predisposition to experience suffering and illness behavior (Costa & McCrae, 1992). Individuals prone to depression are likely to have elevated premorbid neuroticism scores (Hirschfield et al., 1989). Clearly, some degree of discomfort is a prerequisite for seeking psychotherapy. Miller (1991) asserted that, with patients with high neuroticism, it will be important to set clear and attainable goals. The degree of agitation seen in this group can make it difficult for them to sit down to the business of psychotherapy. In addition, their chronic, intense vulnerability to anxiety can make this subgroup particularly susceptible to the *"nocebo" reaction* (adverse treatment response of psychological etiology). The use of sedatives or relaxation techniques prior to an invasive intervention can limit the development of such a response. Frustration intolerance and excessive self-defeating rumination make this group extremely likely to terminate treatment prematurely and against medical advice. This can occur when the inevitable challenge to the patient's defenses takes place in therapy. Therefore, therapy goals for these individuals often need to be modest. Indeed, for patients with high neuroticism, therapy of a supportive or palliative nature might be most appropriate.

In contrast, individuals with low neuroticism will infrequently initiate psychotherapy. Rather, they are likely to come grudgingly to the psychologist or mental health clinic, and they tend to doubt that they really need treatment. Helping them conceptualize their pain using a medical model can increase the likelihood that they will stay in therapy long enough to benefit from treatment. Therefore, rather than using hypnosis or imagery techniques, patients with low neuroticism sometimes prefer biofeedback. Miller (1991) provided preliminary data that neuroticism correlates with treatment (psychotherapy) outcome. It is not clear from these data whether patients with low neuroticism benefited more from the treatment or simply had milder forms of illness at the outset.

Extraversion reflects qualities such as interpersonal energy and possibly the degree of enthusiasm for participation in psychotherapy. Patients with high extraversion are talkative and active but also emotionally labile. Their interest in people suggests that a group treatment format or the use of gestalt techniques, such as the empty chair and role playing, can be particularly useful. Patients with low extraversion are likely to be less talkative and look to the therapist for the "cure."

Openness could be one of the most important of the 5 factors when it comes to treatment outcome. Openness is modestly correlated with IQ and education (Costa & McCrae, 1985). No one likes to become painfully aware of the maladaptive ways in which they cope. Individuals high in openness will be more willing to try new ways to cope with old problems. Their willingness to experiment with new activities and their curiosity for novelty suggest that hypnosis and other alternative approaches might be possible treatment avenues. Very high openness also can suggest relatively fragile ego boundaries. Like the patient with low extraversion, the individual with low openness prefers practical, scientifically based, problem-focused conceptualizations. Biofeedback therefore should be a treatment consideration with these patients.

Individuals with low openness rarely show excitement or enthusiasm. Care must be taken then not to infer a lack of interest in treatment based on resistance to new strategies or experiences.

Individuals high in agreeableness are easy to sit with. These are compassionate, giving individuals who view the glass always as half full. It will be easy for the therapist to form an alliance with these patients. Interpretations will be accepted with mercurial speed. Care must be taken by the therapist not to abuse the patient's uncritical willingness to receive feedback and take on new homework assignments. In contrast, individuals with low agreeableness can be the first to terminate treatment against medical advice and to denigrate the therapist later. The therapist must avoid the trap of trying to convince such patients to reassess emotional, cognitive, or behavioral stances. Power struggles are common.

Like openness, conscientiousness is a critical factor in determining treatment outcome. People high in conscientiousness are likely to follow through with homework assignments, tolerate discomfort, and delay gratification. Possibly as a concomitant of these qualities, conscientiousness is associated with academic and vocational success (Digman & Takemoto-Chock, 1981). Indeed, there are few, if any, treatment pitfalls when working with the individual with high conscientiousness. The converse is probably true as well. Individuals with low conscientiousness do not have the perseverence necessary to buckle down to the business of psychotherapy. They take on life in a half-hearted manner and project responsibility for their dilemmas onto those around them. For these reasons, they fail to profit from experience. Their resistance to change, unwillingness to take any responsibility for the work involved in therapy, impulsivity, and intolerance for discomfort suggest that the patients with low conscientiousness are among the most challenging. Miller (1991) has offered the term *misery triad* to describe the individuals least likely to succeed in psychotherapy or, for that matter, life in general. These people are high in neuroticism, low in extraversion, and low in conscientiousness.

Summary and Conclusion

The goal of pain assessment should be to develop a comprehensive treatment plan that accounts for individual needs. Repeating a subset of the original assessment procedures will clarify treatment efficacy. Clinicians often attempt to clarify treatment efficacy by asking patients directly for feedback. This might involve asking patients to rate pain on a scale of 0 to 10 (with the polls representing extremes of *no pain* and *worst pain*). Alternatively, the clinician might ask patients to estimate the percentage of pain reduction achieved. Both approaches are fraught with methodological weaknesses (e.g., Hawthorne effect, demand characteristics, selective memory problems for the recall of pain).

Understanding an individual's pain experience and evaluating the effects of treatment require explicit recognition that pain is multidimensional and that it has discrete stages. A pain-processing model is conceptualized as representing unique stages with subcomponents. The first stage is the sensory-discriminative dimension, and sensation intensity is most often the focus of treatment. The second stage of the pain model is that of the immediate pain-related unpleasantness. There is typically a close relationship between Stage 1 (pain sensation intensity) and this first stage of emotional processing. Unpleasantness can be viewed as reflecting the extent to which the pain sensation intrudes on or interferes with thought and behavior. Enduring personality traits, memories, and cognitive appraisal of the pain's meaning have only a small moderating influence on the severity of immediate pain-related unpleasantness. In contrast, the latter factors are of overriding importance, and they greatly influence the second component of affective processing, referred to here as "suffering." An appreciation of Stage 3 of pain processing requires an assessment of negative emotions (depression, anxiety, frustration, fear, anger) and negative illness beliefs (hope for cure, ability to endure pain, perceived control over pain reduction, degree of lifestyle interference). Stage 4 of pain processing, illness behavior, is a complex construct that might require the combined use of several assessment methodologies (unobtrusive observation, structured interviews, self-report measures). The 4-stage pain-processing model (Figure 4.1) specifically addresses the fact that personality factors (both normal personality and psychopathology) selectively influence the latter stages of pain processing (excluding the pain sensation itself). Therefore, in evaluating a person with chronic pain it will be critical to understand what the individual "brings to" the pain problem. This involves assessing for the presence of psychopathology and the 5 factors that constitute normal personality structure.

We have reviewed assessment tools with demonstrated reliability and validity for assessing the 4 stages of pain processing. The Medical College of Virginia Pain Questionnaire consists of pain visual analogue scales assessing pain sensation intensity, immediate pain-related unpleasantness, and suffering (both emotional and ideational realms). A questionnaire included in this test battery incorporates a structured clinical interview (Getto & Heaton, 1985), permitting an assessment of illness behavior. We reviewed two objective personality tests that can be used to assess normal personality (NEO PI-R and HPI). Probably, the most popular measure of psychopathology in current use is the MMPI-2 (Piotrowski & Lubin, 1990). Although it is important to include an assessment of psychopathology in a comprehensive pain assessment battery, it is beyond the scope of this chapter to discuss in more detail the relationship between pain and psychopathology. Regardless of which measures the clinician chooses to assess pain and personality dimensions, it is critical that the tools are reliable and valid, and that they are relatively quick to administer and score. The goal of the assessment process should be to establish a treatment plan that incorporates the individual's social and cultural background, pain stage data, and personality functioning. Serial evaluation using a subset of the original test battery facilitates an evaluation of treatment efficacy.

References

Affleck, G., Tennen, H., Urrows, S., & Higgins, P. (1992). Neuroticism and the pain–mood relation in rheumatoid arthritis: Insights from a prospective daily study. *Journal of Consulting and Clinical Psychology, 60*(1), 119–126.

Allport, G. W., & Odbert, H. S. (1936). Trait-names: A psycho-lexical study [Whole of no. 211]. *Psychological Monographs, 47*(1).

Aurelius, Marcus. (1980). Meditations 7:16 (G. Long, Trans.). In C. W. Eliot (Ed.), *The Harvard classics*. Danbury, CT: Grolier.

BenDebba, M., Torgerson, W. S., & Long, D. M. (1997). Personality traits, pain duration and severity, functional impairment, and psychological distress in patients with persistent low back pain. *Pain, 72*, 115–125.

Blumberg, H., Griesser, H. J., & Hornyak, M. (1990). New viewpoints on the clinical picture, diagnosis and pathology of reflex sympathetic dystrophy. *Unfallchirurgie, 16*, 95–106.

Borgatta, E. F. (1964a). The structure of personality characteristics. *Behavioral Science, 9*, 8–17.

Borgatta, E. F. (1964b). A very short test of personality: The Behavioral Self-Rating (BSR) Form. *Psychological Reports, 14*, 275–284.

Boyce, P., & Parker, G. (1985). Neuroticism as a predictor of outcome in depression. *Journal of Nervous and Mental Disease, 173*, 685–688.

Breslau, N., Chilcoat, H. D., & Andreski, P. (1996). Further evidence on the link between migraine and neuroticism. *Neurology, 47*, 663–667.

Brickman, A. L., Young, S. E., Blaney, N. T., Rothberg, S. T., & De-Nour, A. K. (1996). Personality traits and long-term health status: The influence of neuroticism and conscientiousness on renal deterioration in type-1 diabetes. *Psychosomatics, 37*(5), 459–468.

Bush, F. M., Harkins, S. W., Harrington, W. G., & Price, D. D. (1993). Analysis of gender effects on pain perception and symptom presentation in temporomandibular pain. *Pain, 53*, 73–80.

Cattell, R. B., & Eber, H. W. (1964). *Manual for the 16 Personality Factor Test*. Champaign, IL: Institute for Personality and Ability Testing.

Cattell, R. B., Eber, H. W., & Tatsuoka, M. M. (1970). *Handbook for the Sixteen Personality Factor Questionnaire*. Champaign, IL: Institute for Personality and Ability Testing.

Chapman, W. P., & Jones, C. M. (1944). Variations in cutaneous and visceral pain sensitivity in normal subjects. *Journal of Clinical Investigation, 23*, 81.

Costa, P. T. (1987). Influence of normal personality dimension of neuroticism on chest pain symptoms and coronary artery disease. *American Journal of Cardiology, 60*, 20–26.

Costa, P. T., Busch, C. M., Zonderman, A. B., & McCrae, R. R. (1986). Correlations of MMPI factor scales with measures of the five factor model of personality. *Journal of Personality Assessment, 50*, 640–650.

Costa, P. T., & McCrae, R. R. (1976). Age differences in personality structure: A cluster analytic approach. *Journal of Gerontology, 31*, 564–570.

Costa, P. T., & McCrae, R. R. (1985). *The NEO Personality Inventory manual*. Odessa, FL: Psychological Assessment Resources.

Costa, P. T., & McCrae, R. R. (1987). Personality assessment in psychosomatic medicine: Value of a trait taxonomy. In G. A. Fava & T. N. Wise (Eds.), *Advances in psychosomatic medicine: Vol. 17. Research paradigms in psychosomatic medicine* (pp. 71–82). Basel, Switzerland: Karger.

Costa, P. T., & McCrae, R. R. (1988). Personality in adulthood: A six-year longitudinal study of self-reports and spouse ratings on the NEO Personality Inventory. *Journal of Personality and Social Psychology, 54*, 853–863.

Costa, P. T., & McCrae, R. R. (1992). *Revised NEO Personality Inventory (NEO-PI-R) and NEO Five-Factor Inventory (NEO-FFI) manual*. Odessa, FL: Psychological Assessment Resources.

Costa, P. T., Zonderman, A. B., Engel, B. T., Baile, W. F., Brimlow, D. L., & Brinker, J. (1985). The relation of chest pain symptoms to angiographic findings of coronary artery stenosis and neuroticism. *Psychosomatic Medicine, 47*(3), 285–293.

DeVilder, J. (1980). Personality of patients with Sudeck's atrophy following tibial fracture. *Acta Orthopaedica Belgica, 58*, 463–468.

Digman, J. M., & Inouye, J. (1986). Further specification of the five robust factors of personality. *Journal of Personality and Social Psychology, 50*, 116–123.

Digman, J. M., & Takemoto-Chock, N. K. (1981). Factors in the natural language of personality: Re-analysis, comparison, and interpretation of six major studies. *Multivariate Behavioral Research, 16*, 149–170.

Dubreuil, D., & Kohn, P. (1986). Reactivity and response to pain. *Personality and Individual Differences, 7*, 907–909.

Ellermeier, W., & Westphal, W. (1995). Gender differences in pain ratings and pupil reactions to painful pressure stimuli. *Pain, 61*, 435–439.

Eysenck, H. J. (1967). *Biological basis of personality*. Springfield, IL: Charles C Thomas.

Eysenck, H. J. (1991). Dimensions of personality: 16, 5, or 3?: Criteria for a taxonomic paradigm. *Personality and Individual Differences, 12*, 773–790.

Eysenck, H. J. (1992). Four ways five factors are *not* basic. *Personality and Individual Differences, 13*, 667–673.

Eysenck, H. J., & Eysenck, S. B. G. (1975). *Manual of [the] Eysenck Personality Questionnaire*. London: Hodder & Stoughton.

Fagan, P. J., Wise, T. N., Schmidt, C. W., Ponticas, Y., Marshall, R. D., & Costa, P. T., Jr. (1991). A comparison of five-factor personality dimensions in males with sexual dysfunction and males with paraphilia. *Journal of Personality Assessment, 57*, 434–448.

Friedman, H. S., Tucker, J. S., Tomlinson-Keasey, C., Schwartz, J. E., Wingard, D. L., & Criqui, M. H. (1993). Does childhood personality predict longevity? *Journal of Personality and Social Psychology, 65*, 176–185.

Galton, F. (1884). Measurement of character. *Fortnightly Review, 36*, 179–185.

Garron, D., & Leavitt, F. (1979). Demographic and affective covariates of pain. *Psychosomatic Medicine, 41*, 525–534.

Gertrudis, I. J. M., Kempen, M. H., & Ormel, J. (1997). Personality, chronic medical morbidity, and health-related quality of life among older persons. *Health Psychology, 16*(6), 539–546.

Getto, C. J., & Heaton, R. (1985). *Psychosocial Pain Inventory*. Odessa, FL: Psychological Assessment Resources.

Goldberg, L. R. (1981). Language and individual differences: The search for universals in personality lexicons. In L. Wheeler (Ed.), *Review of personality and social psychology* (Vol. 2, pp. 141–165). Beverly Hills, CA: Sage.

Goldberg, L. R. (1982). From ace to zombie: Some explorations in the language of personality. In C. D. Spielberger & J. N. Butcher (Eds.), *Advances in personality assessment* (Vol. 1, pp. 203–234). Hillsdale, NJ: Erlbaum.

Goldberg, L. R. (1990). An alternative "description of personality": The Big-Five factor structure. *Journal of Personality and Social Psychology, 59*, 1216–1229.

Goldberg, L. R. (1992). The development of markers of the Big-Five factor structure. *Psychological Assessment, 4*, 26–42.

Gordon, A., & Hitchcock, E. R. (1983). Illness behavior and personality in intractable facial pain syndromes. *Pain, 17*(3), 267–276.

Gough, H. G. (1957). *California Psychological Inventory manual*. Palo Alto, CA: Consulting Psychologists Press.

Gracely, R. (1979). Psychophysical assessment of human pain. In J. J. Bonica, J. C. Liebeskind, & D. Albe-Fessard (Eds.), *Advances in pain research and therapy* (Vol. 3, pp. 805–824). New York: Raven Press.

Gracely, R. H. (1989). Pain psychophysics. In C. R. Chapman & J. D. Loeser (Eds.), *Advances in pain research and therapy* (Vol. 12, pp. 211–229). New York: Raven Press.

Gracely, R. H., McGrath, P., & Dubner, R. (1978). Ratio scales of sensory and affective verbal pain descriptors. *Pain, 5*, 5–18.

Greene, D. (Trans.) (1957). *Sophocles II*. Chicago: University of Chicago Press.

Greenwald, H. P., Bonica, J. J., & Bergner, M. (1987). The prevalence of pain in four cancers. *Cancer, 60*, 2563–2569.

Haddox, J. D. (1990). Psychological aspects of reflex sympathetic dystrophy. In M. Stanton-Hicks (Ed.), *Pain and the sympathetic nervous system* (pp. 207–224). Boston: Kluwer Academic.

Harkins, S. W., Price, D. D., & Braith, J. (1989). Effects of extroversion and neuroticism on experimental pain, clinical pain, and illness behavior. *Pain, 36*, 209–218.

Harkins, S. W., Price, D. D., & Martelli, M. (1986). Effects of age on pain perception: Thermonociception. *Journal of Gerontology, 41*, 58–63.

Hirschfield, R. M. A., Klerman, G. L., Lavori, P., Keller, M. B., Griffith, P., & Coryell, W. (1989). Premorbid personality assessments of first onset of major depression. *Archives of General Psychiatry, 46*, 345–350.

Hogan, R. (1983). Socioanalytic theory of personality. In M. M. Page (Ed.), *1982 Nebraska Symposium on Motivation: Personality—Current Theory and Research* (pp. 55–89). Lincoln: University of Nebraska Press.

Hogan, R. (1986). *Hogan Personality Inventory manual.* Minneapolis: National Computer Systems.

Joreskeg, K. G. & Sorbom, D. (1976). *LISTREL III: Estimation of linear structural equation systems by maximum likelihood methods: Users guide.* Chicago: International Education Series.

Keefe, F., Brown, G., Wallson, K., & Caldwell, D. (1989). Coping with rheumatoid arthritis pain: Catastrophisizing as a maladaptive strategy. *Pain, 37*, 51–56.

Lander, J., Fowler-Kerry, S., & Hargreaves, A. (1989). Gender effects in pain perception. *Perceptual and Motor Skills, 68*, 1088–1090.

Larsen, R. J. (1992). Neuroticism and selective encoding and recall of symptoms: Evidence from a combined concurrent–retrospective study. *Journal of Personality and Social Psychology, 62*, 480–488.

Lauver, S. C., & Johnson, J. L. (1997). The role of neuroticism and social support in older adults with chronic pain behavior. *Personality and Individual Differences, 23*(1), 165–167.

Leon, B. (1974). Pain perception and extraversion. *Perceptual and Motor Skills, 38*, 510.

Lipton, J. A., & Marbach, J. J. (1984). Ethnicity and the pain experience. *Social Science and Medicine, 19*(12), 1279–1298.

Lynch, M. E. (1992). Psychological aspects of reflex sympathetic dystrophy: A review of the adult and pediatric literature. *Pain, 49*, 337–347.

McCrae, R. R. (1993). Moderated analyses of longitudinal personality stability. *Journal of Personality and Social Psychology, 65*(3), 577–585.

McCrae, R. R., & Costa, P. T. (1983). The five-factor model and its assessment in clinical settings. *Journal of Personality Assessment, 57*, 399–414.

McCrae, R. R., & Costa, P. T. (1985a). Comparison of EPI and psychoticism scales with measures of the five-factor model of personality. *Personality and Individual Differences, 6*, 587–597.

McCrae, R. R., & Costa, P. T. (1985b). Updating Norman's "adequate taxonomy": Intelligence and personality dimensions in natural language and in questionnaires. *Journal of Personality and Social Psychology, 49*, 710–721.

McCrae, R. R., & Costa, P. T. (1987). Validation of the five-factor model of personality across instruments and observers. *Journal of Personality and Social Psychology, 52*, 81–90.

McCrae, R. R., & Costa, P. T. (1989a). More reasons to adopt the five-factor model. *American Psychologist, 44*, 451–452.

McCrae, R. R., & Costa, P. T. (1989b). Reinterpreting the Myers–Briggs Type Indicator from the perspective of the five-factor model of personality. *Journal of Personality, 57*, 17–40.

McMillan, S. C. (1989). The relationship between age and intensity of cancer-related symptoms. *Oncology Nursing Forum, 16*(2), 237–241.

Melzack, R. (1975). The McGill Pain Questionnaire: Major properties and scoring methods. *Pain, 1*, 277–299.

Miller, T. R. (1991). The psychotherapeutic utility of the five-factor model of personality: A clinician's experience. *Journal of Personality Assessment, 57*(3), 415–433.

Mumford, J. M. (1965). Pain perception threshold and adaptation of normal human teeth. *Archives of Oral Biology, 10*, 957.

Muten, E. (1991). Self-reports, spouse ratings, and psychophysiological assessment in a behavioral medicine program: An application of the five-factor model. *Journal of Personality Assessment, 57*, 449–464.

Nagelberg, D. B., Hale, S. L., & Ware, S. L. (1984). The assessment of bulimic symptoms and personality correlates in female college students. *Journal of Clinical Psychology, 40*, 440–445.

Norman, W. T. (1963). Toward an adequate taxonomy of personality attributes: Replicated factor structure in peer nomination personality ratings. *Journal of Abnormal and Social Psychology, 66*, 574–583.

Peabody, D., & Goldberg, L. R. (1989). Some determinants of factor structures from personality-trait descriptors. *Journal of Personality and Social Psychology, 57*, 552–567.

Philips, H. C., & Jahanshahi, M. (1985). The effects of persistent pain: The chronic headache sufferer. *Pain, 21*, 163–176.

Pietri-Taleb, F., Riihimäki, H., Viikari-Juntura, E., & Lindström, K. (1994). Longitudinal study on the role of personality characteristics and psychological distress in neck trouble among working men. *Pain, 58*, 261–267.

Piotrowski, C., & Lubin, B. (1990). Assessment practices of health psychologists: Survey of APA Division 38 clinicians. *Professional Psychology: Research and Practice, 21*(2), 99–106.

Price, D. D. (1988). *Psychological and neural mechanisms of pain.* New York: Raven Press.

Price, D. D., & Harkins, S. W. (1992). Psychological approaches to pain measurement and assessment. In D. C. Turk & R. Melzack (Eds.), *Handbook of pain assessment* (pp. 111–134). New York: Guilford Press.

Price D. D., Harkins, S. W., & Baker, C. (1987). Sensory-affective relationships among different types of clinical and experimental pain. *Pain, 28*, 297–307.

Price, D. D., McGrath, P. A., Rafii, A., & Buckingham, B. (1983). The validation of visual analogue scales as ratio scale measures for chronic and experimental pain. *Pain, 17*, 45–56.

Procacci, P., Bozza, G., Buzzelli, G., & Della Corte, M. (1970). The cutaneous pricking pain threshold in old age. *Gerontology Clinics, 12*, 213.

Rainville, P., Carrier, B., Hofbauer, R. K., Bushnell, M. C., & Duncan, G. H. (in press). Dissociation of sensory and affective dimensions of pain using hypnotic modulation. *Pain.*

Rainville, P., Duncan, G. H., Price, D. D., Carrier, B., & Bushnell, M. C. (1997). Pain affect encoded in human anterior cingulate but not somatosensory cortex. *Science, 277*, 968–971.

Reuter, E. K., Wallbrown, F. H., & Wallbrown, J. D. (1985). 16PF profiles and four-point codes for clients seen in a private practice. *Multivariate Experimental Clinical Research, 7*, 123–147.

Roll, M., & Theorell, T. (1987). Acute chest pain without obvious organic cause before age 40—Personality and recent life events. *Journal of Psychosomatic Research, 31*(2), 215–221.

Rosenstiel, A., & Keefe, F. (1983). The use of coping strategies in chronic low back pain patients: Relationship to patient characteristics and current adjustment. *Pain, 17*, 33–44.

Roy, A., Custer, R., Lorenz, V., & Linnoila, M. (1989). Personality factors and pathological gambling. *Acta Psychiatrica Scandinavica, 80*, 37–39.

Russo, J., Katon, W., Lin, E., Von Korff, Sc. D., Bush, T., Simon, G., & Walker, E. (1997).

Neuroticism and extraversion as predictors of health outcomes in depressed primary care patients. *Psychosomatics, 38*(4), 339–348.

Sherman, E. D., & Robillard, E. (1964). Sensitivity to pain in relationship to age. *Journal of the American Geriatrics Society, 12*, 1037.

Smith, G. M. (1967). Usefulness of peer ratings of personality in educational research. *Educational and Psychological Measurement, 27*, 967–984.

Smith, G. M. (1969). Relations between personality and smoking behavior in pre-adult subjects. *Journal of Consulting and Clinical Psychology, 33*, 710–715.

Smith, T. W., & Williams, P. G. (1992). Personality and health: Advantages and limitations of the five-factor model. *Journal of Personality, 60*, 395–423.

Sorkin, B. A., Rudy, T. E., Hanlon, R. B., Turk, D. C., & Stieg, R. L. (1990). Chronic pain in old and young patients: Differences appear less important than similarities. *Journal of Gerontology, 45*(2), 64–68.

Sternbach, R. A., & Tursky, B. (1965). Ethnic differences among housewives in psychophysical and skin potential responses to electric shock. *Psychophysiology, 1*, 241–246.

Thurstone, L. L. (1934). The vectors of mind. *Psychological Review, 41*, 1–32.

Thurstone, L. L. (1953). *Thurstone Temperament Schedule*. Chicago: Science Research Associates.

Tupes, E. C., & Christal, R. E. (1958). *Stability of personality trait rating factors obtained under diverse conditions* (USAF WADC Tech. Note No. 58-61). Lackland Air Force Base, TX: U.S. Air Force.

Tupes, E. C., & Christal, R. E. (1961). *Recurrent personality factors based on trait ratings* (USAF ASD Tech. Rep. No. 61-97). Lackland Air Force Base, TX: U.S. Air Force.

Wade, J. B. (1999). [Study on age, gender, ethnicity, and medical diagnosis in four parts]. Study in process.

Wade, J. B., Dougherty, L. M., Archer, C. R., & Price, D. D. (1996). Assessing the stages of pain processing: A multivariate analytical approach, *Pain, 68*, 157–167.

Wade, J. B., Dougherty, L. M., Hart, R. P., & Cook, D. B. (1992). Patterns of normal personality structure among chronic pain patients. *Pain, 48*, 37–43.

Wade, J. B., Dougherty, L. M., Hart, R. P., Rafii, A., & Price, D. D. (1992). A canonical correlation analysis of the influence of neuroticism and extraversion on chronic pain, suffering, and pain behavior. *Pain, 51*, 67–73.

Wade, J. B., Price, D. D., & Hamer, R. M. (1990). An emotional component analysis of chronic pain. *Pain, 40*, 303–310.

Weisenberg, M., Kreindler, M. L., Schachat, R., & Werboff, J. (1975). Pain: Anxiety and attitudes in Black, White, and Puerto Rican patients. *Psychosomatic Medicine, 37*, 123–135.

Woodrow, K. M., Friedman, G. D., Siegelaub, A. B., & Collen, M. F. (1972). Pain tolerance: Differences according to age, sex and race. *Psychosomatic Medicine, 34*(6), 548–556.

Zatzick, D. F., & Dimsdale, J. E. (1990). Cultural variations in response to painful stimuli. *Psychosomatic Medicine, 52*(5), 544–557.

Chapter 5
The MMPI-2 AND CHRONIC PAIN

William W. Deardorff

Current theories of the etiology and maintenance of chronic pain emphasize its multidimensional nature. The theories account for the affective, cognitive, behavioral, social, and sensory aspects of the pain experience (Turk & Melzack, 1992; Wall & Melzack, 1984), and the models of pain require detailed assessment of a patient's full range of functioning and pain experience (Turk & Melzack, 1992). Adequate assessment is important for illuminating all aspects of the chronic pain patient's suffering and for developing successful treatment programs (Turk, 1990). As can be seen, such assessments go far beyond traditional medical examinations.

To adequately complete a multidimensional assessment, psychological testing is commonly used. The original Minnesota Multiphasic Personality Inventory (MMPI; Hathaway & McKinley, 1943) was the most commonly used standardized personality test for patients with chronic pain (Keller & Butcher, 1991; Love & Peck, 1987). The original MMPI was revised and released as the MMPI-2 (Butcher, Dahlstrom, Graham, Tellegen, & Kaemmer, 1989). It is likely that the MMPI-2 is now the most commonly used personality test for patients with chronic pain. Of course, any self-report personality test such as the MMPI or MMPI-2 should be just one part of a comprehensive evaluation that includes medical, behavioral, psychosocial, and demographic information. Keller and Butcher (1991) concluded that two goals of chronic pain assessment should be (a) to identify and describe personality and behavioral characteristics of the typical patient, and (b) to identify and describe unique differences among patients. This latter goal is especially important because the individual characteristics of a patient with chronic pain will influence the design of individualized multidisciplinary pain programs and guide predictions about treatment outcome. The MMPI (and now the MMPI-2) can help to achieve these assessment goals.

This chapter specifically reviews the use of the MMPI-2 in the assessment of personality and other characteristics of patients with chronic pain. The use of the original MMPI for this purpose is discussed elsewhere in the volume. Therefore, this chapter limits its focus to the following areas: (a) a discussion of the controversy attendant to the use of the MMPI–MMPI-2 with chronic pain patients, (b) a review of the utility of using the MMPI-2 as part of a chronic pain evaluation, (c) an outline of the development of the MMPI-2, (d) an explanation of some similarities and differences in the two instruments, and (e) a review of some interpretive strategies for the MMPI-2.

MMPI-2 and Chronic Pain Assessment: Controversy

The use of the MMPI or the MMPI-2 as part of a chronic pain assessment is not without controversy. Main and Spanswick (1995a) contended that the use of the test in assessing chronic pain is "understandable but no longer justifiable" (p. 90). Other researchers have taken a similar stand (Fishbain, 1996; Helmes, 1994; Main & Spanswick, 1995a, 1995b; Turk & Fernandez, 1995). These investigators have posited that the MMPI and the MMPI-2 have problems that preclude their usefulness with chronic pain patients. Some of the minor problems with the MMPI were remedied with the development of the MMPI-2, including item content and wording and outdated norms.

Other, more fundamental criticisms have been leveled at both versions of the test. Anyone who uses the MMPI-2 to assess the personality characteristics of chronic pain patients (either clinically or as part of a research project) must be aware of these issues to understand the strengths and weaknesses of the instrument and to avoid its inappropriate use.

First, the point is made by Helmes and Reddon (1993) that the MMPI and MMPI-2 are based on outdated theories of psychopathology. They noted that the concepts that underlie the diagnostic categories used to form the inventory's clinical scales are no longer used in modern theories of psychopathology. Because the original scale names and most items have been retained in the MMPI-2, there remain links with the original diagnostic system that have been called "relics of an antiquated psychiatry" (Cronbach, 1990, p. 539). Critics say that the scales clearly measure something other than what their names imply (Turk & Fernandez, 1995). Various researchers have argued that the outdated approach makes the MMPI-2 less than useful in helping identify personality characteristics and psychopathology among chronic pain patients.

The second major criticism concerns the significant overlap in item content across the clinical and validity scales, which can result in spurious profiles. Critics of the MMPI-2 believe item overlap causes scale elevations that do not accurately reflect what patients experience. For instance, two common profiles among chronic pain patients are the "Conversion V" profile and the "neurotic triad." The first of these is characterized by elevated T scores on Scales 1 (Hypochondriasis) and 3 (Hysteria), with a lower T score on Scale 2 (Depression). The neurotic triad is characterized by elevations on all three of these scales. Critics have pointed out that there is significant item overlap across these and other scales. For instance, the scales for Hypochondriasis and Depression have 20 items in common; other items are scored on as many as six inventory scales. The critics believe this overlap makes it difficult to interpret profiles and to discriminate among different groups. Their argument is summarized by Helmes (1994): "The overlap also makes it more difficult for the test to discriminate among different groups, because the responses to a small set of common items can influence several scales" (p. 5).

It also has been argued that the results of the MMPI-2 profiles are invalid when used with chronic pain patients because of the inclusion of items that reflect features of both a psychiatric disturbance and a chronic illness, such as long-term pain (Pincus, Callahan, Bradley, Vaughn, & Wolfe, 1986). The Hypochondriasis and Depression scales contain several items that reflect general medical or physical condition. Research has shown that elevations on these scales can indicate organic disease rather than psychological status (Pincus et al., 1986). Thus, there is the possibility that having a patient simply report symptoms of his or her medical disorder could lead to the inappropriate conclusion of emotional and psychiatric problems indicated by elevations on these scales (Helmes, 1994).

These criticisms must be weighed against other arguments that substantiate the utility of the MMPI-2 as part of a chronic pain evaluation. In answer to the first criticism, MMPI-2 proponents have argued that sophisticated users understand that the scale names on the MMPI-2 do not necessarily reflect distinct psychopathological disorders in the patient (Bradley, 1995; Keefe, Lefebvre, & Beaupre, 1995; Sanders, 1995). In fact, to avoid erroneous connections being drawn from the original scale meanings, many interpretive guidelines suggest using scale numbers rather than names.

Relative to the second and third criticisms, advocates have argued that the MMPI-2 provides valuable information about persons with chronic pain and that experienced interpreters account for item overlap and medical symptom content as part of their analyses. For example, it will be considered that chronic pain patients will almost automatically have elevated scores on given scales simply because they are reporting medical symptoms (Bradley, Haile, & Jaworski, 1992; Moore, McFall, Kivlahan, & Capestany, 1988; Naliboff, Cohen, & Yellin, 1982; Pincus et al., 1986; Prokop, 1986; Watson, 1982). MMPI-2 users also will use the subscales to help aid in their interpretation of the profiles and to determine exactly what subgroup of items causes scale elevations (Butcher, 1990; Graham, 1990; Greene, 1991; Keefe et al. 1995).

Special issues related to the utility of the MMPI-2 in assessing chronic pain patients are reviewed more fully later in the chapter, but briefly, MMPI–MMPI-2 assessment provides information about individual characteristics of the chronic pain patient that have been found to be correlated to other important pain variables, such as exhibition of pain behaviors, level of emotional distress, difficulty in performing daily activities, and patterns of medication use (Bradley, 1995; Bradley et al., 1992; Keller & Butcher, 1991). Also, individual characteristics, as identified by the MMPI-2, have been used to make predictions regarding patient behavior, such as response to multidisciplinary treatment and likelihood of returning to work (Bradley, 1995; Moore, McCallum, Holman, & O'Brien, 1991).

MMPI-2 and Chronic Pain Assessment: Utility

The specific areas of utility for MMPI-2 assessment of patients with chronic pain can be summarized as follows.

Identification of Psychopathology

One important use of the MMPI-2 in assessing patients with chronic pain is to aid in the identification of psychopathology, including personality disorders (Gatchel, 1997). Research has demonstrated a high prevalence of psychiatric disorders among chronic pain patients. For instance, clinical depression has been found to be at least four times greater in people with chronic back pain than in the general population (Magni, Marchutti, & Moreschi, 1993; Sullivan, Reesor, Mikail, & Fisher, 1992). Sullivan et al. (1992) reported that 32–82% of patients seeking treatment from pain clinics exhibited some type of depressive problem, with an average of 62%.

The prevalence range of personality disorders among chronic pain patients has been shown to be between 37% and 66% across various studies (Fishbain, 1997). One study found that a wide range of personality disorders was identified in a sample of chronic pain patients, with 7 of the 12 possible disorders represented (Reich, Tupin, & Abramowitz, 1983). Another study had indicated that 51% of chronic pain patients met the criteria for one personality disorder, and 30% met the criteria for more than one (Polatin, Kinney, Gatchel, Lillo, & Mayer, 1993). These rates are well above what has been found in the general population—about 6% in a random community sample, according to Samuels, Nestadt, Romanoski, Folstein, and McHugh (1994).

Identifying these psychopathological disorders is extremely important in the management of chronic pain problems. Where significant anxiety or depression are present, specific treatment is a necessary part of a chronic pain treatment (e.g., Sullivan et al., 1992; Turk & Melzack, 1992). An accurate personality disorder diagnosis can help clinicians work with chronic pain patients in many ways. First, the identification of a personality disorder can help clinicians understand that some behavior patterns and psychopathological features are likely to be long-standing and to persist into the future (Weisberg & Keefe, 1997a).

Second, accurate identification of a personality disorder in a chronic pain patient will help improve patient management and treatment planning. For instance, patients with personality disorders often exhibit inadequate coping skills (Gatchel, 1997), which, in turn, has been shown to relate to ineffective pain-coping strategies in chronic pain patients (Kleinke, 1994; Turk & Rudy, 1986). It also will help the treatment team establish realistic goals for treatment outcome. The MMPI-2 can be an important part of a multicomponent assessment for psychiatric diagnoses, including personality disorders (Weisberg & Keefe, 1997a).

As presented by Keller and Butcher (1991), there is "some evidence that the MMPI-2 can identify psychopathology even within this highly homogeneous sample [of chronic pain patients]" (p. 105). However, the authors said, the MMPI-2 scales generally lack specificity for the correlates of psychopathology that were identified. Therefore, the presence of psychopathology seems to be related to a general elevation on the MMPI-2 scales that measure distress and dysphoria. The MMPI-2 has been shown to be able to identify the specific nature of the psychopathology in a more heterogeneous sample, according to Keller and Butcher (1991). In their sample of chronic pain patients, they found that the MMPI-2 scales designed to measure depression, anxiety, and low self-esteem seem to be useful for identifying patients who have difficulty with depression in general. They reported that depressive symptoms seem to be the major dimension along which their sample of chronic pain patients varied.

Keller and Butcher (1991) also stated there was a small group of other correlates that emerged in their data set. For instance, there was a history of various characterologic problems (such as alcohol and drug use, arrest history, and violence) associated with elevations on scales Psychopathic Deviate (PD), Hypomania (Ma; men only), Antisocial Practices, Anger, and MacAndrew alcoholism. The authors suggested that the data support the conclusion that the MMPI-2 can identify these potential problems even within a chronic pain patient population that has been specifically screened to exclude individuals with psychopathic characteristics. They also stated that it was not possible to determine whether the scale elevations reflected current difficulties or past information for the patients in their sample. Other researchers have found MMPI-2 scale correlates with alexithymia in chronic pain patients (Lumley, Asselin, & Norman, 1997).

Personality and Behavioral Characteristics

The identification of personality and behavioral characteristics of chronic pain patients differs from the identification of psychopathology (Weisberg & Keefe, 1997a, 1997b). This is an important distinction to keep in mind: It has been argued that clinicians often "label" chronic pain patients as having personality disorders even when to do so is clearly inaccurate and inappropriate (Weisberg & Keefe, 1997a). The MMPI has a long history of use in identifying personality characteristics in chronic pain patients (see Weisberg & Keefe, 1997a, for a review). The MMPI-2 is now used similarly. Examples of personality characteristics that might be identified by the MMPI-2 include dependent-personality trends, passive–aggressiveness, and obsessive–compulsive behavior. Identification of these characteristics by the MMPI-2 can help in planning treatment for chronic pain patients by indicating a need to develop a time-limited treatment contract (to address the dependent traits), to add assertiveness training to the treatment program (for the passive–aggressive behaviors), or to address obsessive–compulsive behaviors through cognitive behavioral approaches (Weisberg & Keefe, 1997a).

Standardized Scores

Another strength of the MMPI-2 is that its scores are standardized. This allows clinicians to assess the profile of an individual chronic pain patient in an objective way against a set of standards (Keefe et al., 1995). The MMPI-2 includes a new national normative reference group on which all T scores are based. The reference allows for more accurate comparisons with a population that more closely represents the U.S. population as a whole. Of course, the experienced MMPI-2 user will compare a chronic pain patient's profile not only with the normative reference group but also with other profiles and subgroups developed through statistical means (Bradley et al., 1992; Keller & Butcher, 1991).

Treatment Planning and Prediction of Outcome

Many users of the MMPI and MMPI-2 use these instruments to make predictions regarding patient behavior, including response to treatment and treatment outcome (Bradley et al., 1992; Guck, Meilman, Skultety, & Poloni, 1988; Keller & Butcher, 1991). Many studies have shown that MMPI profiles of chronic pain patients can be reliably classified into three or four major subgroups (Bradley et al., 1992; Love & Peck, 1987; Sanders, 1995), which have been found to differ reliably from one another on such variables as pain intensity, medication use, functional disability, and employment status (see Bradley et al., 1992, for a review). Similar results are being found now for the MMPI-2 (Riley, Robinson, Geisser, & Wittmer, 1993; Riley, Robinson, Geisser, Wittmer, & Smith, 1995). Other areas investigated using the MMPI-2 include its ability to predict a poorer rate of return to work (Moore et al., 1991) and surgery outcome (Riley et al., 1995).

In their study, Maruta and colleagues (1997) examined the relationship between MMPI-2 scale elevations and nonorganic signs (measured by a "Waddell" score) of low back pain on physical examination. The Waddell signs are patient responses to standardized physical examination procedures that suggest a nonorganic component of the pain behavior (Waddell, McCulloch, Kummel, & Venner, 1980). The Maruta et al. (1997) study is important because it expands previous research on how well MMPI-2 scales correlate with other pain-related variables. As discussed by Maruta's group, previous research using the MMPI had established a correlation between the first three clinical scales and nonorganic signs of low back pain. The nonorganic signs have been found to be associated with general affective disturbances, ineffective coping, and abnormal illness behavior (Waddell, Pilowsky, & Bond, 1989). Maruta and colleagues investigated the issue by dividing male and female patients into high and low groups, based scores for showing nonorganic physical signs of low back pain. The groups were called High Waddells (HW) and Low Waddells (LW), after the scoring system used. Among male patients, statistically significant differences were found between the HW and LW groups on the MMPI-2 scales for Hypochondriasis = 1, Hysteria = 3, and Schizophrenia = 8. Among female patients, differences between the HW and LW were statistically significant only on 8. The study provides support for the ability of the MMPI-2 to discriminate between patients showing differing levels of nonorganic physical signs of low back pain.

The MMPI also has been used extensively as part of a comprehensive screening evaluation when chronic pain patients are being considered for placement of a spinal cord stimulator (see Burchiel, et al., 1995; North, Kidd, Wimberly, & Edwin, 1996, for reviews). A spinal cord stimulator is an electronic device with leads placed in the spine to help with pain relief. In general, the first three clinical MMPI scales have been found to correlate with outcome from this procedure. Recently, the MMPI-2 was tested as part of a comprehensive evaluation designed to identify a patient population in whom reasonably long-term success could be expected after placement of the spinal stimulators (Burchiel et al., 1995). In a study of 40 patients (85% of whom were diagnosed with a failed-back-surgery syndrome), the MMPI-2 Depression Scale was found to be a prognostic indicator. This seems to substantiate the ability to generalize previous findings from the original MMPI to the MMPI-2 for use in this area.

Development of the MMPI-2

This chapter would be remiss if it did not include at least a brief overview of the development of the MMPI-2, with a special focus on how it relates to assessing chronic pain patients. As explained by Keller and Butcher (1991), the need for a revision of the MMPI had been discussed for some time (Butcher, 1972) when the revision project began in 1982 (Butcher, Dahlstrom et al., 1989; Keller & Butcher, 1991). The development of the MMPI-2 included several significant changes from the original MMPI, summarized here.

Changes in Items

One goal of the MMPI revision was to preserve the established original MMPI clinical correlates while expanding the item pool to cover additional problem areas (Butcher, Dahlstrom et al., 1989; Keller & Butcher, 1991). First, 16 repeated items in the original MMPI were deleted, and items that used sexist wording, had objectionable content, or used confusing syntax either were removed or were rewritten. The rewording did not affect endorsement frequency, according to Ben-Porath and Butcher (1988). New items were added to cover content areas that were underrepresented in the original MMPI. In its final form, the MMPI-2 has 567 items; the original instrument has 566. Item membership of the basic validity and clinical scales is largely equivalent to the original MMPI, although some scales are shorter. As such, there can be slight shifts in raw-score patterns from the MMPI to the MMPI-2, and comparisons must be made carefully.

New Normative Data

One major change in the MMPI-2 was the inclusion of a new national normative reference group on which all T scores are based. The original MMPI uses norms developed more than 50 years ago that no longer represent the general population (Pancoast & Archer, 1989). The contemporary normative sample was developed with an effort to match data from the 1980 census (Butcher, Dahlstrom et al., 1989). This was largely successful, although the sample tends to be biased toward higher socioeconomic and education status than that of the U.S. population at large. Hispanic and Asian subpopulations are underrepresented as well. These issues should be considered in the interpretation of clinical profiles.

New Psychiatric Sample Comparison Group

As part of the revision, a new sample of psychiatric patients was used as a comparison group. The sample group was used to provide information about the performance of the MMPI-2 with a clinical sample as well as to help refine the new content scales (Butcher, Graham, Williams, & Ben-Porath, 1989; Keller & Butcher, 1991). The use of the new psychiatric comparison group should help clinicians achieve more accurate identification of psychopathology and personality characteristics in chronic pain patients.

Development of New Norms

As discussed by Keller and Butcher (1991), the largest differences between the MMPI and the MMPI-2 are likely to result from differences in the norming procedures. The MMPI normative sample is outdated and even originally was limited. This is in contrast with the norms for the MMPI-2, which are based on a large national sample. Scores from this sample provide the raw score distributions used to develop T scores for each scale. On the MMPI, scales were converted to standardized T scores using a linear transformation with a mean of 50 and a standard deviation of 10 relative to the original normative sample. Because of problems in using linear T score transformations (see Keller & Butcher, 1991, for a discussion of these issues), "uniform" T score transformations were used on the MMPI-2 (see Butcher, Dahlstrom et al., 1989, for a review).

The details of these issues are unimportant for the current discussion except to note that the new uniform T scores result in somewhat lower profile elevations as compared with the linear transformations. This could affect interpretive strategies based on scale elevations or code type patterns (Butcher & Keller, 1991). For instance, it could result in substantially fewer pain patients being classified as psychologically distressed (Butcher, Dahlstrom et al., 1989; Keller & Butcher, 1991). The issue has been addressed somewhat by the shift in the level of critical scale elevations, a T score of 70 on the MMPI and 65 on the MMPI-2 (Keller & Butcher, 1991). A comprehensive study of using the MMPI-2 with chronic pain patients has substantiated the validity of this lower critical T score level on the MMPI-2 (Keller & Butcher, 1991).

MMPI-2 Content Scales

The MMPI-2 includes new content scales that could prove useful for assessing chronic pain patients (Butcher, Dahlstrom et al., 1989; Keller & Butcher, 1991). Among these content scales, the Health Concerns, Work Interference, Negative Treatment Indicators, and MacAndrew Alcoholism Scale-Revised could be particularly useful. They are discussed later.

MMPI-2 Validity Scales

Another strength of the MMPI-2 is that it provides several validity scales beyond those in the MMPI to assess the test-taking attitudes of the patient. The MMPI-2 contains the original validity scales—L, F and K—and several new ones: Back Page Infrequency, True Response Inconsistency, and Variable Response Inconsistency. The new scales assess response consistency, acquiescence–response bias, and random response styles (Butcher, Dahlstrom et al., 1989; Graham, 1990; Keller & Butcher, 1991). The validity pattern on the MMPI-2 is among some of the most valuable information that can be obtained about chronic pain patients (Butcher & Harlow, 1987).

Using the MMPI-2 With Chronic Pain Patients: Comparisons With the MMPI

There are two important questions that must be answered about using the MMPI-2 with patients with chronic pain. First, it must be determined what research and clinical findings are generalizable from the MMPI to the MMPI-2 in this patient population. Literally hundreds of studies have been done using the original MMPI in assessing patients with chronic pain. It is imperative that the generalization from the MMPI to the MMPI-2 can be made with confidence. Second, it is important to determine how the new features of the MMPI-2 might make it more useful in the assessment of patients.

Examining Overall Profile Height in Patient Profiles

Mean profiles for chronic pain patients have been compared for the MMPI-2 and the MMPI (Keller & Butcher, 1991). The new norms and T score conversions on the MMPI-2 resulted in generally lower profiles, even though the overall shape of the profiles was maintained between the two instruments. This problem is addressed by using an interpretive range that is 5 T score points lower on the MMPI-2 than on the MMPI. This appears to be a valid approach for assessing chronic pain patients (Keller & Butcher, 1991).

Subgrouping by Code Type

Research in this area has focused on how MMPI-2 code types compare with those found with the MMPI in this patient population. It is also looks at how unique MMPI-2 code types might be useful in providing information about chronic pain patients.

Keller and Butcher (1991) examined these issues in a large (502) sample of chronic pain patients. They first compared patients with the highest clinical scale in each profile, regardless of elevation (1-point code type). Correspondence was measured by the percentage of profiles with a given high-point elevation using MMPI-2 norms versus the original MMPI norms. It was determined that 64% of the men and 78% of the women would have obtained the same highest-scale elevation had the original MMPI been used. Of course, this means that 36% of men and 22% of women received a different high-point elevation on the MMPI-2 than they would have with the original instrument.

In the same study, there also was an investigation of the consistency of 2-point codes. Using appropriate critical T score criteria, it was found that 56% of the men and 67% of the women would have obtained exactly the same 2-point code type across the MMPI and the MMPI-2. These results support only a moderate level of consistency from the MMPI to the MMPI-2 relative to chronic pain patients. An important conclusion from these data is that the "configuration of scales [Hysteria, Depression, and Hypochondriasis] should not be automatically assumed to correspond to previous research on the scales" (Keller & Butcher, 1991, p. 109). The investigators warned that, when using the MMPI-2, a larger difference between the first three scales should be required before a strong interpretation of the Conversion V profile—as opposed to the neurotic triad or reactive depression profiles—is made. They also concluded that chronic pain patients will look somewhat less depressed and less characterologic (Scale 4, Pd elevation relative to other scales) on the MMPI-2 than on the MMPI. Conversely, patients who obtain high scores on the MMPI-2 scales would have obtained even higher scores on the MMPI.

The Keller and Butcher (1991) study also examined correlates of various scale elevations among patients in their sample group. It was determined that several traditional MMPI clinical scales (D and Pt) and the new MMPI-2 content scales (ANX = anxiety, DEP = depression, LSE = low self-esteem) were associated with depressive symptoms. Also, the Ma and Pd clinical scales, the MacAndrew Alcoholism Scale-Revised (MAC-R) scale and the new Antisocial Practices and Anger content scales were found to be associated with impulse control, characterological, and "acting out" problems, such as alcohol or drug abuse or arrest history. Keller and Butcher (1991) concluded that the general consistency in profile classification between the MMPI and MMPI-2 allows for generalization of previously determined behavioral correlates of these code types as determined using the MMPI with chronic pain patients. Any generalizing of these MMPI findings should be done keeping the previous discussion in mind.

Identifying Subgroups by Cluster Analysis

Initial interest in the identification of MMPI profile subtypes in chronic pain patient populations probably started with Sternbach (1974), who initially described homogeneous subgroups within the chronic pain patient population that were based on his clinical observation of his patients. He then identified four distinct MMPI profile subtypes and concluded that they would require different treatment approaches.

Subsequently, Sternbach's ideas were tested using multivariate cluster analytic techniques to analyze MMPI profiles. Relatively simple code-typing rules will use 1- or 2-point codes to assign chronic pain patients to different subgroups. In contrast, cluster analysis uses information from all of the scales in the profile to classify 100% of the patients in the sample. Many studies have identified either three or four cluster profiles (Bradley et al., 1992; Costello, Hulsey, Schoenfeld, & Ramamurthy, 1987; Keller & Butcher, 1991). Moreover, these subgroups have been validated by identifying cluster differences across patient variables, such as pain duration and intensity, pain-related disruption of activities, number of surgeries, number of hospitalizations, history of mental health treatment, and effectiveness of pain-coping strategies (Bradley, 1995; Bradley et al., 1992; Keller & Butcher, 1991).

This research was furthered by Costello et al. (1987), who used a metaclustering technique to combine the results of 10 previous cluster analysis studies using the MMPI. These researchers concluded that a four-cluster typology was most appropriate. Their system, called P-A-I-N, is organized as follows: "P" corresponds to a depressed–pathological or generally elevated profile; "A" is a Conversion V profile, characterized by elevations on Hypochondriasis and Hysteria at least 10 points above Depression; "I" is a neurotic triad profile, in which the first three scales are all elevated; and "N" is a within-normal-limits profile. Costello et al. (1987) asserted that these four clusters were common to men and women alike. This assertion, as well as the existence of the four clusters, supported work by McGill, Lawlis, Selby, Mooney, and McCoy (1983), who had found similar results previously.

Given the extensive and important cluster analysis findings with the MMPI, it is important to determine that similar subgroups of profiles can be found on the MMPI-2 for chronic pain patients. This issue has been addressed by many researchers since the development of the MMPI-2. Using an experimental form, Cohen (1987) found the same general patterning of the four clusters of Costello et al. (1987). Although Keller and Butcher (1991) could not determine a clearly defined number of clusters, they tested solutions from two to six. They found that only a three-cluster solution could be replicated across two cohorts (general elevation, neurotic triad, and within normal limits). Although Keller and Butcher (1991) concluded that their results support the comparability of the MMPI and MMPI-2, the reasons for their unique finding of three clusters is not clear. Other authors have suggested either that it was a methodology issue (use of the experimental MMPI-AX form, screening criteria that eliminated many chronic pain patient referrals) or that Keller and Butcher (1991) described the correct cluster solution when using the MMPI-2 (Riley et al., 1993).

Riley et al. (1993) investigated whether MMPI-2 cluster solutions would replicate those found by previous researchers with the MMPI specifically in patients with chronic low back pain. Another goal of the study was to help determine which cluster solution was most appropriate with the MMPI-2: the four-cluster solution identified by Costello et al. (1987), Cohen (1987), and many previous researchers using the MMPI; or the three-cluster solution found by Keller and Butcher (1991) using the MMPI-AX form. Riley et al. (1993) found that the four-cluster solution was the more appropriate. These researchers found the same four clusters previously identified consistently on chronic pain patient MMPI profiles (general elevation, neurotic triad, Conversion V, and within normal limits). Significant group differences across these subtypes were found for variables of time from injury to evaluation, the number of previous back surgeries, and preinjury psychiatric treatment. Also, the within-normal-limits and the neurotic triad subgroups had a significantly shorter time from injury to evaluation than did the depressed–pathological subgroup and a significantly fewer number of surgeries than did the V-type subgroup. The depressed–pathological subgroup was significantly more likely to have a reported psychiatric history than were the normal or V-type subgroups. Riley et al. (1993) concluded that "clinical application of MMPI-2 with [chronic low back pain] patients affords little loss in interpretation when compared with the MMPI. Furthermore, although additional studies are certainly warranted, they show that much of the MMPI empirical database with [these] patients is also applicable to the MMPI-2" (p. 252).

In a follow-up study, Riley et al. (1995) investigated how MMPI-2 cluster profiles might predict surgical outcome in a subgroup of their sample that ultimately underwent spine surgery. Similar to findings with the original MMPI (see Riley et al., 1995, for a review) these researchers found that cluster subgroupings of MMPI-2 profiles were predictive of several surgical outcome measures. For instance, the study found that patients in the within-normal-limits or neurotic triad subgroups reported significantly more satisfaction with postsurgical improvement than did patients in the depressed–pathological or V-type subgroups. In addition, the triad subgroup also gave a more favorable subjective rating of surgical outcome than did the depressed–pathological or V-type subgroups.

Identifying Patient Characteristics Through Factor Analysis

One method of improving the utility of the MMPI and MMPI-2 is to identify cluster subgroups. Another method is factor analysis, the objective of which is to identify distinct, relatively independent characteristics of the chronic pain syndrome as assessed by the MMPI. The study completed by Schmidt and Wallace (1982) of the original MMPI analyzed the clinical scales and subscales in a group of 25 chronic pain patients (with a cross-validation sample of 25). Three factors were identified: "Severity of Symptomatology," "Anger and Aggression," and "Psychogenic Components." This study must be viewed with caution because of the small sample size relative to the number of variables being analyzed.

Deardorff, Chino, and Scott (1993) sought to replicate the findings of Schmidt and Wallace (1982) using the MMPI-2. In the Deardorff et al. (1993) study, MMPI-2 profiles of 114 chronic pain patients from two treatment centers were subjected to factor analysis. The analysis included the clinical scales and the Harris and Lingoes subscales for the Hypochondriasis, Depression, and Hysteria scales. Four interpretable factors were identified and labeled: "Psychological Dysfunction," "Interpersonal Isolation," "Psychomotor Retardation," and "Physical Dysfunction." The difference in the findings of Deardorff et al. (1993) and Schmidt and Wallace (1982) could arise from differences in the patient populations (low back versus heterogeneous pain group), factor-loading criteria for variable inclusion (.5 versus .3), and the use of different subscales for analysis.

Interpretative Strategies for MMPI-2 and Chronic Pain Patients

Current research suggests that the MMPI-2 validity, clinical, and supplementary scales will provide the same type of symptom and personality information about the chronic pain patient as was given by the original MMPI scales (Keller & Butcher, 1991; Riley et al., 1993, 1995). Preliminary cluster analysis and factor analysis studies also suggest the comparability of the two instruments. Some caution must be used, however, when generalizing 1- and 2-point code type research and clinical data from the MMPI to the MMPI-2.

Keller and Butcher (1991) summarized an interpretive strategy based on their research and on strategies developed for the original MMPI, especially by Sternbach (1974), Fordyce (1979), Costello et al. (1987), and Love and Peck (1987). These guidelines are summarized here, augmented with information from more recent research.

As with any MMPI-2 interpretive strategy, careful evaluation of the validity scales is the initial step. Keller and Butcher (1991) believed that this is particularly important with chronic pain patients because of the multitude of variables that can influence presentation of pain and disability (compensation–litigation issues, medication use, family reinforcement patterns). They pointed out that the validity configuration can indicate possible drug or alcohol toxicity or cognitive impairment. The validity scales also can help clinicians determine how "comfortable" the patient is in the sick role. The validity pattern can give the interpreter an idea of the patient's typical defense mechanisms (such as denial) and an idea of how the patient views his or her own resources for managing the problem.

A study by Dush, Simons, Platt, Nation, and Ayres (1994) underscored Keller and Butcher's (1991) recommendation about the importance of assessing validity scales in the chronic pain population. Dush et al. (1994) examined chronic pain patients who were in the midst of litigation over financial compensation for their injuries. They compared MMPI-2 profiles from two similar groups of patients—one group in litigation and the other, not. Significant differences between the groups on various MMPI-2 subscales were found. In addition, a Conversion V profile was more likely for those in litigation than for those who were not.

Several lines of research on the K Scale of the original MMPI suggest that it is particularly useful in identifying psychological contributions to physical conditions (see McGrath, Sweeney, O'Malley, & Carlton, 1998, for a review). It is assumed that if most chronic pain patients do not show psychopathological characteristics before developing pain (although this assumption is not without critics; see Weisberg & Keefe, 1997a, 1997b, for a review of this issue), then an elevated K Scale could indicate an individual who demonstrates superior psychological adjustment to the physical injury. In pursuing this line of research with the MMPI-2, McGrath et al. (1998) concluded

> The K-scale emerges as a useful predictor of the individual's emotional response to the development of chronic pain. Patients with relatively elevated scores . . . seem to have demonstrated better psychological adjustment to their pain. Individuals with low or normal K-scale scores were more likely to be seen as psychologically avoidant, dependent, and self-concerned by the program staff suggesting that the intensity of their pain complaints [is] more likely to be exacerbated by psychological factors. (p. 457)

The new validity scales on the MMPI-2 (Back F Scale = Fb, Variable Response Inconsistency Scale = VRIN, True Response Inconsistency Scale = TRIN) can help in determining the validity of the test. For instance, an elevated Back F Scale can indicate that the patient stopped paying attention to test items later in the booklet and shifted to some type of random responding. The Variable Response Inconsistency Scale can help indicate whether the patient is tending to respond inconsistently to items throughout the test. And the True Response Inconsistency Scale can help identify a patient who is showing a response bias toward true or false answers. These three scales are particularly important in assessing chronic pain patients. As an example, patients who complete the MMPI-2 under duress (e.g., because they are involved in medical–legal issues) might elevate these validity schedules if they are trying to manipulate the results. The scales also might be elevated in the patient who is fatigued or lacks enough endurance to complete the task and so simply starts responding randomly at some point in the test.

Once the validity scales are examined, the overall elevation of the clinical profile should be scrutinized. This provides important information about the patient's degree of distress, disability, and the "cost" of being sick. Cluster analysis research has shown that increasing profile elevations are associated with increasing disability in the patient's life and with poorer outcome from traditional, unilateral treatment interventions.

Next, the profile can be examined for specific code type. General personality characteristics and symptom descriptors can be found for specific code types in the interpretative texts that summarize empirical findings for specific populations (Butcher, 1990; Butcher, Dahlstrom et al., 1989; Graham, 1990; Greene, 1991). Beyond that, there are some common code types that occur in chronic pain sample groups. For instance, various combinations of the Hypochondriasis, Depression, and Hysteria scales are probably the most common. According to Keller and Butcher (1991), the interpretive guidelines Fordyce (1979) developed on the MMPI apply as well to the MMPI-2.

It is beyond the scope of this chapter to present the entire interpretive strategy, and readers are referred to the original reference for more information. But as a brief example, Fordyce (1979) suggested that the Hypochondriasis Scale indicates a general readiness to emit pain behaviors. Further, the relative elevation of the Depression Scale compared with Hypochondriasis and Hysteria can suggest the "cost" to the individual for remaining in the sick role. Elevations on the first and third scales with a low score for Depression can indicate a low cost or distress associated with the condition. Thus, the patient might find that some aspects of the sick role are reinforcing. Alternatively, elevations on all three scales can indicate a readiness to emit pain behaviors and a great deal of distress over the situation. Elevations on the first four scales typically describe a passive–dependent person who has a considerable readiness to seek nurturance and support from others. A person with this profile might use pain behaviors to attain support from others and to find shelter from normal responsibilities. Beyond analyzing the profile for code type, the user can evaluate the overall profile shape to determine whether it approximates one of the clusters identified in the research, as discussed previously. Many computer-generated interpretive programs will statistically match the patient's profile to one of the four clusters.

The new MMPI-2 content scales can provide information beyond what was available from the original MMPI (Butcher, Graham et al., 1989). As pointed out by Keller and Butcher (1991), the content scales are interpreted according to the attitudes and themes reflected in the items. For instance, Keller and Butcher (1991) pointed out that the Health Concerns (HEA) Scale might function as a marker of somatic preoccupation and concerns. They also believed the other content scales might be useful for determining different courses of treatment for individual patients. As an example, the Work Interference (WRK) Scale is designed to measure attitudes and behaviors likely to contribute to poor work performance, a lack of ambition, and negative attitudes toward co-workers (Graham, 1990). Assessment of work attitudes is especially important for at least two reasons. First, many chronic pain patients have had their problems start with an occupational injury and are disabled from work. Second, job dissatisfaction has been shown to be an important variable in chronic pain problems that stem from work injuries (Bigos, Battié, & Spengler, 1991; Fordyce, Bigos, Battié, & Fisher, 1992).

The Negative Treatment Indicators (TRT) Scale is designed to measure negative attitudes toward doctors, giving up easily when problems are encountered, and showing poor problem-solving abilities and judgment (Graham, 1990). This scale might be useful in predicting difficulties during treatment for the chronic pain problem so that obstacles can be removed early in the intervention program. Finally, the MAC-R Scale is shown by Keller and Butcher (1991) to be a useful indicator of substance abuse history among chronic pain patients.

References

Ben-Porath, Y. S., & Butcher, J. N. (1988, March). *Exploratory analyses of rewritten MMPI items*. Paper presented at the 23rd Annual Symposium on Recent Developments [in the] Use of the MMPI, St. Petersburg, FL.

Bigos, S. J., Battié, M. C., & Spengler, D. M. (1991). A prospective study of work perceptions and psychological factors affecting the report of back injury. *Spine, 16*, 1–6.

Bradley, L. A. (1995). Biopsychosocial model and the Minnesota Multiphasic Personality Inventory: Even psychologists make cognitive errors. *Pain Forum, 4*, 97–100.

Bradley, L. A., Haile, J. M., & Jaworski, T. M. (1992). Assessment of psychological status using interviews and self-report instruments. In D. C. Turk & R. Melzack (Eds.), *Handbook of pain assessment* (pp. 193–213). New York: Guilford.

Burchiel, K. J., Anderson, V. C., Wilson, B. J., Denison, D. B., Olson, K. A., & Shatin, D. (1995). Prognostic factors of spinal cord stimulation for chronic back and leg pain. *Neurosurgery, 36*, 1101–1111.

Butcher, J. N. (1972). *Objective personality assessment: Changing perspectives.* New York: Academic Press.

Butcher, J. N. (1990). *MMPI-2 in psychological treatment.* New York: Oxford University Press.

Butcher, J. N., Dahlstrom, W. G., Graham, J. R., Tellegen, A., & Kaemmer, B. (1989). *Manual for administration and scoring. MMPI-2.* Minneapolis: University of Minnesota Press.

Butcher, J. N., Graham, J. R., Williams, C. L. & Ben-Porath, Y. S. (1989). *Development and use of the MMPI-2 content scales.* Minneapolis: University of Minnesota Press.

Butcher, J. N., & Harlow, T. (1987). Personality assessment in personal injury cases. In A. Hess & I. Weiner (Eds.), *Handbook of forensic psychology* (pp. 128–154). New York: Wiley.

Cohen, N. (1987). *Response of chronic pain patient to the original and revised versions of the Minnesota Multiphasic Personality Inventory.* Unpublished doctoral dissertation, University of Minnesota, Minneapolis.

Costello, R. M., Hulsey, T. L., Schoenfeld, L. S., & Ramamurthy, S. (1987). P-A-I-N: A four-cluster MMPI typology for chronic pain. *Pain, 30,* 199–209.

Cronbach, L. (1990). *Essentials of psychological testing* (5th ed.). New York: Harper & Row.

Deardorff, W. W., Chino, A. F., & Scott, D. W. (1993). Characteristics of chronic pain patients: Factor analysis of the MMPI-2. *Pain, 54,* 153–158.

Dush, D. M., Simons, L. E., Platt, M., Nation, P. C., & Ayres, S. Y. (1994). Psychological profiles distinguishing litigating and nonlitigating pain patients: Subtle, and not so subtle. *Journal of Personality Assessment, 62,* 299–313.

Fishbain, D. A. (1996). Some difficulties with the predictive validity of Minnesota Multiphasic Personality Inventory. *Pain Forum, 5,* 81–82.

Fishbain, D. A. (1997). Can personality disorders in chronic pain patients be accurately measured? *Pain Forum, 6,* 16–19.

Fordyce, W. E. (1979). *Use of the MMPI in the assessment of chronic pain. Clinical notes on the MMPI, #3.* Nutley, NJ: Hoffman-LaRoche.

Fordyce, W. E., Bigos, S. J., Battié, M. C., & Fisher, L. D. (1992). MMPI Scale 3 as a predictor of back injury report: What does it tell us? *Clinical Journal of Pain, 8,* 222–226.

Gatchel, R. J. (1997). The significance of personality disorders in the chronic pain population. *Pain Forum, 6,* 12–15.

Graham, J. R. (1990). *MMPI-2: Assessing personality and psychopathology.* New York: Oxford University Press.

Greene, R. L. (1991). *The MMPI-2/MMPI: An interpretive manual.* Boston: Allyn & Bacon.

Guck, T. P., Meilman, P. W., Skultety, M., & Poloni, L. D. (1988). Pain-patient Minnesota Multiphasic Personality Inventory (MMPI) subgroups: Evaluation of long-term treatment outcome. *Journal of Behavioral Medicine, 11,* 159–169.

Hathaway, S. R., & McKinley, J. C. (1943). *The Minnesota Multiphasic Personality schedule (revised).* Minneapolis: University of Minnesota Press.

Helmes, E. (1994). What types of useful information do the MMPI and MMPI-2 provide on patients with chronic pain? *American Pain Society Bulletin, 4*(1), 1–5.

Helmes, E., & Reddon, J. R. (1993). A perspective on developments in assessing psychopathology: A critical review of the MMPI and MMPI-2. *Psychological Bulletin, 113,* 453–471.

Keefe, F. J., Lefebvre, J. C., & Beaupre, P. M. (1995). The Minnesota Multiphasic Personality Inventory in chronic pain: Security blanket or sound investment? *Pain Forum, 4,* 101–103.

Keller, L. S., & Butcher, J. N. (1991). *Assessment of chronic pain patients with the MMPI-2.* Minneapolis: University of Minnesota Press.

Kleinke, C. L. (1994). MMPI scales as predictors of pain-coping strategies preferred by patients with chronic pain. *Rehabilitation Psychology, 39,* 123–128.

Love, A. W., & Peck, C. L. (1987). The MMPI and psychological factors in chronic low back pain: A review. *Pain, 28,* 1–28.

Lumley, M. A., Asselin, L. A., & Norman, S. (1997). Alexithymia in chronic pain patients. *Comprehensive Psychiatry, 38,* 160–165.

Magni, G., Marchutti, M., & Moreschi, C. (1993). Chronic musculoskeletal pain and depressive symptoms in the National Health and Nutrition Examination: I. Epidemiological follow-up study. *Pain, 53,* 163–168.

Main, C. J., & Spanswick, C. C. (1995a). Personality assessment and the Minnesota Multiphasic Personality Inventory, 50 years on: Do we still need our security blanket? *Pain Forum, 4,* 90–96.

Main, C. J., & Spanswick, C. C. (1995b). Response to our commentators. *Pain Forum, 4,* 110–113.

Maruta, T., Goldman, S., Chan, C. W., Ilstrup, D. M., Kunselman, A. R., & Colligan, R. C. (1997). Waddell's nonorganic signs and Minnesota Multiphasic Personality Inventory profiles in patients with chronic low back pain. *Spine, 22,* 72–75.

McGill, J. C., Lawlis, G. F., Selby, D., Mooney, V., & McCoy, C. E. (1983). The relationship of Minnesota Multiphasic Personality Inventory profile clusters to pain behaviors. *Journal of Behavioral Medicine, 6,* 77–92.

McGrath, R. E., Sweeney, M., O'Malley, W. B., & Carlton, T. K. (1998). Identifying psychological contributions to chronic pain complaints with the MMPI-2: The role of the K Scale. *Journal of Personality Assessment, 70,* 448–459.

Moore, J. E., McCallum, S., Holman, C., & O'Brien, S. (1991, November). *Prediction of return to work after pain clinic treatment by MMPI-2 clusters.* Paper presented at the meeting of the American Pain Society, New Orleans.

Moore, J. E., McFall, M. E., Kivlahan, D. R., & Capestany, R. (1988). Risk of misinterpretation of MMPI Schizophrenia Scale elevations in chronic pain patients. *Pain, 32,* 207–213.

Naliboff, B. D., Cohen, M. J., & Yellin, A. N. (1982). Does the MMPI differentiate chronic illness from chronic pain? *Pain, 13,* 333–341.

North, R. B., Kidd, D. H., Wimberly, R. L., & Edwin, D. (1996). Prognostic value of psychological testing in patients undergong spinal cord stimulation: A prospective study. *Neurosurgery, 39,* 301–311.

Pancoast, D. L., & Archer, R. P. (1989). Original adult MMPI norms in normal samples: A review with implications for future developments. *Journal of Personality Assessment, 53,* 376–395.

Pincus, T., Callahan, L. F., Bradley, L. A., Vaughn, W. K., & Wolfe, R. (1986). Elevated MMPI scores for Hypochondriasis, Depression, and Hysteria in patients with rheumatoid arthritis reflect disease rather than psychological status. *Arthritis and Rheumatism, 29,* 1456–1466.

Polatin, P. B., Kinney, R. K., Gatchel, R. J., Lillo, E., & Mayer, T. G. (1993). Psychiatric illness and chronic low back pain. *Spine, 18,* 66–71.

Prokop, C. K. (1986). Hysteria Scale elevation in low back pain patients: A risk factor for misdiagnosis: *Journal of Consulting and Clinical Psychology, 54,* 558–562.

Reich, J., Tupin, J. P., & Abramowitz, S. I. (1983). Psychiatric diagnosis of chronic pain patients. *American Journal of Psychiatry, 140,* 1495–1498.

Riley, J. L., Robinson, M. E., Geisser, M. E., & Wittmer, V. T. (1993). Multivariate cluster analysis of the MMPI-2 in chronic low-back pain patients. *Clinical Journal of Pain, 9,* 248–252.

Riley, J. L., Robinson, M. E., Geisser, M. E., Wittmer, V. T., & Smith, A. G. (1995). Relationship between MMPI-2 cluster profiles and surgical outcome in low-back pain patients. *Journal of Spinal Disorders, 8,* 213–219.

Samuels, J. F., Nestadt, M. D., Romanoski, A. J., Folstein, M. F., & McHugh, P. R. (1994). *DSM-III* personality disorders in the community. *American Journal of Psychiatry, 151,* 1055–1062.

Sanders, S. H. (1995). Minnesota Multiphasic Personality Inventory and clinical pain: The baby or the bathwater? *Pain Forum, 4,* 108–109.

Schmidt, J. P., & Wallace, R. W. (1982). Factor analysis of the MMPI profiles of low back pain patients. *Journal of Personality Assessment, 46,* 366–369.

Sternbach, R. A. (1974). *Pain patients: Traits and treatments.* New York: Academic Press.

Sullivan, M. J. L., Reesor, S., Mikail, R., & Fisher, R. (1992). The treatment of depression in chronic low back pain: Review and recommendations. *Pain, 50,* 5–13.

Turk, D. C. (1990). Customizing treatments for chronic pain patients: Who, what, and why. *Clinical Journal of Pain, 6,* 255–270.

Turk, D. C., & Fernandez, E. (1995). Personality assessment and the Minnesota Multiphasic Personality Inventory in chronic pain: Underdeveloped and overexposed. *Pain Forum, 4,* 104–107.

Turk, D. C., & Melzack, R. (1992). *Handbook of pain assessment.* New York: Guilford.

Turk, D. C., & Rudy, T. E. (1986). Assessment of cognitive factors in chronic pain: A worthwhile enterprise? *Journal of Consulting and Clinical Psychology, 54,* 760–768.

Waddell, G., McCulloch, J., Kummel, E., & Venner, R. M. (1980). Non-organic physical signs in low-back pain. *Spine, 5,* 117–125.

Waddell, G., Pilowsky, I., & Bond, M. R. (1989). Clinical assessment and interpretation of abnormal illness in low back pain. *Pain, 39,* 41–53.

Wall, P. D., & Melzack, R. (Eds.). (1984). *Textbook of pain.* New York: Churchill-Livingstone.

Watson, D. (1982). Neurotic tendencies among chronic pain patients: An MMPI item analysis. *Pain, 14,* 365–385.

Weisberg, J. N., & Keefe, F. J. (1997a). Personality disorders in the chronic pain population: Basic concepts, empirical findings and clinical implications. *Pain Forum, 6,* 1–9.

Weisberg, J. N., & Keefe, F. J. (1997b). Methodological considerations for diagnosis of personality disorders in chronic pain patients. *Pain Forum, 6,* 20–21.

Part III

Nonpathological Personality Characteristics of Pain

Chapter 6
RELATIONSHIP OF PAIN-COPING STRATEGIES TO ADJUSTMENT AND FUNCTIONING

Douglas E. DeGood

Psychological interventions seldom cure pain. Rather, the psychology of chronic pain management is mostly about how people manage to cope with pain. It is obvious to any casual observer that, given an identical cause for pain, some individuals become more impaired than others. Not surprising, we find the same individual differences in capacity to cope with pain that we find with all other sources of life stress. For this reason, coping with pain clearly meets the individual-difference criterion defining a personality variable.

The term *coping* falls subject to many nuances of use in the pain literature. Often, it is merely a general descriptor of how well or poorly someone appears to handle his or her physical discomfort. Used in this manner, coping can be inferred from observing the emotional state and level of physical functioning of a person in pain relative to the degree of disruption expected with an identified pain condition. But coping also can be inferred from standardized questionnaire responses, and it can be used synonymously with the adjustment level interpreted from the questionnaire. For example, one empirically established profile from a widely used, standardized self-report inventory, the Multiphasic Pain Inventory (Turk & Rudy, 1988, 1990), is the adaptive coper, an individual with a chronic pain condition who nevertheless reports less emotional and behavioral disruption than might be expected. This adaptive coping profile appears to be similar to a subgroup profile found in a variety of similar pain assessment tools (Jamison, Rudy, Penzien, & Mosley, 1994). In contrast, individuals with profiles characterized by greater emotional distress and more life disruption than displayed by the adaptive copers are considered less adept at coping with pain. Similarly, patients with positive treatment outcomes are often characterized as having improvement in their coping with the pain. Defined in the broadest sense, nearly every chapter in this volume relates to coping with pain. However, in this chapter the term coping is used in a much narrower sense, referring to specific cognitive and behavioral efforts undertaken by the individual in an attempt to restore equilibrium and resolve problems caused by chronic pain. Such efforts can be successful or unsuccessful and, in some instances, can even make matters worse.

Although identification and recognition of cognitive and behavioral coping strategies can be traced back through the ancient writings within many cultural and religious traditions (see Morris, 1991), the scientific effort to quantify and measure coping strategies is recent. Even if one questions whether any assessment technique can ever truly capture the individual human experience of coping with pain, the effort is necessary if the process of coping is to be understood in a manner that provides an empirical basis for determining therapeutic goals and strategies.

Two major comprehensive reviews of the pain-coping research literature are currently available. The first covers the period from 1983 (when studies specific to pain coping first appeared) to 1991 (Jensen, Turner, Romano, & Karoly, 1991); the second updates the literature from 1991 to 1998 (Boothby, Thorn, Stroud, & Jensen,

1999). Rather than duplicating these two excellent existing reviews, I focus in this chapter on the development and current status of some of the important instruments used in coping research. The existing reviews provide conclusions concerning the relationships between these measures and overall adjustment to chronic pain. Issues and problems in this research, especially related to the clinical utility of coping assessment and the relationships between coping and other dimensions of functioning, are considered in some detail. Only by looking carefully at the nature of the key psychometric instruments used in pain-coping research is it possible to get a sense of how clinical observations are turned into empirical assessment procedures. The strengths and weaknesses of these instruments for everyday use by the clinician also are considered here.

Cognitive–Behavioral Therapy and Coping With Pain

The basic rationale underlying cognitive–behavioral interventions for pain is that such interventions can increase coping with the pain sensation and the threat to functioning and reduce associated emotional distress. As outlined by Keefe, Jacobs, and Underwood-Gordon (1997), most cognitive–behavioral interventions for chronic pain patients follow a general format:

1. The intervention typically begins with an educational component that explains the role of situations, thoughts, emotions, and behaviors in the pain experience.
2. Patients are then encouraged to recognize and challenge the dysfunctional thoughts (beliefs, automatic reactive patterns of thinking, motivational attitudes) that might be contributing to their pain and suffering.
3. The patient is then instructed in some combination of specific behavioral skills (self-relaxation, imagery–hypnotic self-analgesia, distraction techniques, exercise, pacing of activities, assertiveness). These skills are first practiced and rehearsed in the treatment session and then tried on the outside. Self-monitoring and self-reinforcement are typically encouraged.
4. Later, patients are urged to identify high-risk situations (pain flare-ups, work and home stressors, emotional upsets) and to plan and rehearse strategies to meet these challenges.
5. The final stage often involves decision making or problem solving in relationship to employment, rehabilitation, or insurance settlements necessary to return to prior daily life or adapt to a new phase of life.

Success with a cognitive–behavioral intervention is synonymous with improvement in coping. More than the cliche "learn to live with it," cognitive–behavioral therapists believe that, if patients can improve their coping skills, the noxious pain experience can be modified, the mood elevated, and the overall quality of life improved. This is the reason so much effort has been expended on trying to better explain the nature of pain-coping strategies.

Coping Theory

Strategies

The current high level of research and clinical, as well as public, interest in pain and stress management owes much to the pioneering advances in stress theory and research of Richard Lazarus (e.g., Lazarus, 1966; Lazarus & Folkman, 1984). More than 35 years ago, Lazarus and associates began a systematic experimental exploration of the cognitive and situational factors that enhance or dampen cognitive, emotional, and physiological reactions to stressful situations. One self-report instrument (described in more detail later) that grew out of this effort is the Ways of Coping (WOC) checklist (Folkman & Lazarus, 1980, Lazarus & Folkman, 1984). Coping is just one aspect of the Lazarus transactional model of adaptation to stressful events. He suggested that stress management involves dispositions, cognitive appraisals, and coping responses. Dispositions are stable biological, personality, and social role characteristics that can influence how a person responds to stress. Appraisals are cognitive processes that influence emotional responses to stress through judgments about the danger posed by an event. Finally, coping responses are "constantly changing cognitive and behavioral efforts to manage specific external and/or internal demands that are appraised as taxing or exceeding the resources of the person" (Lazarus & Folkman, 1984, p. 141).

Lazarus set many of the ground rules that have since been followed by other researchers. He felt it was insufficient simply to ask "How did you cope?" Rather, Lazarus and Folkman (1984) proposed a process-oriented approach in which coping: (a) refers to specific thoughts, feelings, and acts; (b) is examined in the context of encountering a specific source of stress; and (c) is studied in slices of time so that changes can be observed in what is thought, felt, and done as the requirements of the situation change. Researchers were urged to avoid confounding the coping process itself with the outcomes of coping. Good psychological adjustment and maintenance of functioning per se are outcomes of good coping, but outcome alone does not enlighten us about the process of coping. The Lazarus approach to studying the effects of coping, especially cognitive appraisals of danger in response to laboratory-controlled stressors, set a high standard for stress research, which unfortunately is difficult to emulate in the study of naturally occurring stressors, such as chronic pain.

Researchers have classified coping strategies in several ways. Lazarus and Folkman (1984) drew a distinction between problem-focused coping, which is described as an effort to alter the environmental source of stress, and emotion-focused coping, which involves an effort to regulate an emotional reaction to a situation. This distinction is quite similar to that drawn between behavioral coping, which is overt action taken to deal with stress, and cognitive coping, which is the use of mental strategies or ways to use thoughts or feelings to deal with stress. Another distinction found in the coping-research literature concerns the classification of the coping behavior itself as an active or instrumental coping response, in contrast to passive coping strategies (Brown & Nicassio, 1987). Examples of active coping responses to pain might include attempting to maintain regular activities, using distraction to ignore pain, and practicing psychophysiological stress management. Passive activities include restricting activity, resting in bed, or seeking help from others. Jensen, Turner, Romano, and Strom (1995) have added yet another coping dichotomy: illness-focused versus wellness-focused coping behaviors. Illness-focused coping consists of strategies aimed at avoiding pain and illness, such as taking medication, resting, and guarding or bracing sore muscles. Wellness-focused strategies aimed at promoting health include relaxation, task persistence, exercise–stretching, and use of coping self-statements.

Many of the pain-coping behaviors of an individual are difficult to classify: There is a good deal of overlap in the artificial dichotomies. Problem-focused coping is obviously similar to behavioral coping, and emotion-focused coping is similar to cognitive coping. The tendency is to judge active strategies as adaptive and passive strategies as maladaptive, but in the individual case a particular coping response can be paradoxical—for example, self-relaxation, a behaviorally passive technique, is usually considered an active strategy. Even rest, clearly a passive response, might be labeled as active when it is a planned part of pacing to achieve greater total activity. Maes, Leventhal, and DeRidder (1996) have attempted to place coping strategies into a hierarchical order, but it is a hierarchy unlikely to apply uniformly to all individuals in all situations.

Assessment Measures

No matter how crucial coping is to the pain management process, it remains a hypothetical construct represented by a complex set of difficult-to-measure behaviors. Undoubtedly, pain clinicians observe the effects of adaptive and maladaptive coping efforts every day in the mood and functioning of their patients. The coping behaviors that produce these results are directly observed or inferred, but they are largely nonquantifiable. Although there are many useful therapists' materials and self-help books to aid patients in the process of learning to cope with pain, research on coping requires some form of quantifiable measurement. Several of the more popular measures are described here, and their relationships to other indicators of functioning are discussed.

Just as there have been attempts to classify coping strategies, there have been attempts to classify measures of coping as dispositional versus situational (Endler, Parker, & Summerfeldt, 1998; Schwarzer & Schwarzer, 1996). The dispositional instrument looks for coping strategies that are common across different stressful situations. Self-report dispositional coping measures might ask the respondent how he or she characteristically handles stressful situations. By contrast, the situational approach searches for the coping strategies that are used in particular circumstances. A self-report situational measure might ask how a patient responded (or would expect to respond) to a specific stressful situation. This application of dispositional versus situational terminology appears similar to the concept of trait versus state (e.g., Spielberger, Gorsuch, & Lushene, 1983), an approach pervasive in individual assessment of psychopathology as well as normal personality. Some coping measures combine the dispositional and situational approaches. For example, the WOC checklist (Lazarus & Folkman, 1984) is a list of general dispositional coping responses, but the instructions normally ask the respondent to report strategies used in response to a specific stressor. Other investigators find it necessary to have a separate questionnaire designed for each form of stress.

Coping-assessment procedures also have been classified as composite or individual measures (Boothby et al., 1999; Jensen, Turner, & Romano, 1992). Composite scales, either rationally derived or factorially derived measures, combine several related coping strategies into a broader category. These broader categories are often interpreted as corresponding to adaptive versus maladaptive patterns of coping. Because most coping instruments contain this presumed mixture of adaptive and maladaptive strategies, simple calculation of an overall coping score is not feasible, unless one were to try to work out a score from a ratio of the two components. Some composite measures have been singular in format rather than dichotomous, and not all are calculated from existing inventories but can be a composite of unique items combined for a single study. Composite measures have the advantage of capturing more variance under a single rubric and therefore offer a greater chance of demonstrating significant relationships with other measures of functioning. The disadvantage of a composite measure is that one does not know what particular strategies within the coping composite contribute to the relationship and which do not. However, when the composite measure is a higher order factor within a scale composed of individual strategy subscales, composite and individual scale scores alike can be calculated.

Despite the fact that facilitating coping skills is essential to pain management, formal psychometric assessment of coping largely has been limited to research settings and not well-integrated into routine clinical assessment. Reasons for this are considered later. The description of coping measures that follows in the next section focuses on measures that have been subjected to a reasonable degree of psychometric testing for reliability and validity. They are therefore likely to continue to appear in future coping studies and have some potential for more general future clinical use.

The measures detailed here are all composite measures of coping, but they also contain individual scales that can be scored as measures of individual strategies. The first inventory, the WOC checklist, is a general coping measure that has been applied to pain. The second, the Coping with Health Injuries and Problems (CHIP) scale, is a general health-coping measure, which also has been used with chronic pain. The third and fourth exemplify measures designed specifically for the study of pain-coping strategies: the Coping Strategies Questionnaire (CSQ) and the Vanderbilt Multidimensional Pain Coping Inventory (VMPCI).

Ways of Coping Checklist

The WOC checklist is the best known of the general coping measures, and it has been used extensively in the field of stress research. It also was used in some of the early studies of pain coping. Many versions of the checklist are found in the stress-coping literature. The 1984 version (Lazarus & Folkman, 1984) is a 67-item scale consisting of two broad scales, (a) problem-focused coping, which refers to efforts to change the situation, and (b) emotion-focused coping, which refers to efforts to manage internal emotional states. Items loading on the problem-focused coping scale reflect cognitive and behavioral efforts, such as trying different solutions, gathering more information, and making and following a plan of action. The emotion-focused coping scale contains items that reflect seeking emotional support from others, distancing, avoidance, emphasizing the positive aspects of the situation, and self-blame. They include mixtures of strategies judged likely to be both adaptive and maladaptive. The questionnaire asks about the kinds of stressors experienced and for ratings of ability to cope with them.

Vitaliano, Russo, Carr, Maiuro, and Becker (1985) developed a 55-item version of the WOC checklist and sorted the items into 6 subscales:

1. Cognitive restructuring. Sample item: I came out of the experience better than when I went in.
2. Information seeking. Sample item: I spoke to someone to find out more about the situation.
3. Self-blame. Sample item: I realized I brought the problem on myself.
4. Wish-fulfilling fantasy. Sample item: I wished the situation would go away or somehow be over with.
5. Emotional expression. Sample item: I let my feelings out somehow.
6. Threat minimization. Sample item: I made light of the situation; I refused to get too serious about it.

From the sample items, it becomes evident that many of the subscales do not quite fit the chronic pain situation. To remedy this shortcoming, Turner, Clancy, and Vitaliano (1987) added items to the checklist to represent stressors specific to chronic pain and found associations between coping strategies and patient beliefs about their pain. For example, patients who reported using cognitive restructuring and information seeking were more likely to believe they must accept pain and not let their pain hold them back from what they wanted to do. Revenson and Felton (1989) administered a related version of the WOC checklist to a group of patients with rheumatoid arthritis on two occasions separated by 6 months. Increased use of wish-fulfilling fantasy over the period was associated with increased physical disability. Additionally, a decrease in positive affect after 6 months was linked with growing use of self-blame, emotional expression, and wish-fulfilling fantasy and with a decreased use of information seeking. Closely related findings, also with arthritis patient samples, have been reported by others (Manne & Zautra, 1990; Parker et al., 1988; Regan, Lorig, & Thoresen, 1988).

In one of the few studies in the pain-coping literature to consider a normal personality dimension, Buckelew et al. (1990) found a relationship between WOC strategies and locus-of-control orientation measured by the Multidimensional Health Locus of Control (Wallston, Wallston, & DeVellis, 1978). Subtle age and gender differences were found in the relationships in this sample drawn from a multidisciplinary pain rehabilitation program. Women patients, especially those with a high internal locus-of-control orientation, were more likely than men to use cognitive restructuring and information-seeking coping strategies. Women also reported less associated psychological distress than did men.

Because the WOC checklist was developed for wide use with a variety of medical and other stress-related problems, its use with chronic pain patients has been limited. However, many of the coping strategies identified in the checklist reappear in the pain-specific measures, although attached to an altered set of items. From the subscale labels alone one can speculate that some strategies are likely to be more adaptive than others. Lazarus and colleagues established the tradition of studying the coping strategies of successful and unsuccessful copers and argued that, to clarify the process of coping, it was necessary to identify what did and did not work in specific situations. Furthermore, their emphasis on the need to separate coping strategies from coping outcomes has had a lasting influence on the research.

Despite its importance in the emergence of coping research and its extensive use in health research, several researchers have questioned the validity of using instruments like the WOC checklist to study coping strategies in medical populations (e.g., Endler, Parker, & Summerfeldt, 1993; Thomas & Marks, 1995; Wineman, Durand, & McCulloch, 1994). The argument is that the checklist was designed to tap a cross-section of generally stressful situations and, as seen above, many of the scale's items are inapplicable for people coping with particular health problems, especially chronic problems (Endler, Parker, & Summerfeldt, 1998). Many of the items fail to capture the uniqueness of a situation or the quality of the coping required and therefore are not useful clinical tools. With relatively brief questionnaires, it takes only a small number of inapplicable or inappropriate items to significantly reduce a scale's validity and reliability (Waller, 1989).

Coping With Health Injuries and Problems Scale

As a result of the concerns described above, most investigators of pain coping have adopted instruments designed specifically for their work. However, Endler, Parker, and Summerfeldt (1998) opined that the pendulum has swung too far in the direction of specialization. They believe that health-coping research has become so fragmented by the development of instruments specific to every possible health disorder that it is difficult to advance the research through comparisons across conditions. With the recent development of the CHIP scale they offer a compromise between generalization and specialization of measurement. Although it is not a broad generalized or dispositional stress-coping measure, it is nonetheless intended to be applicable to a range of health problems, not just to pain or to any other specific illness or injury.

The CHIP scale is a 32-item questionnaire developed after both a rational and an empirical approach to test construction. For each item, participants respond to a 5-point frequency Likert scale (from 1 = not at all to 5 = very much) with the following instructions:

> The following are ways of reacting to health problems, such as illnesses, sicknesses, or injuries. We are interested in your last illness, sickness, or injury. Please circle a number from 1 to 5 for each of the following items. Indicate how much you engaged in these types of activities when you encountered this health problem. (Endler, Parker, & Summerfeldt, 1998, p. 196)

Several related studies, included in a single report (Endler, Parker, & Summerfeldt, 1998), involving both exploratory and confirmatory factor analyses establish four reliable coping scales:

1. Palliative coping involves a variety of self-help responses aimed at alleviating the unpleasantness of a situation.
2. Instrumental coping involves task-oriented responses, such as actively seeking health information or medical advice.
3. Distraction coping involves attempts to think about other (possibly more

pleasant) experiences, engage in unrelated activities, or seek the company of others.

4. Emotional preoccupation involves fixation with the emotional consequences of the health problem.

As seen in Table 6.1 the rotated factor loadings clearly differentiate the scales as four unique factors. This structure was cross-validated from a large derivation sample of adults to a heterogeneous group of general medical patients and a homogeneous group of patients with low back pain. The intercorrelations between the scales are reported to be low to moderate, which is expected with a multidimensional measure of this nature, and test–retest reliability over 4 weeks (tested with cancer patients) generally was .70 to .79 (Endler, Courbasson, & Fillion, 1998). The CHIP scale also demonstrates a degree of discriminant validity among "normal" adults, the general medical population, and patients with lower back pain, with the pain group giving higher scores on all four coping subscales.

The CHIP scale has not been tested against other measures of personality, psychopathology, or general functioning of medical populations. It has been examined only for construct validity against another coping measure. As part of the initial test construction, 292 "normal" adults completed the Coping Inventory for Stressful Situations (CISS; Endler & Parker, 1990, 1994) as well as the CHIP scale. The CISS is a 48-item general dispositional coping scale that assesses three broad coping styles: task oriented, emotion oriented, and avoidance oriented. Respondents are asked to report on coping behaviors normally used when facing "a difficult, stressful, or upsetting situation." The CHIP scale and the CISS share just one identical item. Results from a path analysis of intercorrelations reveal several expected relationships between this medical situational measure and the more dispositional CISS measure. The CHIP measure of instrumental coping with illness was moderately associated with the CISS task-oriented coping style. Also, a strong association was present between CHIP emotional preoccupation and CISS emotion-oriented coping. Finally, CHIP distraction coping with illness had a strong association with the CISS avoidance-oriented coping style.

Although the relationships between CHIP scale and CISS scores are not surprising, they do illustrate an important point. Participants who demonstrate a general disposition to cope with stress in a particular manner do tend to report a similar pattern of coping behaviors in response to specific health concerns. Thus, at least in this case, individual patterns of pain coping appear to have both trait and state characteristics, typical of many other individual-differences variables studied by personality and psychopathology researchers.

Despite the limited data available, the CHIP scale is included here because it represents a promising new instrument that draws our attention to important theoretical issues that face researchers. As a coping-assessment tool, it represents a compromise between a purely dispositional approach to coping assessment and a highly situational, problem-focused questionnaire. An effort is made by the framers to identify constructs that can bridge a variety of health problems. Although the four constructs might be insufficient to fully satisfy the pain-coping researcher, the scale does encourage one to consider whether investigators concerned with pain coping should try to forge a stronger link with general health-coping research as well as even broader (nonhealth) avenues of coping research.

Table 6.1—*Results of a Principal-Components Factor Analysis of the 32 Coping Items of the CHIP Scale*

Item	Factor 1: Palliative Coping	Factor 2: Instrumental Coping	Factor 3: Distraction Coping	Factor 4: Emotional Preoccupation Coping
2. Stay in bed	**.620**	−.105	.025	.181
6. Rest when tired	**.574**	.082	.145	.040
10. Sleep	**.645**	.053	.116	−.124
14. Conserve energy	**.687**	.002	−.047	.094
18. Stay warm	**.551**	.115	.289	−.015
22. Make surroundings quiet	**.658**	.154	−.044	.078
26. Stay quiet	**.667**	.106	−.180	.095
30. Get comfortable	**.650**	.115	.253	.040
3. Find out more information	−.161	**.632**	.140	.262
7. Seek treatment quickly	.014	**.623**	−.001	.141
11. Focus on getting better	.169	**.423**	.266	.078
15. Learn more	−.088	**.552**	.279	.154
19. Comply with advice	.132	**.801**	.027	−.001
23. Follow doctor's advice	.174	**.806**	.087	−.002
27. Take medications on time	.276	**.638**	.038	.037
31. Find out about treatments	.057	**.678**	.181	.214
1. Think about better times	.059	.175	**.536**	.201
5. Be with others	−.248	.050	**.637**	.020
9. Day dream	.219	.025	**.561**	.180
13. Enjoy attention from people	.120	.024	**.652**	.036
17. Plan for the future	.009	.242	**.623**	.055
21. Listen to music	.115	.062	**.682**	−.067
25. Invite company	−.063	.037	**.675**	.074
29. Have nice things around	.239	.145	**.568**	−.066
4. Wonder "why me"	−.010	.055	.036	**.691**
8. Feel angry	−.004	.040	.051	**.777**
12. Become frustrated	.073	.051	.063	**.679**
16 Think about things I can't do	.253	.006	.092	**.655**
20. Fantasize about being healthy	.264	.005	.258	**.438**
24. Wish it hadn't happened	.011	.148	.078	**.610**
28. Think about being vulnerable	.079	.179	.025	**.664**
32. Worry about my health	−.042	.202	−.025	**.639**
Eigenvalues	6.34	3.18	2.97	2.48
% of variance	19.80	9.90	9.30	7.70

Note. N = 598. Factor loadings greater than 0.35 are in boldface type. CHIP = Coping With Injuries and Problems.

From Endler, N. S., Parker, J. D. A., & Summerfeldt, L. J. (1998). Coping with health problems: Developing a reliable and valid multidimensional measure. *Psychological Assessment, 10*, p. 198. Copyright 1998 by American Psychological Association. Adapted by permission.

Coping Strategies Questionnaire

The CSQ (Rosenstiel & Keefe, 1983) was the first inventory designed to measure coping specific to pain. The initial subscales and items were selected on a rational basis from observations made by clinicians dealing with chronic pain patients. The items are worded so that each completes the sentence "When I feel pain. . . ." The CSQ is heavily weighted toward assessment of cognitive coping strategies. It has 6 cognitive and 2 behavioral coping strategy scales, creating 8 subscales with 6 items each. There are 2 additional self-efficacy-type items, not included in the subscales, which require the respondent to report perceived control over pain and ability to decrease pain. Unlike the wording of the WOC checklist or the CHIP scale, many of the items themselves contain a direct reference to pain (Table 6.2). In completing the CSQ, respondents check a 7-point scale to indicate the frequency with which they use each strategy when experiencing pain (0 = *never*; 3 = *sometimes*; 6 = *always*). The use of coping strategies appears to be relatively stable over time. Gil et al. (1993) reported that, for patients with sickle cell diseases who completed a modified version of the CSQ, the type of coping strategy described was highly constant over 18 months, although the constancy was less for adolescents and children than for adults.

The cognitive subscales of the CSQ (Rosensteil & Keefe, 1983) are listed here.

1. Diverting attention involves thinking of things or paying attention to things that serve to distract one from the pain. Often simply called distraction, it is probably the cognitive strategy that makes the most intuitive sense to the casual observer.
2. Reinterpreting pain sensation is imagining something that would be inconsistent with the experience of pain: Imagining the pain sensation as a dull ache rather than as burning, or even imagining it as a color or sound. There are many versions of imaging, a competing but less noxious sensation.
3. Coping self-statements involve telling oneself that one can deal with the pain, no matter how bad. This is a particular application of a commonplace behavioral technique often called positive self-talk.
4. Ignoring pain sensations is denying that the pain exists or affects one in any way. This strategy is often used in conjunction with diverting attention.
5. Praying or hoping involves telling oneself to hope and pray the pain will get better someday. There is a quality of magical wishful thinking in the items used in this scale. It is not a comprehensive measure of spiritual or inner-resource-based coping.
6. Catastrophizing includes the use of negative self-statements, catastrophizing thoughts, and ideation: "I can't stand it." "My life is ruined." The term is borrowed from Albert Ellis (1962). Catastrophizing is a central theme found in pain literature and a common response for those who are overwhelmed by pain.

The behavioral coping-strategy scales of the CSQ are as follows:

1. Increasing activity level is engaging in active behaviors that divert one's attention from the pain (e.g., household chores). This is similar to diverting attention, but it involves physical, rather than cognitive, activity.

Table 6.2—*Factor Loading, Mean, and Standard Deviation for CSQ–R Items*
(Six-Factor Florida Model)

Item	Loadings	M	SD
Factor 1—Distraction			
3. I try to think of something pleasant.	0.73	3.28	1.80
30. I replay in my mind pleasant experiences in the past.	0.82	2.64	1.97
31. I think of people I enjoy doing things with.	0.96	2.75	2.01
43. I think of things I enjoy doing.	0.84	2.83	1.86
45. I do something I enjoy, such as watching TV or listening to music.	0.53	3.80	1.70
Factor 2—Catastrophizing			
5. It's terrible and I feel it's never going to get any better.	0.70	3.15	2.02
12. It's awful and I feel that it overwhelms me.	0.81	3.14	1.96
14. I feel my life isn't worth living.	0.80	1.31	1.87
28. I worry all the time about whether it will end.	0.65	2.85	2.18
38. I feel I can't stand it anymore.	0.84	3.03	1.91
42. I feel like I can't go on.	0.90	1.96	1.90
Factor 3—Ignoring pain			
20. I don't think about the pain.	0.67	2.82	1.91
24. I don't pay any attention to it.	0.83	1.95	1.84
27. I pretend it's not there.	0.82	1.58	1.84
35. I just go on as if nothing happened.	0.78	2.17	1.96
40. I ignore it.	0.87	1.86	1.81
Factor 4—Distancing from the pain			
1. I try to feel distant from the pain, almost as if the pain was in somebody else's body.	0.66	1.60	1.82
18. I try not to think of it as my body, but rather as something separate from me.	0.89	1.12	1.73
34. I imagine that the pain is outside of my body.	0.98	0.82	1.47
46. I pretend it's not a part of me.	0.90	1.02	1.64
Factor 5—Coping self-statements			
6. I tell myself to be brave and carry on despite the pain.	0.71	4.15	1.77
8. I tell myself that I can overcome the pain.	0.76	3.60	1.79
23. I tell myself that I can't let the pain stand in the way of what I have to do.	0.91	3.87	1.79
37. Although it hurts, I just keep on going.	0.80	3.79	1.81
Factor 6—Praying			
17. I pray to God it won't last long.	0.88	3.88	2.19
32. I pray for the pain to stop.	0.93	4.05	2.13
41. I rely on my faith in God.	0.85	3.52	2.22

Note. CSQ–R = Coping Strategies Questionnaire–Revised.

From Riley, J. L., & Robinson, M. E. CSQ: Five factors or fiction? *Clinical Journal of Pain, 13*, p. 159. Copyright 1997 by Lippincott-Raven Publisher. Adapted by permission.

2.   Increasing pain behaviors involves the use of overt pain behaviors that can reduce pain sensations, such as applying ice or heat or taking medication.

The ratings of perceived effectiveness of pain control are *control over pain* and *ability to decrease pain.*

More than any other pain-coping-research tool, the CSQ has been subjected to repeated efforts to identify its underlying structure and improve its interpretability through factor analysis studies. It is not surprising that, with a test initially based on rational item selection and rational scale identification and containing cognitive, behavioral, and self-efficacy appraisal items, there has been considerable difficulty in establishing its factor structure and therefore, in empirically identifying distinct dimensions of the represented coping responses.

Early studies examining the relationships among the subscales (Keefe et al., 1987; Rosensteil & Keefe, 1983; Turner & Clancy, 1986) failed to find a consistent factor structure. However, Lawson, Reesor, Keefe, and Turner (1990) applied a confirmatory factor analysis and were able to identify three replicable factors across five heterogeneous sample groups of pain patients from five independent sites. This analysis indicated 2 global factors with some consistency: (a) conscious cognitive coping (highest loading on the scales for ignoring pain and coping self-statements) and (b) self-efficacy appraisals (highest loadings on the scales for control over pain and ability to decrease pain). A 3rd factor, pain avoidance (highest loadings on the scales for diverting attention and praying and hoping) was identified, but with less consistency. Catastrophizing and the behavioral coping strategies subscales did not load consistently on any of the three basic dimensions.

Individual-item factor analyses of the CSQ fared somewhat better than have the scale analyses in replicating the original rationally designed scales. Tuttle, Shutty, and DeGood (1991) found, using an exploratory factor analysis with a heterogeneous pain sample, a 5-factor solution supporting (in the order listed): (a) catastrophizing, (b) praying and hoping, (c) reinterpreting pain sensation, and (d) diverting attention. The 5th factor combined the subscales for ignoring pain sensation and diverting attention—similar to a finding of Lawson et al. (1990). Swartzman, Gwadry, Shapiro, and Teasell (1993), using a similar exploratory analysis with a sample of patients with whiplash injuries, also found a 5-factor solution, although the individual items were not in complete agreement with those of Tuttle et al. (1991).

Given the degree of uncertainty created by the factor analyses of relatively small patient samples, Robinson et al. (1997) completed a similar item level factor analysis with a sample of 965 patients with chronic pain. In this principal-components analysis with a varimax rotation, 9 factors were identified, accounting for 54.5% of the variance. Although not overlapping on every item, the first 5 factors are quite similar to subscales of the original CSQ: (a) distraction (or diverting attention), (b) catastrophizing, (c) ignoring pain sensations, (d) reinterpreting pain sensations, and (e) coping self-statements. The items from the CSQ praying and hoping subscale split into separate factors, Factors 6 and 8, respectively. Factor 7 contained two items, representing increasing activity. Factor 9 contained two items from the CSQ reinterpreting pain sensations subscale and one item from the diverting attention subscale. Finally, 13 of the CSQ items were dropped because of insufficient or excessively shared loadings. Internal consistency was then determined for each factor by calculation of coefficient α and was acceptable (>.8), or at least marginal, for the first 6 factors, but insufficient to consider as stable the final 3 factors.

In an even more ambitious undertaking, Riley and Robinson (1997) compared all the prior published exploratory factor solutions through a confirmatory factor analysis using the LISREL-8 structural equation-modeling program (Joreskog & Sorbom, 1993). This was done with a new sample of 472 heterogeneous chronic pain patients. Five separate statistics were calculated to rate goodness-of-fit for each factor model to the observed data. Beginning with a single-factor model, they were able to reject the hypothesis that the CSQ consists of a single underlying construct. A 2-factor solution, consisting of catastrophizing and active coping, proposed by Affleck, Tennen, Urrows, and Higgins (1992), fit considerably better but still was insufficient to account for the variance–covariance in the sample. The 6-factor model generated from their prior study (called the Florida model because of the authors' location) clearly had a much better goodness-of-fit to the data than did the 1- or 2-construct models. The Florida model, although having much in common with the earlier 5-factor models of Tuttle et al. (1991) and Swartzman et al. (1993), did demonstrate a superior goodness-of-fit to the 5-factor models.

In their final factor-based model, Riley and Robinson (1997) retain only 27 of the original 48 items from the CSQ and suggest creation of the Coping Strategy Questionnaire–Revised containing these retained items organized into 6 factorially demonstrated subscales (Table 6.2). Based on all the item level factor studies, Riley and Robinson concluded that: (a) the catastrophizing factor is clearly the most robust across all studies; (b) the distracting attention subscale appears to replicate across most studies; (c) coping self-statements and ignoring sensations are highly associated and will emerge as separate factors only across very large samples; and (d) distancing from pain (or reinterpreting pain sensation), coping self-statements, and ignoring pain are too intercorrelated to be considered separate dimensions and probably are better viewed as a single, higher order composite factor of cognitive coping.

Turner (1991) concluded from a review of the literature that two major relationships between the CSQ and adjustment to chronic pain have emerged consistently: First, patients who report catastrophizing in response to pain also perceive themselves as ineffectual at controlling their pain and appear to be more disabled and depressed at the initial assessment (e.g., Keefe et al., 1987; Rosenstiel & Keefe, 1983; Turner & Clancy, 1986) and at follow-up (Keefe, Brown, Wallston, & Caldwell, 1989). Second, for patients with low back pain, higher endorsement of ignoring pain sensations, reinterpreting pain sensation, diverting attention, and praying and hoping are associated with greater pain and disability levels. Note that what *does not* make for an effective coping strategy is more evident than what *does* constitute effective coping. This ease at finding associations with the negative rather than the positive strategies, as will be seen, is a persistent theme running through the pain-coping-research literature.

M. P. Jensen, Turner, and Romano (1991) presented a somewhat more involved account of the relationship between the CSQ and adjustment, beginning with a summary of the relationships between adjustment and the 3 higher order CSQ composite factors identified by Lawson et al. (1990). They concluded that the composite factor of self-efficacy beliefs (CSQ ability to control and decrease pain subscales) fares quite well and is consistently correlated with pain intensity (six of nine studies), with psychological dysfunction (seven of nine studies), and with physical disability (six of nine studies). However, the second-order composite factors, based on the CSQ subscales of coping self-statements and ignoring pain (conscious cognitive control factor), and the subscales of diverting attention, and praying and hoping (pain avoidance factor) were not found consistently to predict the three targeted outcomes of behavioral functioning and psychological adjustment. An updated review by Boothby et al. (1999) leaves this impression essentially intact.

Early studies of individual subscale correlations, rather than higher order composite factors, reveal an even more inconclusive picture. Keefe and Williams (1990) found coping self-statements and increasing activity level to be associated with less depression; but while controlling for demographic variables, as well as for pain severity and duration, Sullivan and D'Eon (1990) did not find such a relationship. M. P. Jensen and Karoly (1991) also found that the CSQ subscales of ignoring pain, coping self-statements, and increasing activity level were positively correlated with psychological adjustment, even when controlled for pain severity. They likewise found diverting attention, ignoring pain, and coping self-statements to be associated positively with activity level, but only for patients with relatively low levels of pain. This again points out the importance of moderator variables in trying to examine the relationship between coping techniques and other indicators of adjustment and functioning.

How have more recent studies of item level, factor-based CSQ scales fared in relationships with other measures? Tuttle et al. (1991) found the catastrophizing factor to predict global distress, on the Symptom Checklist-90 (Derogatis, 1983) and disability ratings, whereas praying and hoping and diverting attention were positively related to higher levels of pain and greater self-reported disability. Robinson et al. (1997) found that correlations between their modified 6-factor scales were weak to moderate in the same direction as other studies. Those strategies thought to be adaptive (ignoring sensations, coping self-statements) were positively associated with activity. Those strategies thought to be maladaptive (catastrophizing, praying and hoping) were associated positively with affective distress and negatively with activity level. However, they found distraction from pain, normally considered an adaptive response, was instead positively associated with pain severity and life interference. Riley and Robinson's (1997) proposed 27-item revision of the CSQ does not provide any new external validation measure data, but they do offer an "easy-to use" scoring program to interested parties.

The CSQ has had remarkable hueristic value in stimulating interest in pain-coping research. Both its internal structure and its external correlates have been extensively explored. It has been used as a composite instrument with scales built from factor analyses, and for single-strategy analyses, based on its individual coping scales. Catastrophizing has certainly emerged as the most dominant factor in the CSQ, and high scores in this scale appear to reflect a failure to cope. The picture regarding the use of postive coping strategies is less clear. However, the use of coping self-statements as an adaptive strategy certainly comes through consistently enough to justify the cognitive–behavioral therapist's efforts to encourage replacing catastrophizing self-talk with positive coping self-talk.

The CSQ contains a mixture of cognitive items, behavioral items, and self-efficacy appraisal items, making it theoretically unwieldy. In fact, in reading second-hand accounts of some of the CSQ factor studies, it can be difficult to determine which components were included and which were excluded in a given analysis. A risk for pain-coping research is that innovation is lost when research becomes overly reliant on an instrument that has inherent limitations.

Vanderbilt Multidimensional Pain Coping Inventory

The first coping measure of the Vanderbilt group was the Vanderbilt Pain Management Inventory (VPMI; Brown & Niccassio, 1987), a 19-item self-report scale that measures the frequency with which respondents report engaging in various thoughts or behaviors to cope with their pain. The items were partitioned into active coping and passive coping subscales, thus differentiating coping strategies by the amount of effort the patient exerts to function, despite his or her pain, as compared with a patient's tendency to depend on others. Final item selection was based on factor analysis of the responses of 259 patients with rheumatoid arthritis, later replicated using a confirmatory factor analysis. The rigorous analysis resulted in a brief, face-valid measure with a stable subscale structure, which has been shown to be both internally consistent and invariant over a 6-month period.

In the original study (Brown & Niccassio, 1987), active-coping strategies were found to be linked with lower pain intensity, fewer symptoms of depression, and less functional impairment as compared with passive-coping strategies. In a subsequent study (Brown, Niccassio, & Wallston, 1989) involving 287 rheumatoid arthritis patients, passive coping was again found to be associated with increased depressive symptoms and continued to be so 6 months later. In a later study from a multidisciplinary pain program (Snow-Turek, Norris, & Tan, 1996), passive coping once more was strongly associated with general psychological distress and depression, and, to a lesser extent, active coping was associated with greater activity level and less psychological distress. However, the internal consistency of the VPMI proved relatively weak compared with similar factors on the CSQ.

The Vanderbilt group (Smith & Wallston, 1992; Smith, Wallston, Dwyer, & Dowdy, 1997) has questioned the limitations of its own and other scales designed to yield just two broad composite subscales that correspond to active and passive coping. The group concludes that any coping scale that combines several distinct strategies into a single subscale score can obscure and underestimate the true relationship between coping and adjustment. Individual strategies subsumed by a broad composite scale could have opposing effects on adjustment that would tend to cancel each other when combined into a single score. This is particularly true for strategies that can be context specific. Furthermore, broad summary or composite scales that do not permit determination of the contribution of individual coping strategies are less valuable to the clinician who must try to identify specific behavioral coping strengths and weaknesses in the individual. Thus, the Vanderbilt group set out to develop a different type of measure in their effort to design a pain-coping inventory.

The goal in developing the Vanderbilt Multidimensional Pain Coping Inventory (Smith et al., 1997) was to establish individual subscales covering a range of distinct strategies underlying the factor or composite scales of the VPMI or the CSQ. Although the intent was to develop a scale for patients with pain, the goal was also to produce a pain-coping measure that would have considerable overlap with other (nonpain) types of stress-coping measures. A rational scale development approach was the first step, borrowing possible scales and test items from other inventories, including the VPMI, CSQ, WOC checklist, and the Coping Orientation to Problems Experienced (COPE) scale (Carver, Scheier, & Weintraub, 1989). The initial version had 49 items assessing 12 subscales and was administered to two sample groups (171 and 207 rheumatoid arthritis patients). The measure was later reduced to 11 subscales (Table 6.3) by combining problem-solving and information-seeking into a single subscale, called *planful problem-solving*. Eight items demonstrating low internal consistency with their intended subscales were eliminated. Acceptable internal consistencies (α) and 18-month stabilities were found for the remaining items. Correlations between the new subscales range in two samples from near 0 to .69. Some coping strategies clearly tend to be used together (planful problem-solving and positive reappraisal; wishful thinking and disengagement). Nevertheless, the authors concluded that the observed scale relationships do not preclude the individual coping-strategy subscales from demonstrating unique relations to specific external measures.

One early analysis involving the two patient groups used in test construction compared the 11 individual VMPCI subscales with the 2 composite subscales of the VPMI (Smith et al., 1997). The subscales of planful problem-solving, positive reappraisal, distraction, distancing–denial, and stoicism all demonstrated positive correlations with the VPMI active-coping dimension. Conversely, the disengagement subscale was highly correlated ($r = .80$) with passive coping. The wishful thinking, confrontative coping, self-isolation, and self-blame subscales had moderately high correlations with the passive-coping composite. Religion was not strongly associated either with active or with passing coping. Except for the relationship between the disengagement subscale and passive coping, all correlations are moderate and varied enough to refute the notion that all variance is completely explained by the VPMI

Table 6.3—*Sample Items for the Subscales of the VMPCI*

Subscale	Sample Item
Stem for all items	When my pain is at a moderate level of intensity or greater, I . . .
Subscale 1. Planful Problem-Solving	take direction action to try and improve matters.
Subscale 2. Positive Reappraisal	tell myself things that help me to feel better.
Subscale 3. Distraction	keep myself busy so I won't have to think about what is going on.
Subscale 4. Confrontative Coping	lash out physically or verbally.
Subscale 5. Distancing/Denial	go on as if nothing has happened.
Subscale 6. Stoicism	keep others from knowing how bad things are.
Subscale 7. Use of Religion	pray more than usual.
Subscale 8. Self-Blame	criticize or lecture myself.
Subscale 9. Self-Isolation	get as far away from other people as I can.
Subscale 10. Wishful Thinking	hope a miracle will happen.
Subscale 11. Disengagement	realize the situation is hopeless and give up.

Note. VMPCI = Vanderbilt Multidimensional Pain Coping Inventory.

From Smith, C. A., Wallston, K. A., Dwyer, K. A., & Dowdy, S. W. (1997). Beyond good and bad coping: A multidimensional examination of coping with pain in persons with rheumatoid arthritis. *Annals of Behavioral Medicine, 19*, 11–21. Copyright 1997 by the Society of Behavioral Medicine. Adapted by permission.

active–passive construct. Finally, the power of the VMPCI, relative to the VPMI, to account for individual differences in rheumatoid-arthritis-related impairment and psychological adjustment was examined. In no case did the subscales of the VPMI account for variance above and beyond that captured by the VMPCI. On most measures, the VMPCI significantly accounted for variance beyond that captured by the VPMI, thus confirming the added utility of the individual coping measures.

In the last step with the two developmental samples (Smith et al., 1997), the 11 VMPCI subscales were correlated with external measures of general impairment, life satisfaction, positive affect, negative affect, depressive symptoms, and physical functioning. These correlations are low to moderate. The planful problem-solving, positive reappraisal, and distraction subscales were moderately correlated with positive affect and life satisfaction. The less-adaptive-strategy subscales of self-blame, self-isolation, wishful thinking, and disengagement were associated with greater impairment, more negative affect, and greater numbers of depressive symptoms. The weak correlation of all subscales with physical functioning is disappointing, but with pain level statistically controlled there could have been insufficient remaining variance to obtain meaningful correlations.

The external correlations were all cross-sectional, precluding any inference regarding direction of cause. Therefore, further analyses were completed in an attempt to prospectively examine the ability of the VMPCI coping scales to predict future changes in adjustment (Smith et al., 1997). Outcome measures were obtained approximately 18 months after the initial assessment. Both pain severity and adjustment at the initial assessment were controlled in this prospective analysis. As was true for the CSQ, it was easier to predict poor outcomes (more impairment, more depression) from an initial VMPCI predominance of maladaptive coping strategies than it was to predict positive outcomes from what are considered to be adaptive strategies. Nevertheless, there was some modest degree of association found between better outcome functioning and the more active VMPCI forms of coping, namely positive reappraisal, planful problem-solving, distraction, and distancing–denial. Unusual in this VMPCI study is the finding that the avoidant coping strategies of distancing and denial were associated with better outcome adjustment, whereas in the general coping literature avoidant strategies are typically found to be associated with poorer adjustment (e.g., Affleck & Tennen, 1991; Carver, Pozo, Harris, & Noriega, 1993). The authors (Smith et al., 1997) suggested that, in severe cases of rheumatoid arthritis, where little can be done to control the pain, the use of distancing and denial actually could be beneficial. Clearly, the effect of any given coping strategy is not cast in stone, but is shaped by the person and by the variables of circumstance. As stressed by Lazarus (1993), virtually any coping strategy can be either adaptive or maladaptive given a particular situation.

Although the VMPCI is a relatively new pain-coping inventory, it has generated few new data. Nevertheless, it is built on the tradition of an earlier pain-coping instrument, the VPMI, used in several studies with rheumatoid arthritis patients. It demonstrates several features that reflect recent trends in coping measurement. It limits itself to cognitive coping strategies and does not attempt to mix behavioral and self-efficacy items into a single measure. It does, however, attempt to measure a range of cognitive coping strategies that are not narrowly focused on pain. This creates a potential for use in comparative studies of coping with other, non-pain-specific stressful medical conditions. A current limitation of the VMPCI, as with the

VPMI, is that the research has been entirely restricted to one group of patients, leaving it unclear how well the results might generalize to patients with other pain conditions.

Pain Coping and Adjustment

Coping and Adjustment Studies Before 1991

Several conclusions regarding the relationships of coping measures to external measures of adjustment can be drawn from the M. P. Jensen, Turner, Romano, and Karoly (1991) review of pain coping research prior to 1991:

1. Coping strategies identified as active (exercise, ignoring pain, finding distracting activities) tend to be associated with better psychological and physical functioning.
2. Strategies considered passive (withdrawal, resting, taking medication, wishful thinking) are associated with higher negative affect and poorer physical functioning.
3. Responding to pain with catastrophizing (excessive and exaggerated negative self-statements) is consistently associated with poorer psychological adjustment and poorer physical functioning.
4. Adjustment relationships tend to be stronger with composite coping measures than with individual measures of specific coping strategies.
5. Although there appears to be a general association between coping strategy use and adjustment in patients with chronic pain, problems in methodology limit conclusions regarding the strength and nature of this relationship.

In addition, M. P. Jensen, Turner, Romano, and Karoly (1991) made several recommendations for improving coping research:

1. There should be measures that are more conceptually pure and that do not confound dimensions such as coping, beliefs−appraisals, and adjustment within the same category.
2. More assessment of specific coping constructs rather than combining several coping strategies into a composite measure would be useful.
3. The psychometric soundness of coping measures needs improvement.
4. Less dependence should be placed on self-report questionnaires and more on direct observation of coping behaviors.
5. Greater reliance on testing coping models with true experimental designs and single-subject experimental designs would strengthen research.
6. Further examination of moderating factors, such as pain severity and duration, differences between men and women, and type of diagnosis, is required.

Regarding recommendation 5 above, the experimental model-testing designs the authors have in mind are model-driven research programs similar to those found for learned helplessness (Abramson, Seligman, & Teasdale, 1978; Seligman, 1975), stress and coping (Lazarus & Folkman, 1984), social learning theory (Bandura, 1977, 1986), cognitive models of depression (Beck, 1967, 1976; Ellis, 1962), and control theory (Rotter, 1966).

Coping and Adjustment Studies Since 1991

The conclusions and recommendations of M. P. Jensen, Turner, Romano, and Karoly (1991) provide a convenient marker for comparing the content of the comprehensive review of Boothby et al. (1999).

Composite Measures

Despite dozens of additional studies between 1991 and 1999, the general conclusions regarding the use of composite measures of coping remain virtually unchanged. Coping measures that reflect a composite of apparently adaptive-coping strategies, as indicated by an association with better concurrent and future functioning, continue to include categories labeled as active coping, coping attempts, and pain control and rational thinking. Strategies that continue to appear maladaptive include categories with labels such as passive coping, negative thinking (various catastrophizing composites), and pain avoidance. The composite research continues to affirm that general categories of coping operate in the adaptation to chronic pain, although the prediction of poor functioning from maladaptive composite strategies remains stronger than is the link between the adaptive strategies and better functioning. Also, the interaction with severity of pain remains unclear. Adaptive-coping strategies undoubtedly work for most patients with mild to moderate chronic pain, but how much of an adaptive function they serve with severe pain is less clear, and existing studies are inconsistent on this point.

Individual Measures

Studies since 1991 leave the picture regarding the individual strategy as confusing as before. Most individual measures of coping continue to show inconsistent relationships with adjustment. Only catastrophizing continues to be highly predictive of external measures of maladaptive functioning. Catastrophizing is nearly universally associated with higher levels of pain sensation, psychosocial distress, and impairment in functioning. But even with this maladaptive-coping strategy there are exceptions. Jensen et al. (1992) found that catastrophizing did not predict disability in a group of patients with chronic pain when pain intensity, site, duration, and all the other ratings and scales of the CSQ were statistically controlled. Likewise, in a treatment outcome study (M. P. Jensen et al., 1994), changes in catastrophizing did not predict changes in disability. This raises the question of how much of the variance in predicting functioning is actually unique to catastrophizing and how much is shared with a wide range of other personal and situational factors.

Catastrophizing has fared well in recent studies when measured as a treatment outcome variable. Cognitive–behavioral treatments for chronic pain have been demonstrated to produce a pre-to-post-treatment reduction in catastrophizing (James, Thorn, & Williams, 1993; ter Kuile, Spinhoven, Linssen, & van Houwelingen, 1995; Vlaeyen, Haazen, Schuerman, Kole-Snijders, & van Eck, 1995). In fact, of several measures evaluating a group multimodal treatment for fibromyalgia patients, Bennett et al. (1996) found a greater change for catastrophizing than for any other outcome variable, and this change was maintained at the 2-year follow-up. Because of its known association with poor functioning, the posttreatment degree of catastrophizing could prove to be among the most sensitive indicators of the degree of treatment success or failure. If so, it could become a useful measure, despite its negative connotation, for clinicians to track treatment progress.

Even though positive-coping self-statements often appear as part of the blend of adaptive-coping composite measures, when standing alone the picture is mixed. Boothby et al. (1999) concluded that when significant relationships are found with functioning they tend to be positive, but this relationship appears not to hold from study to study. An identical conclusion is reported regarding engaging in distracting activities. In the largest study of coping-change scores after pain treatment, changes in the use of positive-coping self-statements were unrelated to changes in disability, depression, or number of physician visits (M. P. Jensen et al., 1994).

Boothby et al. (1999) likewise concluded that praying and hoping, as measured by the CSQ, continues to be inconsistently related to measures of adjustment. When correlations are positive they tend to link praying and hoping with greater dysfunction. However, changes in praying and hoping proved to be unrelated to changes in disability (M. P. Jensen et al., 1994). Generally, the frequency with which praying and hoping is used as a coping measure seems to be unaffected by treatment programs. This particular CSQ measure does not measure spirituality as a component of inner resourcefulness, but seems to function more as a measure of passive wishful thinking.

Coping strategies consisting of reinterpreting pain, ignoring pain, and distraction–diversion of attention are judged by Boothby et al. (1999) to be inconsistent from study to study and generally to have only a slight effect if any on adjustment to pain. Several studies suggest that these strategies are, in fact, more useful for acute pain than they are for pain that stems from chronic conditions. Likewise, pre-to-post-treatment changes in these coping responses appear unrelated to improvement.

On balance, the recent research confirms that there are composites of positive and negative coping strategies that can be related to psychological adjustment and physical functioning of patients with chronic pain. But when one attempts to break down the composite measures into individual strategies, with the exception of catastrophizing, they tend to be unreliable from study to study. This suggests that moderator variables, which often vary from sample to sample, are more powerful than are individual strategies, making it necessary to consider combinations of individual coping behaviors if we are to successfully predict functioning from knowledge of a patient's coping behaviors.

Recent Trends in Coping Research

Between 1991 and 1998, some of the recommendations listed in the prior section for improving the quality of pain-coping research were partially met, others hardly at all. This section considers current trends in pain-coping research in light of past concerns.

Psychometric Improvements in Older Measures

There have been some psychometric improvements made with the two most popular measures, the CSQ and the VMPCI. The large factor sample used by the Florida group (Robinson et al., 1997), followed by a confirmatory factor analysis (Riley & Robinson, 1997), provides as much internal construct validity for the resulting version of the CSQ as can possibly emerge from the original CSQ item pool. The new VMPCI (Smith et al., 1997) fulfills the recommendation to develop measures of individual coping constructs rather than to rely on composite scales that combine several individual strategies into one measure. Of course, the unavoidable problem with the recommendation for greater specificity of measurement is that global psychometric measures of any phenomenon will nearly always capture more variance than will specific measures. Thus, individual measures of coping are less likely to demonstrate concurrent and predictive validity with a criterion measure than is a more global measure. This is a Catch-22: The need for psychometric soundness is at odds with the needs of the clinician for specific behavioral information relevant to intervention planning.

Psychometric Improvements in New Measures

The recommendation for development of coping measures that are based on behavioral observation has received some attention. Following their own recommendations, Jensen et al. (1995) constructed a measure targeted at observable behavioral coping strategies as opposed to the cognitive strategies favored by the WOC checklist, CSQ, and VMPCI. Their goal was to quantify the behaviors that are most often the targets of change in multidisciplinary pain programs. After some preliminary refinements, they produced a 65-item measure, the Chronic Pain Coping Inventory (CPCI), which assesses 11 pain-coping dimensions covering two broad categories of coping behaviors. The broad categories are illness-focused coping and wellness-focused coping. A version of the CPCI (Jensen et al., 1995) designed for significant others' ratings of patient coping also was developed, permitting calculation of inter-rater reliabilities between self-report and direct observer scales.

The illness-focused coping dimension of the CPCI contains 6 scales: guarding, resting, asking for assistance, opioid medication use, nonsteroidal medication use, and sedative–hypnotic medication use. The wellness-focused coping dimension contains 4 scales: relaxation, task persistence, exercise–stretch, and coping self-statements. An additional scale, lying outside the two dimensions, is called seeking social support. The illness-focused scales target behaviors that are normally discouraged in multidisciplinary programs. Eight scales (guarding, opioid medication use, nonsteroidal anti-inflammatory medication use, sedative–hypnotic medication use, resting, asking for assistance, exercise–stretch) demonstrated moderate-to-strong relationships between patient and significant-other versions. Correlations with external measures of mood and activity demonstrated that higher amounts of wellness-focused coping were associated with less depression and with more normal activity; the opposite was true for illness-focused coping. Individual scales showed acceptable internal consistency (α) coefficients and fair test–retest reliability. The internal structure and external predictability have not been cross-validated in other settings.

Some limited effort also has followed the recommendation to take a more ideographic approach to coping assessment. Large (1985) attempted to put an old measure, the repertory grid, to use in a new way. Repertory grid measures are efforts to quantify Personal Construct Theory (Kelly, 1963), which proposes that people make sense of their world by forming constructs by which they can predict the behavior of those around them. Large and Strong (1997) had volunteers with nonclinical low back pain complete a repertory grid with eight given elements signifying various self- and illness-related roles. Several constructs emerged to characterize the perception of those who cope successfully with pain. The characterizations included authenticity, the limitations of being a coper, mastery, active stoicism, cheerfulness, acceptance, and maintaining acceptable social interactions and appearances. This unique approach to exploring coping has considerable intuitive appeal in that it allows the patient to define his or her own perception of coping relative to his or her own ideal of a person who copes well with pain. The preliminary findings, the authors stressed, should be explored further in community and patient groups.

Another noteworthy fledging line of pain-coping research represents an attempt to study the emergence of pain coping from a developmental–motivational perspective (e.g., Karoly & Lecci, 1997; Karoly & Ruehlman, 1996; Leventhal, 1993). The study by Karoly and Lecci (1997) provides an example. A sample group of 127 college students, reporting persistent (but nonclinical) pain, completed the Goal System Assessment Battery (Karoly & Ruehlman, 1996). It was found that the "pattern of goal construal produced by this young and generally healthy group of college students reflects cognitive–motivational dysfunctions possibly presaging pain-schemes in later life" (p. 104). Although difficult to critique at this stage, this is a direction that offers considerable potential for merging pain-coping research with personality and developmental psychopathology research. We need to know more about how coping skills develop during the life of the individual.

Finally, a relatively new measure has appeared in studies with acute pain, the Cognitive Coping Strategies Inventory (Butler, Damarin, Beaulieu, Schwebel, & Thorn, 1989), although it has not been used in studies with chronic pain. Similarly, although the 72-item Coping Strategies Inventory (Tobin, Holroyd, Reynolds, & Wigal, 1989) has not been put to sufficient test to judge its merit, its large number of individual-strategy subscales has appeal for the clinician.

Moderating Factors

It is not surprising that the effectiveness of a coping strategy varies from person to person and situation to situation. Of all the suggestions of M. P. Jensen et al. (1991), the recommendation to sample across a broader range of chronic pain problems and consider the interacting effects of age, gender, and duration and severity of pain have received the most attention.

Most of the studies done in the 1980s either used rheumatoid arthritis populations or heterogeneous, multidimensional pain center populations. Each group has unique features that could generate cohort effects that can restrict generalization of results.

Arthritis patients, as a group, are somewhat older, have clear-cut physical diagnoses, and experience their most severe pain in the form of acute flare-ups. Multidisciplinary pain center populations have the advantage of greater heterogeneity, but the characteristics of the samples are by no means uniform from clinic to clinic, potentially reducing reliability of findings. Also, multidisciplinary pain centers as providers of last resort tend to have high percentages of patients with very severe problems, more psychopathology, and poorer overall functioning than is characteristic of chronic pain patients in the general population.

Many studies have examined coping in a wide range of special populations beyond individuals in the widely used sample groups, for example, children with sickle cell disease (Gil, Abrams, Phillips, & Williams, 1992; Gil et al., 1993; Thompson, Gil, Abrams, & Phillips, 1992); breast cancer patients (Jacobsen & Butler, 1996); patients with other cancers (Arathuzik, 1991; Wilkie & Keefe, 1991); patients with fibromyalgia (Martin et al., 1996; Nicassio, Schoenfeld-Smith, Radojevic, & Schuman, 1995); patients with temporomandibular disorder (Turner, Whitney, Dworkin, Massoth, & Wilson, 1995); and patients with phantom limb pain (Hill, 1993; Hill, Niven, & Knussen, 1995).

Other moderators, such as age (e.g., Ruth & Coleman, 1996; Strack & Feifel, 1996), gender (e.g., Jensen, Nygren, Gamberale, Goldie, & Westerholm, 1994; Weir, Browne, Tunks, Gafni, & Roberts, 1996), and duration (e.g., Newman & Revenson, 1993) and severity (e.g., M. P. Jensen & Karoly, 1991; Smith et al., 1997; Sullivan & D'Eon, 1990; Zautra, Sheets, & Sandler, 1996) of pain also have received greater attention. The consequence, however, is a growing awareness that individual coping strategies and adjustment are inconsistent among patients and circumstances.

Finally, still understudied as moderators of coping are socioeconomic circumstances. Two critical factors that interact with chronic pain are the effect on job functioning (and associated economic security) and the availability of social–physical support systems. The former concern is, of course, greatest in a working-age sample and the latter in an elderly population. Although such variables have received widespread scrutiny in the general literature on pain, few studies have considered how they might interact with the use of coping strategies.

New Research Designs

Only a very small amount of research effort has gone into pursuit of new research paradigms. Fledgling efforts to study coping in nonclinical populations (Karoly & Lecci, 1997; Large & Strong, 1997), mentioned previously, represent important efforts to develop a new paradigm.

There is a general view that a laboratory model for acute pain cannot give us much information relevant to chronic pain. However, Gil et al. (1997) demonstrated that this might not always be true. These investigators applied a controlled-pressure stimulation device to the fingers of children and adolescents with sickle cell disease to determine pain perception thresholds under controlled conditions. The laboratory session was completed during a dormant period in the disease cycle. The 41 patients also completed an 80-item version of the CSQ, modified for use with sickle cell patients and scored on three previously developed empirically derived composite-factor scales (Gil, Williams, Thompson, & Kinney, 1991): coping attempts, negative thinking, and illness-focused strategies. Hierarchical regression analysis controlling for age indicated that children who reported using active cognitive and behavioral coping strategies had less tendency to report pain during the laboratory pain task. Additionally, the laboratory sensory thresholds for pain correlated significantly ($r = .46$) with later painful episodes of sickle cell disease and lowered laboratory pain thresholds with more depression and more parent-reported externalization problems. The results certainly suggest a disposition to cope with pain episodes that can be measured by a questionnaire and objectively verified with a controlled acute pain stimulus. Such a paradigm awaits further testing with other chronic pain conditions.

Longitudinal studies, which are on the increase, involve a paradigm improvement over simple concurrent variable measurement. They can serve to: (a) examine how much stability or change there is in coping strategies over time (e.g., Dozois, Dobson, Wong, Hughes, & Long, 1996; Smith & Wallston, 1992); (b) elucidate coping-strategy use as a predictor of treatment outcome (e.g., James et al., 1993; Parker et al., 1995); (c) examine whether changes in coping strategies correspond to changes (with or without treatment) in adjustment and functioning over time (e.g., Jensen, Turner, & Romano, 1994); and (d) determine whether coping interacts with other moderator variables over time (e.g., Gil et al., 1993). Such studies consume more resources than do simple cross-sectional studies, but the added information is well worth the effort. By definition, treatment outcome studies are longitudinal, and certainly there is a continuing need to demonstrate that coping strategies influence outcome at least as much as they affect concurrent adjustment and functioning.

Study of moderator variables also would benefit from more longitudinal research. Rather than simply treating age and duration and severity of pain cross-sectionally as between-subject variables, these dimensions need to be considered over time. The same patient may use different coping strategies at different points or with different severity of pain. There is ample evidence to hypothesize that active cognitive and behavioral coping strategies are more effective with mild and moderate levels of pain and that passive strategies might, in some cases, be the only alternative for patients with severe pain. It also can be hypothesized that catastrophizing comes into play more frequently as the duration of chronic pain increases, although there is also evidence that catastrophizing is associated with a general personality tendency toward neuroticism. Longitudinal studies could help clarify the picture of how this maladaptive coping strategy emerges.

Under research design issues, it needs mentioning that the reader of the coping-strategy literature, in addition to looking for moderator variables, also must be alert to the types of variables used as external validating or predictor measures. Abstracts and reviews usually classify such external measures as indicators of adjustment or functioning. Scrutiny of complete articles will reveal that these indicators vary greatly from study to study. This introduces method variance among studies, which further clouds the comparative size effects of the relationships that emerge between coping strategies and external measures. A recent study provides a convenient example. In the study of Haythornthwaite, Menefee, Heinberg, and Clark (1998) of 195 chronic pain patients, it was found through stepwise multiple regression that coping self-statements, reinterpreting pain, and number of coping strategies reported were powerful predictors of perception of control over pain, whereas ignoring pain sensation predicted lower perceptions of control. Note that the self-reported use of coping strategies was being used to predict self-reported, perceived self-efficacy in controlling pain. Thus, both the independent and the dependent variables reflect similar self-reported cognitive events collected in the same setting, a format that will tend to maximize method variance. If the dependent variable had been a self-report of overt behavior or an independent observer's report of overt coping behaviors, the odds are, based on method variance alone, the relationships would have been weaker. Although the methodology was perfectly legitimate for the purpose of the study, which was to examine the relationships between coping strategies and perceived self-efficacy, it does illustrate yet another subtle source of difficulty in comparing studies.

Finally, the problem of mixing confounding constructs into coping-strategy measures continues. It is ironic that, regarding our best predictor, catastrophizing, researchers still do not agree whether to call it a coping strategy or a self-efficacy appraisal. One can certainly argue that a self-efficacy appraisal can be a coping strategy, but ultimately this lack of conceptual clarity detracts from building conceptually clear empirical models of how people handle chronic pain.

Conclusions and Considerations

Current Issues

The reader, especially the clinician looking for proven patient assessment tools, will be disappointed with the literature. There is little that can be stated definitely except that catastrophizing as a strategy seems to consistently predict functioning and outcome, although in a negative direction. Thus, we know more about how people cope poorly with pain than how they cope effectively. Effective coping can at best be predicted erratically and usually only with composite measures.

Continuing Problems With the Coping Construct

To put the pain-coping literature into perspective, we must return to the Lazarus truism: Virtually any coping strategy can be either adaptive or maladaptive, given a particular set of conditions. The literature does not suggest that there are no adaptive coping strategies, but merely that a given strategy cannot work consistently for everyone in all circumstances.

For example, the passive-coping behavior of rest or social withdrawal usually is maladaptive, but for someone with continuous severe pain, temporary rest or withdrawal actually can serve as an adaptive pacing strategy. Unfortunately, such highly individualized circuitous causation will never lend itself to simple assessment techniques. In light of the tremendous individual variability facing the researcher, I believe that assessment of pain beliefs and appraisals is more manageable, conceptually sound, and has greater clinical utility than does assessment of coping.

Probably only a very few things consistently matter in adjusting to chronic pain —maintaining a degree of positive affect, sufficient confidence in social and medical support, the motivation to maintain a social role, and the self-esteem stemming from a feeling of purpose and usefulness. At its most basic elements, coping with pain is little different from dealing with many other life challenges. Rather than interpreting the coping literature as disparaging regarding the value of coping assessment, or simply counting on improvement in psychometric measures in the future, we might need to ask some fundamental questions about the nature of coping itself.

Addressing the Problems With the Coping Construct

We should first consider whether more could be done to identify and measure the relevant behaviors that constitute coping strategies. We must always remember that subscales and factors can never be stronger than the underlying item pool. We quickly become bound to testing and refining narrower and narrower measures, and then we become frustrated because they are unreliable predictors. Our current measures are limited in their capacity to measure both inner strengths and outer resources. They are lacking in capacity to capture inner strength and motivation—dimensions such as spiritual resources, courage, heartiness, and sense of place in the world. For some, hoping and praying, no doubt, is a meaningless gesture of futility, but the broader health-coping literature suggests that, for many people, religion is an expression of a deeply felt source of inner strength and comfort (e.g., McFadden, 1996). We run the risk that our brief questionnaires trivialize the human spirit and the range of experiences to such an extent that we miss much that is essential to the coping process. We often try to explain outer resources by statistically controlling for demographic factors, but factors such as living conditions, employability, and financial resources can be primary shapers of the form taken by coping and adjustment and therefore essential to understanding the coping process.

Certainly some of the effort to evaluate moderator variables in the link between coping and adjustment is a step in the right direction. Also, unique attempts at idiographic assessment (e.g, Large & Strong, 1997) merit further attention. Furthermore, stronger links must be forged with the broader social psychology fields of personality and coping research. We know remarkably little about normal personality development and coping with pain. Nearly all of the literature on coping with chronic pain has focused on mood and general psychopathology. Even factors such as neuroticism and depression, which have been linked repeatedly with poor coping, have been studied as correlates, not as developmental factors. Locus of control stands as one of the few dimensions of normal personality to be considered. The picture regarding personality and pain is somewhat different for acute pain, which can be studied readily in the laboratory with "normal" participants. But the link between acute pain in the laboratory and chronic pain in medical settings remains tenuous at best.

The problem of measuring the uniqueness of individual coping strategies also extends to the need for uniqueness of external criterion measures. Here the problem goes beyond the frequently mentioned confusion between coping and outcome measures. We also must be concerned that whatever constitutes adequate functioning for a pain patient could be as individualized as what makes up an adaptive-coping response. The issue is of greater concern with measures of functioning than it is for measures of mood state. Is it reasonable to use the same indicators of functioning for an elderly patient in a nursing home and a young person with fibromyalgia? Yet, in many of our multidisciplinary pain center studies one size fits all. In fact, I am unaware of any study that has attempted to study coping in reference to goals appropriately determined for the individual.

It would be helpful to have more studies of nontreatment seekers. Without doubt, there are many people who experience chronic pain but do not seek medical attention, and certainly most of these individuals have never been to a multidisciplinary pain center. Do those who do not seek treatment use the same or different coping strategies? How much do their pain-coping skills relate to the strategies used to manage other life stressors, such as marital or family problems, problems with jobs or finances, time pressure, physical danger, war, natural catastrophes? Are there common links between coping with pain and coping with the major demands and minor hassles of life? It could be that a nearly exclusive focus in past studies with patients characterized by poor adjustment leading to referral to comprehensive pain programs is a primary reason identification of positive coping skills has been so elusive.

More could be done to address the issue of causation in the study of pain coping. In most studies it remains unclear whether the coping strategies that are identified are a cause or a consequence of severity of pain and level of adjustment. Longitudinal studies of the coping strategies and recovery patterns of patients who sustain acute injuries (e.g., in an occupational medicine setting) would facilitate addressing difficult-to-answer developmental and mediational questions.

Because catastrophizing has become such an ingrained cognitive construct in the pain-coping literature, perhaps it would be worthwhile to study more closely those patients who demonstrate a low level of catastrophizing. If high catastrophizing is associated with poor functioning, the inverse also must be true. Are catastrophizing measures truly bidirectional scales? Might further positive correlates of low catastrophizing be identified and worked into a scale that is as successful at measuring adaptive coping as catastrophizing has been for measuring maladaptive coping?

Confusion created by conceptual overlap exists among the constructs of coping, pain beliefs and attitudes, and self-efficacy. This problem, which will be explored in the next section, can be addressed by a greater differentiation of cognitive and behavioral measures.

Future of Pain-Coping Measurement and Research

Over the next decade we should see pain research split into two distinct directions. One will become more theory driven and demonstrate closer ties to the academic psychology traditions of developmental and personality research. The goals will be to better explain pain coping in terms of general personality development and to identify common relationships among pain coping and other types of stress tolerance. What premorbid coping skills, or lack thereof, does the person bring to the pain situation? We know that poor coping is associated with increased psychopathology and decreased physical functioning, but because the vast majority of this evidence is correlational, the direction of the tie with coping is unclear. The required longitudinal research will be difficult, but efforts such as that undertaken by Karoly and Lecci (1997) are a move in the expected direction. For the purpose of linking pain coping with general stress-coping research, one can anticipate expanded use of such general coping measures as the CHIP and COPE scales.

The second direction will remain focused on the patient, but will more directly address the needs of the clinician. Patients' beliefs about their pain, their coping skills, and their moods are the crucial variables to monitor. The trend will continue to move toward beliefs, and coping assessment will become the primary form of routine psychological assessment of patients. Screening for standard psychiatric classifications will become secondary. However, clinicians, whose jobs require conducting cognitive–behavioral interventions, would like a clearer set of guidelines from the coping research than has been available. Currently, the measures used in most of the coping research are seldom administered outside academic medical centers. Much of the measurement remains theory driven and highly individualized to particular research settings. Additional work must refine and make available to clinicians convenient, reliable, and valid measures. Until such measures are well established and readily available, most clinicians will continue to assess their patients' beliefs and coping through interviews and informal behavioral observations.

Clinical assessment of chronic pain patients will become increasingly differentiated into subgroups of cognitive versus behavioral measures. Coping measurement will probably become increasingly behavioral, following the example of M. P. Jensen et al. (1995); cognitive self-report measurement will incorporate pain beliefs and attitudes, self-efficacy appraisals, and outcome expectancies into multidimensional cognitive scales. This division would help reduce the conceptual overlap between existing instruments. Cognitions that underlie both adaptive and maladaptive pain behavior would be clearly identified as such, and coping strategies would be limited to actual behaviors, presumably carried out in response to these cognitions.

Beliefs and Appraisals

Cognitive constructs, such as pain beliefs and appraisals, appear to be easier to measure and to validate than are coping constructs. A belief is always a cognition, but a coping response can be cognition or overt behavior. Arguably, there are probably fewer key pain beliefs that influence coping than there are ways of coping. Additionally, beliefs are easier to assess reliably in a self-report format than are coping strategies. Patients will readily acknowledge their beliefs about their pain and its treatment, whereas we can have less confidence that their self-reported coping responses are in fact the ones they actually use.

Beliefs can take many forms and can include beliefs about self-efficacy in control of pain and specific beliefs and expectations about etiology, medical diagnoses, diagnostic procedures, treatment expectations, and outcome goals (DeGood & Kiernan, 1997). An example helps clarify the operational meaning of the above terms and illustrates how patient beliefs can interact with actual behavior: Picture a patient with musculoskeletal back pain who has been informed that a particular set of stretching exercises can be helpful for managing such pain. The patient might or might not believe the information is accurate (treatment outcome expectancy belief). If he or she believes the information is incorrect, this opinion could be based on the belief that the diagnosis is inaccurate. The belief about diagnosis could stem from the belief that his or her examination was inadequate. Even if the diagnosis is accepted as valid and the recommended exercise as appropriate, he or she may question his or her own ability to perform such exercises (self-efficacy belief). If, after it has been demonstrated to the patient, this stretching is to be transformed into an actual pain-coping behavior, the individual must: (a) believe the prescribed exercise recommendation is reasonable and might be helpful, (b) believe he or she can do it, (c) actually perform the exercise, and (d) experience the perception of pain mastery as an outcome. The actual exercise behavior is of course the critical coping behavior, but the patient's cognitions regarding the behavior can be critical in the pattern of motivation leading even to an attempt at the behavior.

The differentiation between the cognitions' influence on behavior and the actual execution of the behavior appears to overlap with the concepts of "readiness for change" or "stages of change" (Prochaska & DeClemente, 1984), a model that has been successful in predicting response to treatment for several health risk behaviors. Kerns and his colleagues applied this model to chronic pain and developed the Pain Stages of Change Questionnaire (PSOCQ; Kerns, Rosenberg, Jamison, Caudill, & Haythornthwaite, 1997), a 30-item self-report measure with 4 reliable scales that assess stage of readiness to adopt a self-management approach to chronic pain. The scales measure attitudes and beliefs about pain in stages: precontemplation, contemplation, action, and maintenance. Kerns and Rosenberg (1997) did a preliminary study with 88 chronic pain patients who initially agreed to participate in cognitive–behavioral treatment. Of that group, the 37 patients who dropped out of treatment prematurely were found to have significantly higher scores (relative to those who completed treatment) on the precontemplation scale and lower scores on the contemplation scale before treatment. The PSOCQ, which clearly falls under the rubric of cognitive assessment of pain beliefs, appears to capture a dimension of considerable importance to the clinician. Further development of its predictive validity is currently under way.

Beliefs and appraisals have been more consistently related both to concurrent adjustment and to response to treatment than have coping strategies (see reviews by DeGood & Kiernan, 1997; DeGood & Shutty, 1992). Problematic pain beliefs appear to be more than artifacts of chronic pain that can be expected to disappear once correct diagnosis and treatment are found. Instead, maladaptive beliefs regarding diagnosis and treatment can become the internal reality controlling a patient's behavior. This makes assessment of such cognitive variables essential to treatment planning. In one early study of the direct link between pain beliefs and treatment outcome, Shutty, DeGood, and Tuttle (1990) assessed patients' agreement–disagreement with information presented in an educational videotape detailing multidisciplinary pain center strategies for pain management. Analysis of 100 patients indicated that those who did not believe that the information applied to their specific cases reported more pain and disability and were less satisfied with their treatment at a 1-month follow-up than were those who did agree with the personal relevance of the videotape presentation.

The only study to compare belief and coping-strategies measures as predictors of pain treatment outcome was done by M. P. Jensen, Turner, and Romano (1994). They found the correlations between changes in beliefs (before and after treatment) measured by the Survey of Pain Attitudes (SOPA; M. P. Jensen, Karoly, & Huger, 1989) and pre-to-post changes in measures of functioning to be higher and more consistent than were correlations between changes in CSQ-measured coping strategies and functional outcome changes.

This is not to say that one is more important than the other, but to illustrate that beliefs seem easier to measure reliably and with validity than are coping strategies. Beliefs also seem somewhat less influenced than are coping behaviors by moderating variables. Unfortunately, as is seen in research on coping, dysfunctional beliefs are more readily linked to poor adjustment and poor outcomes than adaptive beliefs are connected with good adjustment and outcome. Pain beliefs statistically found to be especially associated with poor treatment outcomes in our research (DeGood & Kiernan, 1997) can be expressed as follows: (a) My pain is someone's fault. (b) I should receive financial entitlements and work disability payments for my pain. (c) Emotion plays no role in my pain. (d) I have received inadequate medical care. Such beliefs must be addressed if treatment outcomes are to be improved.

Clinical Pain Assessment Format

Straightforward belief scales, such as the SOPA (Jensen et al., 1989), the Cognitive Predictors of Pain Treatment Outcome (DeGood & Kiernan, 1997), and the PSOCQ (Kerns et al., 1997), will gradually make their way into routine clinical assessment of pain patients. Cognitive–behavioral therapists eventually will have reliable indicators of which cognitions must be addressed and modified if treatment is to succeed. In the future, coping assessment will become more focused on specific behavioral coping strategies measured by self-report and systematic observation alike.

The existing instruments, such as the CSQ and the VMPCI, might continue to be used as research tools, but if they have a future in routine clinical assessment, it will be simply as checklists for providing clues to clinicians in planning interventions. For example, if a person reports a high level of catastrophizing, along with use of primarily passive or illness-focused coping strategies, a therapist may wish to explore this. How are these strategies helping or hindering the individual patient, given his or her unique circumstances? However, for all the reasons that have already been discussed, judgments about the quality of coping will not be made on the basis of the questionnaire alone in isolation from information about the person and circumstances.

One area in which existing coping strategies could continue as research tools is in the assessment of cognitive-treatment effects. Catastrophizing, and to a lesser extent the passive strategy composite from the CSQ, has been demonstrated to be reduced after cognitive–behavioral treatments, and such changes generally appear to be a correlate of improved functioning (Bennett et al., 1996; James et al., 1993; Jensen, Turner, & Romano, 1994; ter Kuile et al., 1995). Clearly, the reduction of the global helplessness that is so much a part of catastrophizing is an important goal for an intervention program. However, considering that catastrophizing could just as well be considered a cognitive appraisal as a coping strategy, it might better be incorporated into a cognitive beliefs–appraisal instrument.

Summary

This chapter describes the development of several measures used in the assessment of pain coping. For each measure, the degree of relationship demonstrated with psychological and physical functioning is discussed. On balance, composite measures of coping (scales that include several specific coping responses) are better at predicting functioning than are individual strategy measures, but composite measures are difficult to interpret and use for treatment planning. The pain-coping research has been more successful at identifying coping efforts that do not work well than at identifying what does work well. The most consistent finding concerning individual cognitive-coping strategies has been the relationship between high levels of catastrophizing and poor overall functioning. Other passive-coping strategies, such as praying and hoping and reinterpreting pain sensations, have not been proven particularly effective. Behavioral strategies of pain-contingent rest, guarding, and use of sedative–hypnotic medication similarly are of limited value. The most effective cognitive strategies appear to be the use of coping self-statements and, sometimes, engaging in distracting activities. The behavioral strategies of regular exercise, seeking social support, and task persistence tend to have some value when combined with other strategies, such as activity pacing.

For individual patients, the value of coping strategies is subject to many moderator variables. Almost any coping strategy will be useful for some individuals under a particular set of circumstances. This makes problematic the use of the current pain-coping-research instruments for individual clinical assessment. Several suggestions are made for strengthening the research, and speculations are made regarding the future of assessment in clinical and research settings. It is proposed that pain-coping research will become more closely linked with other types of stress-coping research. For purposes of clinical assessment, some of the confusion surrounding the construct of pain coping could be reduced by maintaining a sharper demarcation between cognitive measures (beliefs, attitudes, appraisals) and overt behavioral measures of coping efforts.

References

Abramson, L. Y., Seligman, M. E. P., & Teasdale, J. D. (1978). Learned helplessness in humans: Critique and reformulations. *Journal of Abnormal Psychology, 87,* 49–74.

Affleck, G., & Tennen, H. (1991). Appraisal and coping predictors of mother and child outcomes after newborn intensive care. *Journal of Social and Clinical Psychology, 10,* 424–447.

Affleck, G., Tennen, H., Urrows, S., & Higgins, P. (1992). Neuroticism and pain–mood relation in rheumatoid arthritis: Insights from a prospective daily study. *Journal of Consulting and Clinical Psychology, 60,* 119–126.

Arathuzik, D. (1991). Appraisal of pain and coping in cancer patients. *Western Journal of Nursing Research, 13,* 714–731.

Bandura, A. (1977). Self-efficacy: Toward a unifying theory of behavioral change. *Psychological Review, 84,* 191–215.

Bandura, A. (1986). *Social foundations of thought and action: A social cognitive theory.* Englewood Cliffs, NJ: Prentice-Hall.

Beck, A. T. (1967). *Depression: Causes and treatment.* Philadelphia: University of Pennsylvania Press.

Beck, A. T. (1976). *Cognitive therapy and the emotional disorders.* New York: International Universities Press.

Bennett, R. M., Burckhardt, C. S., Clark, S. R., O'Reilly, C. A., Wiens, A. N., & Campbell, S. M. (1996). Group treatment of fibromyalgia: A 6-month outpatient program. *Journal of Rheumatology, 23,* 521–528.

Boothby, J. L., Thorn, B. E., Stroud, M. W., & Jensen, M. P. (1999). Coping with pain. In R. J. Gatchel & D. C. Turk (Eds.), *Psychosocial factors in pain* (pp. 343–359). New York: Guilford Press.

Brown, G. K., & Nicassio, P. M. (1987). Development of a questionnaire for the assessment of active and passive coping strategies in chronic pain patients. *Pain, 31,* 53–63.

Brown, G. K., Nicassio, P. M., & Wallston, K. A. (1989). Pain coping strategies, and depression in rheumatoid arthritis. *Journal of Consulting and Clinical Psychology, 57,* 652–657.

Buckelew, S. P., Shutty, M. S., Hewett, J., Landon, T., Morrow, K., & Frank, R. G. (1990). Health locus of control, gender differences and adjustment to persistent pain. *Pain, 42,* 287–294.

Butler, R. W., Damarin, F. L., Beaulieu, C. L., Schwebel, A. I., & Thorn, B. E. (1989). Assessing cognitive coping strategies for acute pain. *Psychological Assessment, 1,* 41–45.

Carver, C. S., Scheier, M. F., & Weintraub, J. K. (1989). Assessing coping strategies: A theoretical based approach. *Journal of Personality and Social Psychology, 65,* 375–390.

Carver, C. S., Pozo, C., Harris, S. D., & Noriega, V. (1993). How coping mediates the effect of optimism on distress: A study of women with early stage breast cancer. *Journal of Personality and Social Psychology, 65,* 375–390.

DeGood, D. E., & Kiernan, B. D. (1997). Pain related cognitions as predictors of pain treatment outcome. *Advances in Medical Psychotherapy, 9,* 73–90.

DeGood, D. E., & Shutty, M. S. (1992). Assessment of pain beliefs, coping, and self-efficacy. In D. C. Turk & R. Melzack (Eds.), *Handbook of pain assessment* (pp. 214–234). New York: Guilford Press.

Derogatis, L. R. (1983). *SCL-90-R: Administration, scoring, and procedures manual* (2nd ed.). Towson, MD: Clinical Psychometric Research.

Dozois, D. J. A., Dobson, K. S., Wong, M., Hughes, D., & Long, A. (1996). Predictive utility of the CSQ in low back pain: Individual vs. composite measures. *Pain, 66,* 171–180.

Ellis, A. (1962). *Reason and emotion in psychotherapy.* New York: Lyle Stuart.

Endler, N. S., Courbasson, C. M. A., & Fillion, L. (1998). Coping with cancer: The evidence for the temporal stability of the French-Canadian version of the Coping with Health Injuries and Problems (CHIP). *Personality and Individual Differences, 25,* 711–717.

Endler, N. S., & Parker, J. D. A. (1990). *Coping Inventory for Stressful Situations (CISS): Manual.* Toronto: Multi-Health Systems.

Endler, N. S., & Parker, J. D. A. (1994). Assessment of multidimensional coping: Task, emotion, and avoidance strategies. *Psychological Assessment, 6,* 50–60.

Endler, N. S., Parker, J. D. A., & Summerfeldt, L. J. (1993). Coping with health problems: Conceptual and methodological issues. *Canadian Journal of Behavioral Science, 25,* 384–399.

Endler, N. S., Parker, J. D. A., & Summerfeldt, L. J. (1998). Coping with health problems: Developing a reliable and valid multidimensional measure. *Psychological Assessment, 10,* 195–205.

Folkman, S., & Lazarus, R. S. (1980). An analysis of coping in a middle-aged community sample. *Journal of Health and Social Behavior, 21,* 219–239.

Gil, K. M., Abrams, M. R., Phillips, G., & Williams, D. A. (1992). Sickle cell disease: 2. Predicting health care use and activity level at 9-month follow-up. *Journal of Consulting and Clinical Psychology, 60,* 267–273.

Gil, K. M., Edens, J. L., Wilson, J. J., Raezer, L. B., Kinney, T. R., Schultz, W. H., & Daeschner, C. D. (1997). Coping strategies and laboratory pain in children with sickle cell disease. *Annals of Behavioral Medicine, 19,* 22–29.

Gil, K. M., Thompson, R. J., Jr., Keith, B. R., Tota-Faucette, M., Noll, S., & Kinney, T. R. (1993). Sickle cell disease pain in children and adolescents: Change in pain frequency and coping strategies over time. *Journal of Pediatric Psychology, 18,* 621–637.

Gil, K. M., Williams, D. A., Thompson, R. J., & Kinney, T. R. (1991). Sickle cell disease in children and adolescents: The relation of child and parent pain coping strategies to adjustment. *Journal of Pediatric Psychology, 16,* 643–663.

Haythornthwaite, J. A., Menefee, L. A., Heinberg, L. J, & Clark, M. R. (1998). Pain coping strategies predict perceived control over pain. *Pain, 77,* 33–39.

Hill, A. (1993). The use of pain coping strategies by patients with phantom limb pain. *Pain, 55,* 347–353.

Hill, A., Niven, C. A., & Knussen, C. (1995). The role of coping in adjustment to phantom limb pain. *Pain, 62,* 79–86.

Jacobsen, P. B., & Butler, R. W. (1996). Relation of cognitive coping and catastrophizing to acute pain analgesic use following breast cancer surgery. *Journal of Behavioral Medicine, 19,* 17–29.

James, L. D., Thorn, B. E., & Williams, D. A. (1993). Goal specification in cognitive behavioral therapy for chronic headache pain. *Behavior Therapy, 24,* 305–320.

Jamison, R. N., Rudy, T. E., Penzien, D. B., & Mosley, T. H. (1994). Cognitive–behavioral classifications of chronic pain: Replication and extension of empirically derived patient profiles. *Pain, 57,* 277–292.

Jensen, I., Nygren, A., Gamberale, F., Goldie, I., & Westerholm, P. (1994). Coping with a long-term musculoskeletal pain and its consequences: Is gender a factor? *Pain, 57,* 167–172.

Jensen, M. P., & Karoly, P. (1991). Control beliefs, coping efforts, and adjustment to chronic pain. *Journal of Consulting and Clinical Psychology, 59,* 431–438.

Jensen, M. P., Karoly, P., & Huger, R. (1989). Development and preliminary validation of an instrument to assess patients' attitudes toward pain. *Journal of Psychosomatic Research, 31,* 393–400.

Jensen, M. P., Turner, J. A., & Romano, J. M. (1991). Self-efficacy and outcome expectancies: Relationship to chronic pain coping strategies and adjustment. *Pain, 44,* 263–269.

Jensen, M. P., Turner, J. A., & Romano, J. M. (1992). Chronic pain coping measures: Individual vs. composite scores. *Pain, 51,* 273–280.

Jensen, M. P., Turner, J. A., & Romano, J. M. (1994). Correlates of improvement in multidisciplinary treatment of chronic pain. *Journal of Consulting and Clinical Psychology, 62,* 172–179.

Jensen, M. P., Turner, J. A., Romano, J. M., & Karoly, P. (1991). Coping with chronic pain: A critical review of the literature. *Pain, 47,* 249–283.

Jensen, M. P., Turner, J. A., Romano, J. M., & Strom, S. E. (1995). Chronic Pain Coping Inventory: Development and preliminary validation. *Pain, 60,* 203–216.

Joreskog, K., & Sorbom, D. (1993). *LISTREL-8: Structural equation modeling with the SIMPLIS command language.* Chicago: Scientific Software Inc.

Karoly, P., & Lecci, L. (1997). Motivational correlates of self-reported persistent pain in young adults. *Clinical Journal of Pain, 13,* 104–109.

Karoly, P., & Ruehlman, L. S. (1996). Motivational implications of pain: Chronicity, psychological distress, and work goal construal in a national sample of adults. *Health Psychology, 15,* 1040–1048.

Keefe, F. J., Brown, G. K., Wallston, K. A., & Caldwell, D. S. (1989). Coping with rheumatoid arthritis pain: Catastrophizing as a maladaptive strategy. *Pain, 37,* 51–56.

Keefe, F. J., Caldwell, D. S., Queen, K. T., Gil, K. M., Martinez, S., Crisson, J. E., Ogden, W., & Nunley, J. (1987). Pain coping strategies in osteoarthritis patients. *Journal of Consulting and Clinical Psychology, 55,* 208–212.

Keefe, F. J., Jacobs, M., & Underwood-Gordon, L. (1997). Biobehavioral pain research: A multi-institute assessment of cross-cutting issues and research needs. *The Clinical Journal of Pain, 13,* 91–103.

Keefe, F. J., & Williams, D. A. (1990). A comparison of coping strategies in chronic pain patients in different age groups. *Journal of Gerontology, 45,* 161–165.

Kelly, G. A. (1963). *A theory of personality: The psychology of personal constructs.* New York: W. W. Norton.

Kerns, R. D., & Rosenberg, R. (1997, August). *Pain stages of change as predictors of pain treatment outcome*. Paper presented at the annual meeting of the American Pain Society, New Orleans.

Kerns, R. D., Rosenberg, R., Jamison, R. N., Caudill, M. A., & Haythornthwaite, J. (1997). Readiness to adopt a self-management approach to chronic pain: The Pain Stages of Change Questionnaire (PSOCQ). *Pain, 72*, 227–234.

Large, R. G. (1985). Self-concepts and illness attitudes in chronic pain: A repertory grid study of pain management programme. *Pain, 23*, 113–119.

Large, R., & Strong, J. (1997). Personal constructs of coping with chronic low back pain: Is coping a necessary evil? *Pain, 73*, 245–252.

Lawson, K. C., Reesor, K. A., Keefe, F. J., & Turner, J. A. (1990). Dimensions of pain-related cognitive coping: Cross-validation of the factor structure of the Coping Strategies Questionnaire. *Pain, 43*, 195–204.

Lazarus, R. S. (1966). *Psychological stress and the coping process*. New York: McGraw-Hill.

Lazarus, R. S. (1993). Coping theory and research: Past, present and future. *Psychosomatic Medicine, 55*, 234–247.

Lazarus, R. S., & Folkman, S. (1984). *Stress, appraisal, and coping*. New York: Springer.

Leventhal, H. (1993). Pain system: A multilevel model for the study of emotion and motivation. *Motivation and Emotion, 17*, 139–146.

Maes, S., Leventhal, H., & DeRidder, D. T. (1996). Coping with chronic disease. In M. Zeidner & N. S. Endler (Eds.), *Handbook of coping: Theory, research, and applications* (pp. 221–251). New York: Wiley.

Manne, S. L., & Zautra, A. J. (1990). Couples coping with chronic illness: Women with rheumatoid arthritis and their healthy husbands. *Journal of Behavioral Medicine, 13*, 327–342.

Martin, M. Y., Bradley, L. A., Alexander, R. W., Alarcon, G. S., Triana-Alexander, M., Aaron, L. A., & Albers, K. R. (1996). Coping strategies predict disability in patients with primary fibromyalgia. *Pain, 68*, 45–53.

McFadden, S. H. (1966). Religion, spirituality, and aging. In J. E. Birren & K. W. Schaie (Eds.), *Handbook of the psychology of aging* (4th ed., pp. 162–177). San Diego: Academic Press.

Morris, D. B. (1991). *Culture of pain*. Berkeley: University of California Press.

Newman, S. P., & Revenson, T. A. (1993). Coping with rheumatoid arthritis. *Bailliere's Clinical Rheumatology, 7*, 259–280.

Nicassio, P. M., Schoenfeld-Smith, K., Radojevic, V., & Schuman, C. (1995). Pain coping mechanisms in fibromyalgia: Relationship to pain and functional outcomes. *Journal of Rheumatology, 22*, 1552–1558.

Parker, J., McRae, C., Smarr, K., Beck, N., Frank, R., Anderson, S., & Walker, S. (1988). Coping strategies in rheumatoid arthritis. *Journal of Rheumatology, 15*, 1376–1383.

Parker, J. C., Smarr, K. L., Buckelew, S. P., Stucky-Ropp, R. C., Hewett, J. E., Johnson, J. C., Wright, G. E., Irvin, W. S., & Walker, S. E. (1995). Effects of stress management on clinical outcomes in rheumatoid arthritis. *Arthritis and Rheumatism, 38*, 1807–1818.

Prochaska, J. O., & DeClemente, C. C. (1984). *Transtheoretical approach: Crossing traditional boundaries of change*. Homewood, IL: Dow Jones/Irwin.

Regan, C. A., Lorig, K., & Thoresen, C. E. (1988). Arthritis appraisal and ways of coping: Scale development. *Arthritis Care Research, 3*, 139–150.

Revenson, T. A., & Felton, B. J. (1989). Disability and coping as predictors of psychological adjustment to rheumatoid arthritis. *Journal of Consulting and Clinical Psychology, 57*, 344–348.

Riley, J. L., & Robinson, M. E. (1997). CSQ: Five factors or fiction? *Clinical Journal of Pain, 13*, 156–162.

Robinson, M. E., Riley, J. L., Myers, C. D., Sadler, I. J., Kvaal, S. A., Geisser, M. E., & Keefe, F. J. (1997). Coping Strategies Questionnaire: A large sample, item level factor analysis. *Clinical Journal of Pain, 13*, 43–49.

Rosenstiel, A. K., & Keefe, F. J. (1983). The use of coping strategies in chronic low back pain patients: Relationship to patient characteristics and current adjustment. *Pain, 17*, 33–44.

Rotter, J. B. (1966). Generalized expectancies for internal versus external control of reinforcement. *Psychological Monographs, 80* (Whole No. 609).

Ruth, J. E., & Coleman, P. (1996). Personality and aging: Coping and management of the self in later life: In J. E. Birren & K. W. Schaie (Eds.), *Handbook of the psychology of aging* (4th ed., pp. 308–322). San Diego: Academic Press.

Schwarzer, R., & Schwarzer, C. (1996). A critical survey of coping instruments. In M. Zeider & N. S. Endler (Eds.), *Handbook of coping: Theory, research, application* (pp. 107–132). New York: Wiley.

Seligman, M. E. P. (1975). *Helplessness.* San Francisco: W. H. Freeman.

Shutty, M. S., DeGood, D. E., & Tuttle, D. H. (1990). Chronic pain patients' beliefs about their pain and treatment outcomes. *Achives of Physical Medicine and Rehabilitation, 71*, 128–132.

Smith, C. A., & Wallston, K. A. (1992). Adaptation in patients with chronic rheumatoid arthritis: Application of a general model. *Health Psychology, 11*, 151–162.

Smith, C. A., Wallston, K. A., Dwyer, K. A., & Dowdy, S. W. (1997). Beyond good and bad coping: A multidimensional examination of coping with pain in persons with rheumatoid arthritis. *Annals of Behavioral Medicine, 19*, 11–21.

Snow-Turek, A. L., Norris, M. P., & Tan, G. (1996). Active and passive coping strategies in chronic pain patients. *Pain, 64*, 455–462.

Spielberger, C. D., Gorsuch, R. L., & Lushene, R. E. (1983). *Manual for the State–Trait Anxiety Inventory.* Palo Alto, CA: Consultant Psychologists Press.

Strack, S., & Feifel, H. (1996). Age differences, coping, and the adult life span. In M. Zeider & M. S. Endler (Eds.), *Handbook of coping: Theory, research, and applications* (pp. 485–504). New York: Wiley.

Sullivan, M. J. L., & D'Eon, J. L. (1990). Relation between catastrophizing and depression in chronic pain patients. *Journal of Abnormal Psychology, 99*, 260–263.

Swartzman, L. C., Gwadry, F. G., Shapiro, A. P., & Teasell, R. W. (1993). The factor structure of the Coping Strategies Questionnaire. *Pain, 57*, 311–316.

ter Kuile, M. M., Spinhoven, P., Linssen, A. C. G., & van Houwelingen, H. C. (1995). Cognitive coping and appraisal processes in the treatment of chronic headaches. *Pain, 64*, 257–264.

Thomas, S. F., & Marks, D. F. (1995). The measurement of coping in breast cancer patients. *Psycho-Oncology, 4*, 231–237.

Thompson, R. J., Jr., Gil, K. M., Abrams, M. R., & Phillips, G. (1992). Stress, coping, and psychological adjustment of adults with sickle cell disease. *Journal of Consulting and Clinical Psychology, 60*, 433–440.

Tobin, D. L., Holroyd, K. A., Reynolds, R. V., & Wigal, J. K. (1989). Hierarchical factor structure of the Coping Strategies Inventory. *Cognitive Therapy and Research, 13*, 343–361.

Turk, D. C., & Rudy, T. E. (1988). Toward a comprehensive assessment of chronic pain patients: Integration of psychological assessment data. *Journal of Consulting and Clinical Psychology, 56*, 233–238.

Turk, D. C., & Rudy, T. E. (1990). Robustness of an empirically derived taxonomy of chronic pain patients. *Pain, 43*, 27–35.

Turner, J. A. (1991). Coping and chronic pain. In M. R. Bond, J. E. Charlton, & C. J. Woolf (Eds.), *Proceedings of the VIth world congress on pain* (pp. 219–227). New York: Elsevier.

Turner, J. A., & Clancy, S. (1986). Strategies for coping with chronic low back pain: Relationships to pain and disability. *Pain, 24*, 355–364.

Turner, J. A., Clancy, S., & Vitaliano, P. P. (1987). Relationship of stress, appraisal and coping, to chronic low back pain. *Behaviour Research and Therapy, 25*, 281–288.

Turner, J. A., Whitney, C., Dworkin, S. F., Massoth, D., & Wilson, L. (1995). Do changes in patient beliefs and coping strategies predict temporomandibular disorder treatment outcomes? *Clinical Journal of Pain, 11*, 177–188.

Tuttle, D. H., Shutty, M. S., & DeGood, D. E. (1991). Empirical dimensions of coping in chronic pain patients: A factorial analysis. *Rehabilitation Psychology, 36*, 179–188.

Vitaliano, P., Russo, J., Carr, J., Maiuro, R., & Becker, J. (1985). Ways of Coping Checklist: Revision and psychometric properties. *Multivariate Behavioral Research, 20*, 3–26.

Vlaeyen, J. W. S., Haazen, I. W. C. J., Schuerman, J. A., Kole-Snijders, A. M. J., & van Eck, H. (1995). Behavioral rehabilitation of chronic low back pain: Comparison of an operant treatment, an operant-cognitive treatment and an operant-respondent treatment. *British Journal of Clinical Psychology, 34*, 95–118.

Waller, N. G. (1989). The effect of inapplicable item responses on the structure of behavioural checklist data: A cautionary note. *Multivariate Behavioural Research, 24*, 125–134.

Wallston, K. A., Wallston, B. S., & DeVellis, R. (1978). Development of the Multidimensional Health Locus of Control (MHLC) scales. *Health Education Monographs, 6*, 160–170.

Weir, R., Browne, G., Tunks, E., Gafni, A., & Roberts, J. (1996). Gender differences in psychosocial adjustment to chronic pain and expenditures for health care services used. *Clinical Journal of Pain, 12*, 277–290.

Wilkie, D. J., & Keefe, F. J. (1991). Coping strategies of patients with lung cancer-related pain. *Clinical Journal of Pain, 7*, 292–299.

Wineman, N. M., Durand, E. J., & McCulloch, B. J. (1994). Examination of the factor structure of the Ways of Coping Questionnaire with clinical populations. *Nursing Research, 43*, 268–273.

Zautra, A. J., Sheets, V. L., & Sandler, I. N. (1996). An examination of the construct validity of coping dispositions for a sample of recently divorced mothers. *Psychological Assessment, 8*, 256–264.

Chapter 7
LOCUS OF CONTROL IN THE PATIENT
WITH CHRONIC PAIN

Janette L. Seville and Amy B. Robinson

Although chronic pain can lead to emotional and physical dysfunction for many individuals, other people appear to adjust relatively well to persistent pain. Social scientists have tried to isolate the demographic factors and individual differences that could predict who best learns to live with chronic pain and who has more difficulty accepting and managing pain. Stress and coping models propose that strategies of cognitive appraisal of stressors (perceptions of stressors) are linked to preferred coping styles (Lazarus & Folkman, 1984). Identifying these appraisal strategies and coping styles has been found to be useful in exploring differences in adjustment within pain populations (Turner, 1991). Using a model such as Lazarus and Folkman's as a theoretical base, researchers have focused on the perception of and response to pain as key parts of understanding how people cope with pain (Turk, Meichenbaum, & Genest, 1983).

Some effective psychologically and behaviorally based pain management interventions aim to alter the cognitive appraisal of pain and to improve coping style. Despite the efficacy of these treatments, not all patients respond well to them. Therefore, the examination of a variety of cognitive factors, and their interaction, continues in hopes of finding what might predict treatment success or failure. These complex factors include cultural norms for the expression of pain, the personal meaning of pain, pain-coping style, and the degree of control patients believe they have over pain. This chapter focuses on one area of this complex appraisal process: the perception of *locus of control* (LOC) related to chronic pain, that is, a patient's belief that he or she has some control over pain rather than the belief that pain can be controlled only by external factors such as fate, medication, or treatment by physicians.

Locus of Control Construct

The LOC construct was not originally applied to pain or physical symptoms. Rotter (1966) described the theoretical concept to better explain individual differences in learning processes (social learning theory). The method used to measure LOC was originally unidimensional, based on a 29-item, forced-choice self-report test. An individual's score represented the total number of external choices. Therefore, a low score would represent the belief that the respondent has control over his or her life and is considered to have a strong "internal" attribution or sense of control. Those with high scores believe their lives are controlled primarily by external factors, in-

The authors especially thank Tim Ahles, PhD, for his comments and suggestions in improving this chapter.

cluding chance, luck, the actions of other people, or other factors outside of their control. Rotter suggested that persons who view reinforcement as contingent on their own behavior ("internal control") are better adjusted than are those who see reinforcements as determined by fate, chance, or powerful others ("external control"). Specifically, Rotter (1966) stated that those who have a strong internal LOC are likely to

> (a) Be more alert to those aspects of the environment which provide useful information for his future behavior; (b) take steps to improve his environmental condition; (c) place greater value on skill or achievement reinforcements and be generally more concerned with his ability and failures; and (d) be resistive to subtle attempts to influence him. (p. 25)

These observations have important implications for chronic pain patients whose treatment usually focuses on learning more effective coping styles and new pain management skills.

The LOC scale was further developed by Levenson (1974), among others, who revised the Rotter internal–external scale to be multidimensional and yield three independent scales related to general beliefs about control over life situations. The three independent factors are: (a) *internality*, the belief that an individual's behavior influences his or her health status; (b) *powerful others*, the belief that the actions of other people, such as health care providers, influence health status; and (c) *chance*, the belief that fate or luck influences health status. Levenson's scale has been revised to specifically relate to perceptions of health (Wallston, Wallston, Kaplan, & Maides, 1976; Wallston, Wallston, & DeVellis, 1978).

Measurement of Health Locus of Control

Since its development, the LOC construct has been widely studied and applied to many clinical and research populations (Lefcourt, 1981). Rotter's original construct was recognized as potentially useful to explain individual differences in adjustment to chronic illness, but the unidimensional nature of the measure and the general wording of items did not apply adequately to medical populations. Wallston and colleagues (1976) created the Multidimensional Health Locus of Control (MHLC) scales, which specifically assess health-related beliefs across the same three independent dimensions used in Levenson's (1974) scale.

Patients whose scores on the MHLC reflect an internal LOC are likely to believe that health and illness are directly related to their own behaviors. Individuals with an external LOC, however, believe they personally have little control over their health, and they endorse items on the chance or powerful others scales. Wallston and colleagues described the MHLC as having greater usefulness for understanding and predicting health behaviors than the earlier, more general, LOC questionnaires. A debate exists, however, regarding the usefulness of two distinct external LOC scales. Umlauf and Frank (1986), for example, found that the MHLC scales for chance and powerful others were highly correlated—and therefore not necessarily representative of two discrete categories.

Although studies are not conclusive, health outcomes are thought to be more positive in persons who have strong internal control beliefs (Wallston & Wallston,

1982). Because attribution of control beliefs can vary according to different physical conditions, several health-related scales have been constructed for these beliefs in specific chronic conditions, including rheumatoid arthritis (Nicassio, Wallston, Callahan, Herbert, & Pincus, 1985), cancer (Dickson, Dodd, Carrieri, & Levenson, 1985), and heart disease (O'Connell & Price, 1985).

Measurement of Pain Locus of Control

Although many studies investigating chronic pain use the MHLC to measure LOC, there have been some that use questions specific to beliefs about pain control. One frequently used measure is the Pain Locus of Control (PLOC) scale (Appendix A) developed by Toomey, Mann, Abashian, and Thompson-Pope (1991), who modified the MHLC to represent pain rather than general medical health. The PLOC scale is a 36-item questionnaire that uses a 6-point Likert format with 12 items representing each of the three scales: internality, powerful others, and chance. The PLOC scale is scored by adding the item responses for each of the three scales. Split-half reliability has been found to be .89 (Penzien et al., 1989).

Another instrument was developed by Ter Kuile, Linssen, and Spinhoven (1993), who modified Engstrom's (1983) Locus of Pain Control scale to create the Multidimensional Locus of Pain Control (MLPC) questionnaire. The instrument contains 27 items rated on a visual analogue scale. A factor analysis of responses from Dutch patients who completed the MLPC questionnaire yielded four dimensions: (a) *internal*, (b) *chance*, (c) *physician*, and (d) *medication*. Internal consistency estimates of reliability ranged from .72 to .82 for the four subscales. Ter Kuile et al. (1993) acknowledged that, even though their population was limited to patients with chronic headache, they viewed the MLPC as "a generic measure of LOC for chronic pain patients in general" (p. 401).

The Headache-Specific Locus of Control (HSLC) scale (Martin, Holroyd, & Penzien, 1990) was designed specifically for the measurement of LOC in headache patients. The HSLC is a 33-item scale derived from the MHLC scale with items added by headache experts. Factor-analytic evaluation revealed three factors: (a) *internal*, (b) *healthcare professional*, and (c) *chance*. Internal reliabilities range from .84 to .88.

Other pain-specific LOC measures have been developed as researchers continue to adapt and modify earlier scales to improve the measures. In addition to the ever-changing measures, studies are often limited by the participant pool with which the measure was standardized. For example, Ter Kuile et al. (1993) used headache patients to represent a chronic pain population, and Martin et al. (1990) used college students with head pain. Although there are many LOC measures, there is currently no standard either for general chronic pain or for the various subtypes of pain (headache, back pain). Regardless of the lack of a standard measure, much research has attempted to better define the relationship between LOC and adjustment to chronic pain.

Locus of Control in Pain Populations

Theoretically, individuals with strong internal LOC perceive that they have control over their own pain and therefore function better than those with an external LOC, who perceive their pain to be related to chance, medication, or physicians. Those with an internal LOC would be expected to engage in more effective pain-coping strategies and self-management methods, and they could be expected to be less emotionally distressed than those who believe they have no control over pain. In fact, chronic pain patients who acknowledge a strong sense of personal control over their pain have been found to report less functional impairment (Spinhoven, Ter Kuile, Linssen, & Gazendam, 1989), less intense pain (Toomey et al., 1991), and less depression (Rudy, Kerns, & Turk, 1988) than do individuals who do not have a primarily internal LOC.

The research findings across studies, however, are not entirely consistent with this reasonable but oversimplified view. Several factors can interact with and influence the appraisal of control, including coping style, the pattern of the different control dimensions in relation to one another (a person can rate both high internal and chance beliefs), gender, and cultural factors. The following sections will address the factors believed to interact with the appraisal of LOC.

Coping Style

Based on Rotter's original theory, one would expect that persons who report an internal LOC would report less psychological distress and adapt better to chronic pain than would those with a high external LOC. There is some evidence to support this hypothesis (Harkapaa, Jarvikoski, & Vakkari, 1996), but not all positive findings are related specifically to the internal scale. For example, Crisson and Keefe (1988) found that chronic pain patients with higher external LOC, as measured by scales on the MHLC, reported more psychological distress and relied more heavily on previously demonstrated maladaptive pain-coping strategies (hoping and praying versus problem-focused coping) than did patients with low perceived external control. However, there was no relationship between either distress or coping style and the internal control factor. Buckelew et al. (1990) also found that pain patients' patterns of reporting control did not fit the expected pattern of having only one primary LOC. For example, one might expect that patients with high scores on the internal scale would likely have low scores on the external scales, or vice versa. Instead, Buckelew and her colleagues found that patients who endorsed both high internal and high external loci were less likely to use cognitive self-management techniques than were persons who reported only a strong internal sense of control. According to the authors, these findings support the use of a pattern analysis of LOC rather than just assuming the highest scale score is the primary attribution of LOC.

Predicting Pain Treatment Response

There are few controlled studies that investigate either health LOC or PLOC as a predictor of multidisciplinary treatment outcome. Those that do assess LOC tend to find that patients with a greater sense that their efforts can make a difference in their health tend more to engage in treatment and report better treatment outcomes. For example, in treatment outcome research by Harkapaa, Jarvikoski, Mellin, Hurri, and Luoma (1991), patients with stronger internal control beliefs had better treatment outcomes—as measured by better learning and more frequent practice of physical exercises during treatment follow-up—than did patients with lower internal LOC. Patients who did not follow through with the exercises reported greater psychological distress. In a subsequent study, Harkapaa, Jarvikoski, and Estlander (1996) found that patients with low pretreatment belief in powerful others reported significant positive changes in their physical functioning at a 12-month follow-up. Other research in multidisciplinary pain treatment found that positive treatment outcome (lower pain ratings) was associated with a concomitant decreased attribution to external control of pain and an increased internal sense of control (Lipchik, Milles, & Covington, 1993).

Culture and Gender Differences

Research investigating differences in culture and between genders generally supports the finding that both factors can affect responses to pain and illness (Lipton & Marbach, 1984; Riley, Robinson, Wise, Myers, & Fillingim, 1998; Tait, DeGood, & Carron, 1982; Zborowski, 1952). Few studies, however, explore these potential influences in relation to LOC and chronic pain. Bates and Rankin-Hill (1994) reported findings from a series of studies that qualitatively and quantitatively assessed LOC and pain in six ethnic groups across New England and Puerto Rico. They found significant quantitative and qualitative differences between ethnic groups and within those groups in LOC and pain reports. Their complex data cannot be fully described here, but one example of their findings was that 82% of a New England Latino group reported an external LOC, in contrast to a New England Polish group, in which 90% endorsed an internal LOC. Within the Polish group, however, those individuals who endorsed internality did not report less pain than did their counterparts who endorsed externally as one might have expected. In fact, the trend for pain reports was in the opposite direction. The "Old American" group (those who identified themselves as Yankees or New Englanders) was the only group in which those who endorsed a primarily internal LOC reported significantly higher pain than did those who endorsed an external LOC. Overall, Bates and Rankin-Hill reported that, across cultures, an internal LOC style is associated with lower pain intensity—except for the Polish and Old American groups.

Beyond ethnic or cultural differences, at least one study also has found gender differences in LOC (Tait et al., 1982). In New Zealand and U.S. samples they found that women in both countries reported less perceived personal control over their health than did men on the MHLC. The researchers concluded that "in both countries, however, women rated themselves as having less personal control over health than men, a finding that suggests men felt less helpless in dealing with their pain" (p. 59). Despite this conclusion, the only pain measure included in the study was pain duration, reported as a demographic variable. There were no other measures of pain or physical functioning reported in the study, so one cannot discern whether gender differences in LOC were actually related to more pain or less physical function. In contrast, Lipchik et al. (1993) found no differences between men and women on the PLOC scale in their treatment outcome study. Therefore, there is insufficient evidence to make generalizations about gender effects on LOC. Further exploration and understanding of gender and cultural effects on perceived control over pain is important because it could guide treatment considerations and inform clinicians about how to best tailor treatments to make them both culturally appropriate and personally relevant.

External Locus of Control

Many theorists hypothesize that it is important to have a strong internal sense of control, but much of the literature finds no strong relationship between an attribution of internal personal control and reduced pain and psychological distress (Crisson & Keefe, 1988; Toomey, Finneran, & Scarborough, 1988). However, there does appear to be a particularly detrimental relationship between a strong fatalistic attribution (high chance score) and the pain experience (Pastor et al., 1993). For example, chronic pain patients who view their outcome as primarily influenced by chance factors such as fate or luck tend to rely on maladaptive coping strategies such as catastrophizing or hoping (Crisson & Keefe, 1988). Moreover, an external LOC orientation has been shown to relate to increased levels of psychological distress, disease conviction, and pain report (Toomey et al., 1991). And when patients report a fatalistic attribution to their pain control (high chance score) they also report significantly higher pain ratings, less effective ability to use self-control coping methods, and poorer psychological adjustment than do patients who have low chance scores (Toomey, Seville, & Mann, 1995).

One explanation for the reason internality alone is not consistently related to improved coping is that, in many of the pain samples, the internal scores are generally low. Internal LOC scores have been found to be significantly lower than the internal scores of medical patients without pain, according to a study by Toomey, Mann, Abashian, Carnrike, and Hernandez (1993). They reported a significantly lower mean internal LOC score for pain clinic patients than for medical clinic patients without pain ($\bar{x} = 31.96$, $SD = 12.13$ vs $\bar{x} = 46.86$, $SD = 13.53$, respectively). This could indicate that there is a critical level, or strength of belief in personal control, that must be present to have a positive influence on a person's appraisal of the pain or to activate a patient into a more positive coping mode.

Beliefs, Learned Helplessness, and Depression

Depression is a frequent problem in chronic pain populations (see Fishbain, Cutler, Rosomoff, & Rosomoff, 1997, for a review of depression and pain literature) and could be linked, in part, to feelings of learned helplessness (Seligman, 1975) and loss of control associated with pain and physical limitations. The potential for developing learned helplessness (Abramson, Seligman, & Teasdale, 1978) is high in chronic pain patients because of the high probability that they will repeatedly experience situations in which they perceive little or no control over their pain. There also are several other stressful factors, such as financial concerns, decreased ability to work, and reduced ability to fulfill family expectations, that can add to the perception of low control over one's life situation.

Major depression is clearly prevalent in clinical pain populations, but some investigators have observed that pain and depression are sometimes mistaken for one another (Fordyce, 1978) and that there is not always a concordance between clinical impressions of mood during a clinical interview and scores on standardized depression inventories (Crown & Crown, 1973). Skevington (1983) suggested that one explanation for this lack of concordance is that "those in pain are reporting learned helplessness rather than a fully blown depressive syndrome (Becker, 1977)" (p. 309). She also noted that pain patients who feel "universally" helpless report more pain and depression. Patients can certainly develop a clinical depression after enduring pain for a period of time and feeling helpless over its control. Evidence for this causal assumption (depression most often develops after pain begins) is outlined by Fishbain and colleagues (1997) in their review article. A further consideration for LOC researchers is that when patients are already depressed they sometimes report low internal LOC in relation to most life factors, including pain.

Even if patients who feel they have little control do not develop depression there can be other detrimental effects. Learned helplessness theory would predict that as chronic pain patients feel less control and more helplessness they will have decreased motivation to learn cognitive or behavioral ways of controlling their pain and engage less in physical reactivation activities. This is supported, in part, by research indicating that patients who feel little personal control tend to rely on maladaptive pain-coping strategies (Crisson & Keefe, 1988). Furthermore, high internality is associated with increased adherence to physical training programs and preventive behavior (Dishman, Ickes, & Morgan, 1980; Harkapaa, Jarvikoski, & Hurri, 1989; O'Connell & Price, 1982).

Locus of Control Stability

Changing Locus of Control with Multidisciplinary Interventions

Some view appraisal of control as a stable adult personality trait (Rotter, 1966), but there is evidence that pain LOC can be altered through multidisciplinary intervention. Lipchik and colleagues (1993) assessed patients before and after treatment in a 3–4 week inpatient program and found that all three dimensions of control were changed in the expected direction after treatment (Table 7.1). That is, patients reported increases in internal PLOC scores and decreases in the chance and powerful others scales. Patients' LOC can change for naturalistic reasons as well during the course of the pain experience.

Other Factors Influence Locus of Control

Beyond the changes in LOC that can result from multidisciplinary pain interventions, there are apparently other factors that influence the stability of LOC reports. More specifically, LOC can change naturalistically over time for several reasons. Qualitative research by Bates and Rankin-Hill (1994) found a pattern in the retrospective reports of pain patients:

> The majority of patients reported that the first 6–24 months of the chronic pain experience necessitated severe changes in lifestyle, and often involved a sense of having lost control of one's life. However, after this initial period, the patients seemed to diverge into two groups. (p. 638)

Table 7.1—*PLOC and Pain Scores Before and After Inpatient Pain Treatment*

Measure	Control Group		Treatment Group	
	Before Treatment	After Treatment	Before Treatment	After Treatment
PLOC Internal				
M	31.63	31.15	33.26	47.02*
SD	8.76	9.16	9.94	9.26
PLOC Powerful Others				
M	30.91	33.02	28.72	21.40*
SD	7.45	8.73	8.40	7.31
PLOC Chance				
M	31.85	32.43	28.70	21.58*
SD	7.13	7.91	7.99	7.08
Pain Intensity				
M	6.52	6.03	7.05	4.15*
SD	2.08	2.10	2.13	2.82

Note. PLOC = Pain Locus of Control Scale; pain intensity = 0–10 (Likert scale).

*$p < .001$. From Lipchik, G., Milles, K., & Covington, E. (1993). Effects of multidisciplinary pain management treatment on locus of control and pain beliefs in chronic nonterminal pain. *Clinical Journal of Pain, 9*, 49–57. Copyright 1993.

One group was identified as those who gradually regained a sense of control and tried to return to work, stopped taking pain medication, and tried to use adaptive-coping strategies. The other group apparently continued to struggle with managing life with pain. These naturalistic and longitudinal changes in perception of control have yet to be adequately understood in relation to positive adjustment to chronic pain. Many researchers (e.g., Crisson & Keefe, 1988), however, have suggested that early cognitive and behavioral interventions to increase perceived control over pain is the key to effective management of chronic pain.

There could be experience-based mediating factors that influence individual perceptions of LOC. For example, chronic pain patients with a history of abuse (sexual and physical) have been found, in at least one study, to have significantly higher PLOC chance scores, increased psychological distress, and higher frequency of emergency room visits over the course of a year than did pain patients without an abuse history (Toomey, Seville, Mann, Abashian, & Grant, 1995). In addition, the patients with a history of abuse reported significantly less self-rated "resourcefulness" (ability to cope) than did nonabused patients. However, the abused patients, when compared with the nonabused, chronic pain patients, did not report significantly higher pain ratings or functional interference with daily activities. Taken together, these results indicate that individuals with trauma histories might not rate their pain or disability as any worse than would individuals without trauma histories, but they report feeling less control over pain, they seek emergency health care more often, and they are much more emotionally distressed. Based on the findings of this study and others (e.g., Bolstad & Zinbarg, 1997), it can be hypothesized that previous unpredictable negative experiences, such as abuse, are likely to shape perceptions of personal control over many life experiences, including pain.

Although not addressed in the current literature, it is also likely that self-report of LOC is influenced by the quality of care patients receive for their pain. For example, patients who experience poor communication with their physicians could be more likely (at the time of a visit) to endorse an external LOC (chance or powerful other). This could be especially true if patients believe the physicians are stating that nothing can be done for the pain or that there is "nothing physically wrong" with them. One cannot assume that patients are well-educated about their conditions or that treatment options are always explained adequately to allow patients to be active participants in their health care and thereby to increase their sense of control and ability to effect change.

Implications for Research and Clinical Practice

The investigation of LOC has significantly added to the understanding of the effect of chronic pain on individuals' perception of personal control. It has also led to improvements in effective pain management for persons with chronic pain. The complex interaction of cognition and behavior has yet to be clearly understood, but the appraisal of personal control is likely to be an important factor in this pain model. Better understanding of individual differences influencing LOC will likely inform clinicians how to effectively help patients reduce their physical and affective distress and help predict treatment outcome.

A further step in the direction of improving our understanding of the role of perceived LOC includes the development of standardized pain LOC measures that are demonstrated to be valid and reliable across different pain populations as well as between genders, cultures, and races. It is difficult to make inferences across studies when each researcher uses a different measure of LOC. Measurement problems are not isolated to the LOC construct. Main and Waddell (1991) compared several cognitive measures of control and coping in a sample of pain patients and found considerable intercorrelation of the measures. They concluded that there are "a number of psychometric weaknesses in current cognitive measures (p. 296)." Even the most frequently used measure of control, the MHLC, was not found to have a replicable factor structure. Therefore, the development of a "gold standard" of measurement is needed that is relevant to chronic pain patients. It would be particularly valuable for it to be sensitive to treatment effects as well as to changes over time because of the natural course of changing appraisal of pain and associated disability. As better assessment measures are established and applied in clinical situations, treatment effectiveness also will improve. If the role of perceived control can be understood better, more effective individualized treatments can be developed to help patients shift their view of pain control to a more adaptive and personally relevant way.

Another area of research that would be useful is that of determining the nature of the interaction between cognitive factors. Although the research data generally support that an internal LOC is associated with positive pain-coping efforts, there are no studies that specifically test the causal direction of this relationship. Given that multidisciplinary interventions often focus on encouraging problem-focused coping rather than passive types of coping, it could be that the process of engaging in new coping behaviors is the catalyst needed to shift the LOC. It also could be that multidisciplinary treatments improve self-efficacy in physical function, reduce depressive feelings, or reduce pain that results in changes in LOC. All of these physical and coping-style changes could either precede or follow a change in LOC. More research is needed to explain and use this complex interaction for assessment and treatment of clinical pain populations.

References

Abramson, Y., Seligman, M., & Teasdale, J. (1978). Learned helplessness in humans: Critique and reformulation. *Journal of Abnormal Psychology, 87,* 49–74.

Bates, M. S., & Rankin-Hill, L. (1994). Control, culture and chronic pain. *Social Science and Medicine, 39*(5), 629–645.

Becker, J. (1977). *Affective disorders.* Morristown, NJ: General Learning Press.

Bolstad, B. R., & Zinbarg, R. E. (1997). Sexual victimization, generalized perception of control, and posttraumatic stress disorder symptom severity. *Journal of Anxiety Disorders, 11*(5), 523–540.

Buckelew, S. P., Shutty, M. S., Hewett, J., Landon, T., Morrow, K., & Frank, R. G. (1990). Health locus of control, gender differences and adjustment to persistent pain. *Pain, 42,* 287–294.

Crisson, J. E., & Keefe, F. J. (1988). Relationship of locus of control to pain coping strategies and psychological distress in chronic pain patients. *Pain, 35,* 147–154.

Crown, S., & Crown, J. M. (1973). Personality in early rheumatoid disease. *Journal of Psychosomatic Research, 17,* 189–196.

Dickson, A. C., Dodd, M. J., Carrieri, W., & Levenson, H. (1985). Comparison of a cancer-specific locus of control and the multidimensional health locus of control scales in chemotherapy patients. *Oncology Nursing Forum, 12,* 49–54.

Dishman, R. K., Ickes, W., & Morgan, W. P. (1980). Self-motivation and adherence to habitual physical activity. *Journal of Applied Social Psychology, 10,* 115–132.

Engstrom, D. (1983). Cognitive–behavioral therapy methods in chronic pain treatment. In J. J. Bonica, L. E. Jones, & C. Benedetti (Eds.), *Advances in pain research and therapy* (pp. 829–838). New York: Raven Press.

Fishbain, D. A., Cutler, R., Rosomoff, H. L., & Rosomoff, R. S. (1997). Chronic pain-associated depression: Antecedent or consequence of chronic pain? A review. *Clinical Journal of Pain, 13*(2), 116–137.

Fordyce, W. (1978). Learning processes in pain. In R. A. Sternbach (Ed.) *Psychology of pain* (pp. 49–72). New York: Raven Press.

Harkapaa, K., Jarvikoski, A., & Estlander, A. (1996). Health optimism and control beliefs as predictors for treatment outcome of a multimodal back treatment program. *Psychology and Health, 12,* 123–134.

Harkapaa, K., Jarvikoski, A., & Hurri, H. (1989). Health locus of control beliefs in low back pain patients. *Scandinavian Journal of Behavior Therapy, 18,* 107–118.

Harkapaa, K., Jarvikoski, A., Mellin, G., Hurri, H., & Luoma, J. (1991). Health locus of control beliefs and psychological distress as predictors for treatment outcome in low-back pain patients: Results of a 3-month follow-up of a controlled intervention study. *Pain, 46,* 35–41.

Harkapaa, K., Jarvikoski, A., & Vakkari, T. (1996). Associations of locus of control beliefs with pain coping strategies and other pain-related cognitions in back pain patients. *British Journal of Health Psychology, 1,* 51–63.

Lazarus, A., & Folkman, S. (1984). *Stress, appraisal and coping*. New York: Springer.

Lefcourt, H. (Ed.) (1981). *Research with the locus of control construct*. New York: Academic Press.

Levenson, H. (1974). Activism and powerful others: Distinctions within the concept of internal–external control. *Journal of Personality Assessment, 38,* 377–383.

Lipchik, G., Milles, K., & Covington, E. (1993). Effects of multidisciplinary pain management treatment on locus of control and pain beliefs in chronic non-terminal pain. *Clinical Journal of Pain, 9,* 49–57.

Lipton, J. A., & Marbach, J. J. (1984). Ethnicity and the pain experience. *Social Science and Medicine, 19,* 1279–1298.

Main, C. J., & Waddell, G. (1991). Comparison of cognitive measures in low back pain: Statistical structure and clinical validity at initial assessment, *Pain, 46,* 287–298.

Martin, N. J., Holroyd, K. A., & Penzien, D. B. (1990). Headache-specific locus of control scale: Adaptation to recurrent headaches. *Headache, 30,* 729–734.

Nicassio, P. M., Wallston, K. A., Callahan, L. F., Herbert, M., & Pincus, T. (1985). Measurement of helplessness in rheumatoid arthritis: The development of the Arthritis Helplessness Index. *Journal of Rheumatology, 12,* 462–467.

O'Connell, J. K., & Price, J. H. (1982). Health locus of control of physical-fitness program participants. *Perceptual and Motor Skills, 5,* 925–926.

O'Connell, J. K., & Price, J. H. (1985). Development of a heart disease locus of control scale. *Psychological Reports, 56,* 159–164.

Pastor, M., Salas, E., Lopez, S., Rodriguez, J., Sanchez, S., & Pascual, E. (1993). Patients' beliefs about their lack of pain control in primary fibromyalgia syndrome. *British Journal of Rheumatology, 32,* 484–489.

Penzien, D., Moseley, T., Knowlton, G., Slipman, C., Holm, J., & Curtis, K. (1989). Psychometric characteristics of the Pain Locus of Control Scale [Abstract]. *Proceedings of the American Pain Society, 8,* 68.

Riley, J. L., Robinson, M. E., Wise, E. A., Myers, C. D., & Fillingim, R. B. (1998). Sex differences in the perception of noxious experimental stimuli: A meta-analysis. *Pain, 74*(2–3), 181–187.

Rotter, J. (1966). Generalized expectancies for internal versus external control of reinforcement. *Psychological Monographs, 80*(1, Whole No. 609).

Rudy, T. E., Kerns, R. D., & Turk, D. (1988). Chronic pain and depression: Toward a cognitive behavioral mediation model. *Pain, 35,* 129–140.

Seligman, M. E. P. (1975). *Helplessness: On depression, development and death*. San Francisco: Freeman.

Skevington, S. (1983). Chronic pain and depression: Universal or personal helplessness. *Pain, 15,* 309–315.

Spinhoven, P., Ter Kuile, M., Linssen, A., & Gazendam, B. (1989). Pain coping strategies in a Dutch population of chronic low back pain patients. *Pain, 37,* 77–83.

Tait, R., DeGood, D., & Carron, H. (1982). A comparison of health locus of control beliefs in low-back patients from the U.S. and New Zealand. *Pain, 14,* 53–61.

Ter Kuile M., Linssen, A., & Spinhoven, P. (1993). The development of the Multidimensional Locus of Pain Control Questionnaire (MLPC): Factor structure, reliability, and validity. *Journal of Psychopathology and Behavioral Assessment, 15*(3), 387–404.

Toomey, T., Finneran, J., & Scarborough, W. (1988). Clinical features of health locus of control beliefs in chronic facial pain patients. *Clinical Journal of Pain, 3,* 213–218.

Toomey, T. C., Mann, J. D., Abashian, S., Carnrike, C. L., & Hernandez, J. T. (1993). Pain locus of control scores in chronic pain patients and medical clinic patients with and without pain. *Clinical Journal of Pain, 9,* 242–247.

Toomey, T. C., Mann, J. D., Abashian, S., & Thompson-Pope, S. (1991). Relationship between perceived self-control of pain, pain description and functioning. *Pain, 45,* 129–133.

Toomey, T. C., Mann, J. D., Abashian, S., & Thompson-Pope, S. (1993). Pain locus of control scale. Unpublished.

Toomey, T. C., Seville, J. L., & Mann, J. D. (1995). Pain Locus of Control scale: Relationship to pain description, self-control skills and psychological symptoms. *Pain Clinic, 8*(4), 315–322.

Toomey, T., Seville, J., Mann, J. D., Abashian, S., & Grant, J. (1995). Relationship of sexual and physical abuse to pain description, coping, and psychological distress in a chronic pain sample. *Clinical Journal of Pain, 11,* 307–315.

Turk, D., Meichenbaum, D., & Genest, M. (1983). *Pain and behavioral medicine: A cognitive–behavioral perspective.* New York: Guilford Press.

Turner, J. A. (1991). Coping and chronic pain. In M. Bond, J. E. Charlton, & C. J. Woolfe (Eds.), *Pain research and clinical management* (Proceedings of the VI World Congress on Pain, Vol. 4, pp. 219–227). New York: Elsevier.

Umlauf, R. L., & Frank, R. G. (1986). Multidimensional health locus of control in a rehabilitation setting. *Journal of Clinical Psychology, 42,* 126–128.

Wallston, K. A., & Wallston, R. F. (1982). Who is responsible for your health? The construct of health locus of control. In G. Sanders & J. Suls (Eds.), *Social psychology of health and illness* (pp. 65–95). Hillsdale, NJ: Erlbaum.

Wallston, K. A., Wallston, R. F., & DeVellis (1978). Development of the Multidimensional Health Locus of Control (MHLC) scales. *Health Education Monographs, 6,* 160–170.

Wallston, K. A., Wallston, R. F., Kaplan, G., & Maides, S. A. (1976). Development and validation of the Health Locus of Control Scale. *Journal of Consulting and Clinical Psychology, 44,* 580–585.

Zborowski, M. (1952). Cultural components in responses to pain. *Journal of Social Issues, 8,* 16–32.

APPENDIX 7.A

Pain Locus of Control Scale

This is a questionnaire designed to determine the way in which different people view pain and what makes it worse of better (relieves it). Each item is a brief statement with which you may agree or disagree. Beside each statement is a scale which ranges from *strongly disagree* (1) to *strongly agree* (6). For each item we would like you to circle the number that represents the extent to which you disagree or agree with the statement. The more strongly you disagree with a statement, the lower will be the number you circle. Please make sure that you answer every item and that you circle *only one* number per item. This is a measure of your personal beliefs; obviously, there are no right or wrong answers.

Please answer these items carefully, but do not spend too much time on any one item. As much as you can, try to respond to each item independently. When making your choice, do not be influenced by your previous choices. It is important that you respond according to your actual beliefs and not according to how you feel you should believe or how you think we want you to believe.

Modified by T. C. Toomey, J. D. Mann, S. Abashian, & S. Thompson-Pope (1993). Printed by permission of surviving senior author, J. D. Mann.

	Strongly Disagree	Moderately Disagree	Slightly Disagree	Slightly Agree	Moderately Agree	Strongly Agree
1. If my pain gets worse, it is my own behavior which determines how soon I will get relief.	1	2	3	4	5	6
2. No matter what I do, if my pain is going to get worse, it will get worse.	1	2	3	4	5	6
3. Having regular contact with my physician is the best way for me to avoid my pain getting worse.	1	2	3	4	5	6
4. Most things that affect my relief of pain happen to me by accident.	1	2	3	4	5	6
5. Whenever my pain gets worse, I should consult a medically trained professional.	1	2	3	4	5	6
6. I am in control of relieving my pain.	1	2	3	4	5	6
7. My family has a lot to do with my pain getting worse or better.	1	2	3	4	5	6
8. When my pain gets worse I am to blame.	1	2	3	4	5	6
9. Luck plays a big part in determining how soon my pain is relieved.	1	2	3	4	5	6
10. Health professionals control relief of pain.	1	2	3	4	5	6
11. When my pain is relieved, it is largely a matter of good fortune.	1	2	3	4	5	6
12. The main thing that affects relief of my pain is what I myself do.	1	2	3	4	5	6
13. If I take care of myself, I can relieve my pain.	1	2	3	4	5	6
14. When my pain is relieved, it's usually because other people (for example, doctors, nurses, family, friends) have been taking good care of me.	1	2	3	4	5	6
15. No matter what I do, my pain is likely to get worse.	1	2	3	4	5	6
16. If it's meant to be, I will have relief from pain.	1	2	3	4	5	6
17. If I take the right actions, I can relieve my pain.	1	2	3	4	5	6
18. Regarding relief of my pain, I can only do what my doctor tells me to do.	1	2	3	4	5	6
19. If my pain gets worse, I have the power to relieve it.	1	2	3	4	5	6
20. Often I feel that no matter what I do, if pain is going to get worse, it will get worse.	1	2	3	4	5	6

	1	2	3	4	5	6
21. If I see an excellent doctor regularly, my pain is less likely to get worse.	1	2	3	4	5	6
22. It seems that relief from pain is greatly influenced by accidental happenings.	1	2	3	4	5	6
23. I can only relieve my pain by consulting health professionals.	1	2	3	4	5	6
24. I am directly responsible for relief of my pain.	1	2	3	4	5	6
25. Other people play a big part in whether my pain gets better or worse.	1	2	3	4	5	6
26. Whatever makes my pain worse is my own fault.	1	2	3	4	5	6
27. When my pain gets worse, I just have to let nature run its course.	1	2	3	4	5	6
28. Health professionals relieve my pain.	1	2	3	4	5	6
29. When I have relief from pain, I'm just plain lucky.	1	2	3	4	5	6
30. My relief from pain depends on how well I take care of myself.	1	2	3	4	5	6
31. When my pain gets worse, I know it is because I have not been taking care of myself properly.	1	2	3	4	5	6
32. The type of care I receive from other people is what is responsible for how much my pain is relieved.	1	2	3	4	5	6
33. Even when I take care of myself, it's easy for my pain to get worse.	1	2	3	4	5	6
34. When my pain gets worse, it's a matter of fate.	1	2	3	4	5	6
35. I can pretty much relieve my pain by taking good care of myself.	1	2	3	4	5	6
36. Following doctor's orders to the letter is the best way for me to relieve pain.	1	2	3	4	5	6

Note. The score on each subscale (Internal, Chance, Powerful Other) is the sum of all items endorsed on that subscale.

Internal Items: 1 + 6 + 8 + 12 + 13 + 17 + 19 + 24 + 26 + 30 + 31 + 35
Chance Items: 2 + 4 + 9 + 11 + 15 + 16 + 20 + 22 + 27 + 29 + 33 + 34
Powerful Others Items: 3 + 5 + 7 + 10 + 14 + 18 + 21 + 23 + 25 + 28 + 32 + 36

Chapter 8
EXTRAVERSION–INTROVERSION
AND CHRONIC PAIN

Jennifer M. Phillips and Robert J. Gatchel

This chapter discusses the way clinical researchers have examined the effects of the *extraversion–introversion* personality factor on chronic pain. The early research in this area focused on laboratory-induced pain, and although different researchers report different results, the consensus indicated that extraverted individuals are more tolerant of pain and have a higher threshold for pain than do more introverted people. Later studies began to examine pain—either acute pain (such as postoperative pain) or chronic pain—in clinical situations. Although variable results also are reported in those studies, the general findings have suggested that, even though extraverted individuals are more prone to complain about pain, they also paradoxically have a higher tolerance for pain and experience less pain in given conditions than do introverts. This would imply that extraverted patients are not at all shy in complaining about discomfort, even that which could be considered tolerable. It should be pointed out that, as pain becomes chronic, patients are more prone to develop social introversion, which then sensitizes them more to pain sensations. This chapter examines possible reasons for these relationships, and it reviews the importance of considering extraversion–introversion in the clinical management of patients with pain.

Early Research

Over the years, researchers have demonstrated that, although pain often has an organic, physiological basis, there are many other factors that contribute to the experience of pain and a person's reaction to it. These can include environmental and social factors, gender, age, race, marital status, and social support, as well as religious, cultural, and social beliefs. For example, one early review (Bond, 1971) cites the work of several investigators, such as Exton-Smith (1961), who found that older people tend to experience less pain than do younger people who have similar conditions; Merskey and Spear (1967) found that race affects both the threshold for pain and the degree of complaining associated with pain. They also found that the threshold for pain appears to be generally higher in men than in women. Bond and Pilowsky (1966) reported that, in clinical settings, the attitudes that nursing staff members have toward a patient's pain appear to affect complaint behavior. Finally, social support affects pain, with postsurgical patients who have supportive families showing lower pain associated with surgery (Gil, Ginsberg, Muir, Sullivan, & Williams, 1992). People seem to recover more quickly when they are able to call on family members and friends for support (Williams, 1996).

Emotional state and innate personality characteristics also affect individual re-

The writing of this chapter was supported in part by National Institutes of Health grants DE 10713-05 and MH 46452-05 to the second author.

sponses to pain, according to the early research (Bond & Pearson, 1969). Beecher (1956) reported that soldiers wounded in battle often did not experience pain until later, and then the intensity of the pain seemed to be related to how significant the person believed the wound to be. In addition, in studies by Kennard (1952) and Masson (1966), it is noted that when a person is anxious, there is an increase in pain. Cole (1965) indicated that some of the factors that appear to be related to the presence of persistent pain are anxiety, depression, and a lack of confidence in the doctor.

The above findings all suggest that pain is a biopsychosocial process, with biological, psychological, and social components all interacting in the experience of pain. Indeed, Turk (1996) has emphasized the heuristic value of a biopsychosocial perspective in better explaining the etiology, assessment, and treatment of chronic pain. It is because of the biopsychosocial nature of pain that people experience it in different ways. There is no common point at which every individual will experience pain in relation to a specific painful stimulus, and different people tolerate different levels of pain to different degrees. In addition, in diseases that are known to involve a certain degree of pain, some people will complain more, whereas others will complain less (Baum, Gatchel, & Krantz, 1997).

As one aspect of this biopsychosocial perspective, personality factors have long been thought significant in an individual's perception, experience, and response to pain. Researchers have investigated this relationship many ways over the years. Studies have examined the contribution of personality to pain that is either experimentally induced or measured in clinical settings. Clinically, researchers have studied pain that is more acute, such as postoperative pain, as well as chronic pain, including back pain, headache, and pain from cancer. There has been research on the relationship of personality to pain tolerance, pain thresholds, complaint behavior, and the perceived severity and intensity of pain.

Personality Theory and Pain

Theoretical Perspectives

A common theoretical perspective used to discuss personality is that originally proposed by H. J. Eysenck (1960), who divided personality into two main factors: extraversion–introversion and neuroticism–stability. He identified these factors as independent and uncorrelated, and he indicated that, together, they account for most of the variance in personality. Eysenck chose to break personality into the two factors rather than into many separate subvariables, because dividing personality into more factors leads to high intercorrelations (Stone, 1985). Both factors have been demonstrated to be significant in pain. The focus of this chapter, however, is on the unique workings of extraversion–introversion in the pain process. As defined by Eysenck, that dimension reflects social tendencies: People who are more extraverted are more outgoing, uninhibited, and socially active; introverts are quieter, more introspective, and more reserved (Stone, 1985).

Extending his theory of personality to pain perception, Eysenck hypothesized that extraverts have higher pain thresholds and are more tolerant of pain than are introverts. He explained this by suggesting that introverts operate at higher levels of cortical "excitation" than extraverts do, making them more sensitive and reactive to pain. In addition, he theorized that extraverts develop more reactive inhibition to pain. As a result, he hypothesized that exposure to prolonged pain leads to more adaptation or inhibited response to pain by extraverts than by introverts (Lynn & Eysenck, 1961). Beecher (1959) theorized that pain is accompanied by the fear of future pain—a conditioned fear response. It is thought that extraverts develop conditioned responses to a lesser degree than introverts do and, if so, this would apply to the development of conditioned fear responses. As a result, extraverts would not show the same response to pain that introverts show.

Measuring Extraversion and Introversion

Eysenck developed three self-report inventories to measure the factors defined in his theory of personality, each reflecting refinements in his theory and improving on previous measures. The first instrument—the Maudsley Personality Inventory (MPI; Eysenck, 1959)—provided a measure of the two personality dimensions of extraversion and neuroticism. The second inventory is the Eysenck Personality Inventory (EPI; Eysenck & Eysenck, 1968) updated questions and provided a Lie scale in addition to the measurement of extraversion and neuroticism. The Eysenck Personality Questionnaire (EPQ; Eysenck & Eysenck, 1975) measured extraversion and neuroticism as well as an additional dimension, psychoticism, reflecting the continued research and refinement of Eysenck's theory. Eysenck's tests have been reported to have moderate to good test–retest and concurrent validity (Drummond, 1985; Friedman, 1984; Stone 1985). Critics such as Stone (1985) and Drummond (1985) have noted, however, that because they measure just two broad personality factors, the tests are neither global nor comprehensive, and they should not be considered similar to multivariable measures, such as the Minnesota Multiphasic Personality Inventory (MMPI; Butcher, Dahlstrom, Graham, Tellegen, & Kaemmer, 1989) and the Myers–Briggs Type Indicator (Myers, 1977).

The Eysenck inventories have been the most widely used for examining extraversion–introversion in pain research, but others have been used as well. The Social Introversion Scale (Scale 0) of the MMPI measures the tendency to withdraw from social contact. Items deal with social participation and "general neurotic maladjustment and self-depreciation [sic]" (Graham, 1993, pp. 77–78). People who score high on this scale are socially insecure and uncomfortable; low scorers are outgoing, sociable, and extraverted (Graham, 1993). In a study by Jess and Bech (1994), scores from the MMPI were compared with scores on the EPQ in people with pain from duodenal ulcers. The researchers found that the Depression, Psychasthenia, Hypochondriasis, Hysteria, Schizophrenia, and Social Introversion scales of the MMPI all contribute to the dimension of neuroticism on the EPQ. It is likely that this finding reflects items on the MMPI Social Introversion Scale that address more neurotic features, rather than items referring to social participation, which would reflect the extraversion dimension on the EPQ. This finding supports Eysenck's argument against multivariable measures, as his dimension of neuroticism appears to contribute to many scales of the MMPI, indicating intercorrelations among the scales. It is argued, however, that with multiple variables, one is able to develop a richer picture of an individual's personality and so will have a better chance of understanding the subtle factors that contribute to the overall profile.

The MMPI and Eysenck's measures are the inventories used most commonly for assessing the personality dimension of extraversion–introversion in the pain literature, but others also have been used. For example, the Pittsburgh Scale of Social Extraversion–Introversion and Emotionality (PIT; Bendig, 1962) was used by Davidson and McDougall (1969a) in a study of experimentally induced pain. When compared with participants' scores on the MPI, however, the PIT was found to vary in its correlation with extraversion scores on the more commonly used measure. The Toronto Alexythymia Scale (TAS; Taylor, Ryan, & Bagby, 1986) was used by Millard and Kinsler (1992), whose results indicate a moderate reliability on this measure with the factors of social introversion and proneness to fantasy in a study group of people with chronic, nonmalignant pain. When comparing scores with the MMPI-2, the most significant correlation was with the Social Introversion Scale, indicating that this measure does appear to capture some aspect of that dimension of personality. The Marke–Nyman Temperament (MNT) inventory (Baumann & Angst, 1972) is another measure that has been used in several studies to measure personality factors, including extraversion (Schalling, 1970; Schalling, Rissler, & Edman, 1970). The Solidity Scale of the MNT is an indicator of extraversion-impulsivity.

The Revised NEO Personality Inventory (NEO PI–R) (Costa & McCrae, 1992) measures five major dimensions of personality based on the five-factor model of personality: Neuroticism, Extraversion, Openness, Agreeableness, and Conscientiousness (Digman, 1990). The authors defined extraverts as sociable, assertive, active, and talkative (Costa & McCrae, 1992). Several studies (Wade, Dougherty, Hart, & Cook, 1992; Wade, Dougherty, Hart, Rafii, & Price, 1992) have examined personality factors in chronic pain patients using the NEO PI–R and an earlier version, the NEO–PI (Costa & McCrae, 1985). A more thorough review of the use of the NEO–PI with chronic pain patients is presented in chapter 4 of this volume.

Finally, the Millon Behavioral Health Inventory (MBHI; Millon, Green, & Meagher, 1982) was originally developed for patients undergoing evaluation or treatment in medical settings for physical disorders. The MBHI provides information related to behavioral assessments and treatment decisions about people with physical problems. Scale 1 of the MBHI is the Introversive Style. For high scorers, it is suggested that health care professionals provide clear directions and not expect these patients to take the initiative in following a treatment plan (Millon et al., 1982). Obviously, this trait can have significant implications for the way a pain patient responds to a pain management treatment plan.

Laboratory-Induced Pain and Personality

Many of the original studies investigating the role of personality in pain, summarized in Table 8.1, used experimentally induced pain procedures. These included radiant heat (Davidson & McDougall, 1969a, 1969b; Haslam, 1967; Lynn & Eysenck, 1961), cold pressor (Davidson & McDougall, 1969a, 1969b), electric shock (Bartol & Costello, 1976; Davidson & McDougall, 1969a; Schalling et al., 1970), and pressure techniques (Davidson & McDougall, 1969a). All were designed to provide a painful stimulation that could be quantitatively measured in the laboratory and extrapolated

Table 8.1—*Studies Evaluating Laboratory-Induced Pain and Personality*

Study	N	Personality Measure	Pain Stimulus	Pain Measure	Results	Significance
Petrie, Collins, & Solomon (1960)*	61	MPI	Clinical pain; radiant heat	Tolerance	Extraverts had higher tolerance	$p < 0.05$
Poser (1960)*	8 F	MPI	Ischemic pain	Tolerance	Extraverts had higher tolerance	$r = 0.53$
Lynn & Eysenck (1961)*	30 F	MPI	Radiant heat	Tolerance	Extraverts had higher tolerance	$r = 0.69$ $p < 0.01$
Schalling & Levander (1964)*	20 M	MPI	Electric shock	Tolerance, threshold	No significant relationship	*NS*
Martin & Inglis (1965)*	48 F	MPI	Cold pressor	Tolerance	No significant relationship	*NS*
Levine, Tursky, & Nichols (1966)*	52 F, 29 M	MPI	Electric shock	Tolerance, threshold	No significant relationship	*NS*
Haslam (1967)*	16 F, 19 M	MPI	Radiant heat	Threshold	Introverts had lower thresholds	$p < 0.002$
Davidson & McDougall (1969a)	65 F	MPI, PIT	Pressure, radiant heat, electric shock, cold pressor	Tolerance, threshold	Extraverts had higher tolerance to shock, higher threshold to pressure	$p < 0.05$
Davidson & McDougall (1969b)*	60 F	MPI	Cold pressor, radiant heat	Tolerance, threshold	No significant relationship	*NS*
Vando (1969)*	80 F	EPI	Pressure	Tolerance	Introverts had lower tolerance	$p < 0.01$

(table continues)

Table 8.1—(*Continued*)

Study	N	Personality Measure	Pain Stimulus	Pain Measure	Results	Significance
Schalling, Rissler, & Edman (1970)	50	MNT	Electric shock	Tolerance, threshold	Extraverts had higher tolerance, threshold	—
Schalling (1970)*	18 F, 8 M	MNT	Electric shock	Tolerance, threshold	Extraverts had higher tolerance, threshold	$r = 0.40$ $p < 0.05$
Brown, Fader, & Barber (1973)*	52 F	EPI	Cold pressor, pressure	Tolerance, threshold	No significant relationship	NS
Bartol & Costello (1976)	24 M	EPI	Electric shock	Tolerance	Extraverts had higher tolerance	$p < 0.08$
Barnes (1975)				Tolerance, threshold	With probability pooling of studies,* extraverts had higher tolerance and threshold	tolerance $p < 0.001$, threshold $p < 0.05$

Note. *Cited in Barnes (1975); — = not reported; F = female; M = male; *NS* = not significant; EPI = Eysenck Personality Inventory; MNT = Marke–Nyman Temperament Inventory; MPI = Maudsley Personality Inventory; PIT = Pittsburgh Scale of Social Extraversion–Introversion and Emotionality.

to pain in clinical situations. However, different techniques were found to have different results in terms of pain reactions. For example, Davidson and McDougall (1969a) evaluated all four pain techniques and found a great deal of variability among different measures of pain tolerance. They pointed out that, when different techniques are used, different results are likely to be found. This ultimately led to variability in the literature, and these techniques were later used less frequently, or in conjunction with more clinical research.

Laboratory studies typically have focused on the measurement of pain threshold and pain tolerance. Pain threshold is the point during the administration of a painful stimulus at which it is responded to by the person as "painful." Pain tolerance is the point at which a person is no longer able to tolerate a painful stimulus, or the maximum amount of pain a person can tolerate. Each person's pain threshold appears to be relatively constant, but pain tolerance appears to be more susceptible to change and more likely to be affected by psychological factors (Sternbach, 1975).

One early study investigating the influence of extraversion and introversion on pain was conducted by Lynn and Eysenck (1961). This study used the MPI and a radiant-heat technique of experimentally induced pain. They found that extraverts were able to endure pain for a longer period of time than were introverts ($p = 0.01$), with the highest pain tolerance seen in people with high extraversion and low neuroticism scores. Similar results were found by Petrie (1960), who looked at "Reducers" and "Augmentors" and found that Reducers (equated with extraverts) have the greatest tolerance for pain. Bartol and Costello (1976) found that extraverts, as measured by the EPI, could tolerate more pain from electric shock than introverts could.

In a study of pain threshold using the MPI and a radiant-heat technique, Haslam (1967) found that pain threshold was significantly lower in introverts ($p < 0.002$). She explained this finding in terms of level of arousal, citing the finding of Shagass and Kerenyi (1958) that introverts tend to be more aroused than extraverts. Following this line of reasoning, if introverts characteristically function at a different level of arousal than extraverts, this could account for the difference in pain threshold noted between the two groups. Furthermore, if pain is perceived less at the extremes of arousal (sleep and excited states) and most during normal wake, then, as arousal increases, pain threshold will decrease.

Schalling et al. (1970) used the MNT inventory to study personality, pain tolerance, and pain threshold after continuous increase of electric shock. Both pain tolerance and pain threshold were significantly related to extraversion–impulsiveness and psychopathy scores on the MNT, with higher extraversion indicating higher tolerance and threshold for pain. In a similar study, which examined both continuous and discrete increases of electric shock, Schalling (1970) demonstrated that more extraverted and impulsive participants had higher pain tolerance and pain thresholds, replicating the previous findings.

Davidson and McDougall (1969a) examined tolerance to pain induced by shock, pressure, heat, and cold-pressor techniques. Using the MPI and the PIT, they found a positive correlation between extraversion and electric shock tolerance on the MPI, but not on the PIT. Pain threshold for pressure was significantly correlated with extraversion on both the MPI and PIT. The authors did not, however, replicate Lynn and Eysenck's (1961) findings using the radiant-heat technique. In a second study,

Davidson and McDougall (1969b), using cold-pressor and radiant-heat techniques, found no significant relationship between extraversion and pain tolerance.

Other studies also have failed to report a significant relationship between extraversion–introversion and laboratory-induced pain (Brown, Fader, & Barber, 1973; Levine, Tursky, & Nichols, 1966; Martin & Inglis, 1965; Schalling & Levander, 1964). Barnes (1975) reviewed the literature and found evidence that Eysenck's theory is inconclusive: Some studies support it and some refute it. By using the Fisher (1938) method of probability pooling (converting reported significance levels to chi-square values and running an overall test of significance) to compare studies, however, he found that the hypothesized relationship is, in fact, supported by the literature. The review of studies that examined the relationship between pain threshold and extraversion shows that the overall significance of the studies supports the relationship Eysenck hypothesized ($p < 0.05$). The overall significance of studies of extraversion and pain tolerance also supports the hypothesis that extraverts are more tolerant of pain than are introverts ($p < 0.001$).

Despite this positive finding, Sternbach (1975) noted that the problem with most experimental laboratory research on pain is that it lacks clinical usefulness. Beecher (1959) reported that most studies are not comparable to clinical situations because they fail to elicit the same emotional response. In addition, most use short-term pain despite the realtiy that clinical situations occur when pain is generally longer lasting or even chronic in nature.

Acute Clinical Pain Conditions and Personality

To address the above concern, researchers began to focus less on the artificial conditions of the laboratory and experimentally induced pain and more on pain in actual clinical settings. One way is to evaluate acute pain after surgery, with research focusing on the expression of pain, the amount of complaint associated with pain, and the use of analgesics. Studies have demonstrated that the expression of pain and pain complaints are at least partly associated with extraversion–introversion, in addition to other factors, such as ethnicity and cultural attitudes (Bond, Glynn, & Thomas, 1976; Sternbach, 1975). Pain expression, both acute and chronic, appears to be associated with extraversion; more introverted people tend to express pain less. Pain complaints, a more clinically relevant index of pain, appear to follow a similar pattern, with extraverts complaining of pain more frequently (Bond et al., 1976). Studies also have examined the need for analgesics postoperatively in relation to extraversion–introversion and found that analgesic requirements depend on several factors, including the type of surgery, anxiety, depression, and personality factors such as neuroticism and extraversion (Taenzer, Melzack, & Jeans, 1986). Table 8.2 summarizes these studies.

In the study by Bond et al. (1976), patients who were relatively more extraverted, as measured by the EPI, and who were undergoing back surgery were found to have significantly higher levels of postoperative pain ($p < 0.05$) than were more introverted patients, as measured by the self report of pain using a visual analogue scale, (VAS; Huskisson, 1983) in which the patient assigns a point on a 10 cm line to his or her pain according to severity. However, results of Dalrymple, Parbrook, and Steel (1972) did not demonstrate a significant relationship between extraversion and post-

Table 8.2—*Studies Evaluating Acute Clinical Pain Conditions and Personality*

Study	N	Personality Measure	Pain Condition	Pain Measure	Results	Significance
Dalrymple, Parbrook, & Steel (1972)	50 F	EPI	Cholecystectomy surgery	VAS, threshold (using pressure)	No significant relationship	NS
Bond, Glynn, & Thomas (1976)	26 M	EPI	Back surgery	VAS	Extraverts reported higher postoperative pain	p < 0.05
Tan (1980)	—	EPI	Postsurgery	—	No significant relationship	NS
Taenzer, Melzack, & Jeans (1986)	28 F, 12 M	EPI	Gallbladder surgery	VAS, McGill Pain Questionnaire, analgesic intake	Extraverts had higher analgesic intake; no relationship between pain and extraversion	NS

Note. — = not reported; F = female; M = male; *NS* = not significant; EPI = Eysenck Personality Inventory; VAS = Visual analogue scale (see page 188).

operative reporting of pain. Taenzer, et al. (1986) noted that conflicting results between early studies such as these were the result of several factors. One concern was with the use of different pain scales that had unknown interrelationships and that lacked information on reliability and validity. In addition, studies varied in terms of when the pain occurred in relation to when the psychological assessment took place, and samples both within and between studies were heterogeneous. All of this results in an inability to permit firm conclusions to be drawn from findings.

Taenzer et al. (1986) attempted to rectify some of the previous inconsistencies in their study of personality factors and pain in patients after elective gallbladder surgery, a procedure that produces moderate to severe postoperative pain. Using the EPI, they found that extraversion was related to analgesic requirements, with more extraverted patients receiving more pain medication after surgery. They found no other significant correlations between extraversion and pain using a visual analogue scale to measure pain, and the McGill Pain Questionnaire (Melzack, 1975), a 20-item self-report measure of pain. Tan (1980) reported similar findings: He also found no significant correlation between extraversion and acute pain. Instead, he noted that the two most important factors in predicting postoperative pain were trait anxiety and neuroticism.

Chronic Pain Conditions and Personality

In addition to examining acute postoperative pain, research in clinical settings has considered the effect of personality factors on chronic pain conditions such as pain associated with cancer, headaches, and low back pain. In Table 8.3 we have combined a series of early studies from Bond who examined the association between personality and pain in women diagnosed with advanced cervical cancer (Bond, 1971, 1973; Bond & Pearson, 1969). The first study (Bond & Pearson, 1969) concerned personality factors and pain, the communication of pain, and pain threshold, which they measured using a pressure device similar to those used in other laboratory studies. Using the EPI, they found that extraversion scores were significantly higher for cancer patients than for a control group of other medical patients ($p < 0.05$). They also examined the relationship between patients experiencing no pain, patients experiencing pain who did not receive analgesics, and patients experiencing pain who received analgesics. They found that unmedicated patients with pain had significantly lower extraversion scores on the EPI than did either of the other two groups ($p < 0.02$). When compared with other medical patients, extraversion scores were significantly higher in cancer patients without pain ($p < 0.01$) and in those with pain who received medication ($p < 0.02$).

Patients who experienced pain but did not receive medication also were found to have low extraversion and high neuroticism scores (Bond & Pearson, 1969). Neuroticism has been associated with arousal, with patients scoring low on neuroticism exhibiting low arousability, and those with high scores showing a high degree of arousability. Therefore, low extraversion and high neuroticism indicate introversion and a high level of arousal. Because the patients demonstrated low social participation and failure to communicate pain, they did not receive medication. Patients who did communicate their pain, and therefore did receive analgesics, were found to have high neuroticism and extraversion scores, indicating extraversion and a high

Table 8.3—*Pain and Personality Factors in Women with Advanced Cervical Cancer*

Patient Classification	Other Medical Patients	Patient Classification		
		Cancer Patients With No Pain	Cancer Patients With Pain, No Medication	Cancer Patients With Pain, Took Medication
Other medical patients		E lower in other medical $p < 0.01$	NS	E lower in other medical $p < 0.02$
Cancer patients with no pain	E lower in other medical $p < 0.01$	High E scores	E higher in no-pain group $p < 0.02$	NS
Cancer patients with pain, no medication	NS	E higher in no-pain group $p < 0.02$	Low E, high N	E higher in pain with medication $p < 0.02$
Cancer patients with pain, took medication	E lower in other medical $p < 0.02$	NS	E higher in pain with medication $p < 0.02$	High E, high N

Note. E = extraversion; N = neuroticism; *NS* = no significant difference.

degree of arousal. Millon et al. (1982) suggested that this personality characteristic —the Introversive Style as assessed on the MBHI—can have an important effect on how pain patients respond to pain management situations, including their willingness to communicate about their pain in a study such as that by Bond and Pearson (1969).

Bond and Pearson (1969) hypothesized that their findings could mean that cancer patients who do not report pain could be exhibiting a diminished state of arousal, a poor outlet for emotional discharge, or denial of anxiety about their illness. In addition, these patients, who have higher extraversion scores, also might therefore have high sensory thresholds. In agreement with Millon et al. (1982), Bond and Pearson found that extraverted patients tend to react in an outgoing manner to situations (as opposed to those with an introversive style). This also could apply to their health status and symptoms, leading to a diminished awareness of pain. They also might tend to complain more about pain or health problems. Merskey and Spear (1967) reported that extraverts tend to complain more and that introverts accept less physical pain or react sooner. Neuroticism and extraversion are linked by Claridge (1967), who noted that extraversion governs the psychological and social reaction to the state of arousal, thus linking it to neuroticism.

Bond and Pearson (1969) hypothesized that the presence of pain symptoms is related to neuroticism, whereas extraversion is important in determining the freedom with which those symptoms are communicated. They noted that this is important for analgesic needs, as the lack of a complaint might not necessarily mean that a patient has no pain. Rather, for any given illness at a specified stage and known to be associated with pain, some patients will complain and others will not. In his second study, Bond (1971) summarized his previous findings and noted that extraversion and introversion appear to be related to arousal and the concept of a cortical inhibition–excitation balance (Eysenck, 1967), with introverts exhibiting less cortical inhibition than extraverts. Although the presence or absence of pain in patients with cervical cancer appears to be primarily related to neuroticism in terms of personality, complaint behavior appears to be more related to introversion–extraversion (Bond, 1971).

In Bond's third paper (1973), he noted his previous findings with cervical cancer patients, but added a second study on the effects of surgical relief of severe pain in relation to personality. Patients who were to be surgically treated for chronic pain due to stereotaxic percutaneous cordotomy took the EPI before surgery, and those who noted complete and permanent relief of pain 5 days after surgery completed the EPI again. All patients tended to be introverted both before and after surgery, and the potential for social contact appeared to be unchanged by pain relief. This study, involving the change in personality associated with the surgical relief of severe intractable pain, suggests that changes in neuroticism overshadow introversion–extraversion. Evidence is shown of a divergence from the normal pattern of personality scores for both extraversion and neuroticism before operation, with a change toward normal after the pain was relieved.

Morasso, Costantini, Baracco, Borreani, and Capelli (1996) examined psychological distress in cancer patients. Using the EPQ, they found a positive correlation between psychological distress and neuroticism and a negative correlation with extraversion. The authors suggested that high scores on neuroticism reflect poor adjustment to the stress of having cancer. They further suggested that the lower levels of psychological distress found in patients with higher extraversion scores could be a function of these patients' interpersonal relationships.

Other diseases associated with chronic pain also have been studied (Table 8.4). In a study of women with endometriosis and other gynecological problems, Low, Edelmann, and Sutton (1993) found that women with endometriosis scored higher in terms of psychoticism, introversion, and anxiety than did other pain patients. These findings are in contrast to Bond's high extraversion scores in women with cervical cancer, which could indicate a sampling bias or suggest different personality profiles for different pain disorders (Bond & Pearson, 1969). Woodforde and Merskey (1972) studied patients with chronic pain secondary to neurological disease in comparison with patients with pain of psychological origin. They used the EPI, and their findings also contrasted with those of Bond and Pearson (1969) in that there was a tendency for the extraversion scores to be lower in their patients than in "normal" patients. This finding was demonstrated as well in a study by Robinson, Kirk, Frye, and Robertson (1972) of patients with rheumatoid arthritis, nonrheumatoid arthritis, and other chronic pain conditions with a nondiseased control group. Using the EPI and another measure of personality that does not focus on extraversion–introversion, but instead includes the factor shy–bold, the Sixteen Personality Factor Questionnaire (16 PF; Cattel, 1949), their results indicated that pain patients showed significantly greater introversion than do "normal" control patients. The authors hypothesized that the presence of a painful disease can lead to greater introversion manifested as more self-concern and withdrawal from social contact.

Additional chronic pain conditions of a more benign nature that have been studied have included lower back pain and headache, among others (Table 8.4). Snibbe, Peterson, and Sosner (1980) evaluated individuals who filed workers' compensation claims for head injury, psychiatric "stress and strain," low back pain, and other problems. Their results indicated that all groups showed characteristics of passive dependence, depression, anxiety, and social introversion. Using the MMPI, Ziesat and Gentry (1978) found that, in patients with chronic benign pain of various types, the Social Introversion scale was positively correlated with the Pain Apperception Test (Petrovich, 1973), a semiprojective measure that examines a person's feelings about and response to pain. The authors speculated that their finding could indicate that patients who experience chronic pain become increasingly socially isolated and assume the chronic invalid role as the condition continues.

Millard and Kinsler (1992) used the TAS in a study of patients with chronic, nonmalignant pain of various kinds, most frequently back pain (Table 8.4). They found that the two most significant factors that stood out on the TAS were social introversion and a lack of proneness to fantasy. When comparing MMPI-2 scores and TAS scores, the most significant finding was with the Social Introversion Scale of the MMPI-2 ($r = 0.49$). As people experience chronic pain, they begin to have difficulty recognizing emotions, and they experience constricted affect. One theory to explain this is that these people develop alexythymia, a cognitive deficit in the processing of emotions. In such cases, when an individual experiences any emotional arousal of an unpleasant nature, he or she does not recognize it as such. Instead, it can be experienced in terms of somatic symptoms, such as pain (Lane & Schwartz, 1987).

Several studies have focused specifically on common chronic pain conditions, particularly chronic low back pain. Huncke and McCall (1978) reported that ap-

Table 8.4—*Studies Evaluating Chronic Pain Conditions and Personality*

Study	N	Personality Measure	Pain Condition	Pain Measure	Results	Significance
Bond & Pearson (1969)	85 F	EPI	Advanced cervical cancer	Threshold (pressure), VAS, analgesic intake	Higher E in patients with no pain and with pain who took medication	$p < 0.02$
Bond (1971)	61 F	EPI	Advanced cervical cancer	VAS	(same results as Bond & Pearson, 1969)	$p < 0.02$
Robinson, Kirk, Frye, & Robertson (1972)	42 F, 17 M	EPI, 16 PF	Arthritis	Self-report	I higher in pain patients than normal controls	$p < 0.001$
Bond (1973)	52 F	EPI	Advanced cervical cancer	VAS	(same results as Bond & Pearson, 1969)	$p < 0.02$
	15 F, 15 M	EPI	Surgery, stereotaxic percutaneous cordotomy	(assumed relief of severe pain by surgery)	No significant relationship	NS
Woodforde & Merskey (1972)	22 F, 21 M	EPI	Neurological disease, psychological pain	Self-report	E scores lower in patients than in normals, no difference between types of patients	NS
Philips (1976)	56 F, 12 M	EPQ	Migraine, tension, mixed headache	Presence of medical symptoms	No significant relationship	NS
Ziesat & Gentry (1978)	2 F, 53 M	MMPI	Chronic benign pain	Pain estimate, Tourniquet Pain Test, PAT	High I correlated with high pain report	$p < 0.05$
Snibbe, Peterson, & Sosner (1980)	12 F, 35 M	MMPI	Head injury, back pain, psychiatric stress and strain, other	Self-report	Higher I in all	—

Study	Sample	Personality measure	Pain condition	Pain measure	Findings	Significance
Donham, Mikhail, & Meyers (1984)	40 M	MMPI	Low back pain	Staff ratings	Functional back pain patients rated as more introverted than organic pain patients	$p < 0.05$
Philips & Jahanshahi (1985)	360	EPQ	Headache	McGill Pain Questionnaire, Pain Behavior Checklist	Chronic headache patients that complained more had higher E; overall, headache patients had more avoidance behaviors	$p < 0.001$
Millard & Kinsler (1992)	124 F, 71 M	MMPI-2, TAS	Chronic benign pain	VAS	I associated with alexythymia	$p < 0.001$ $r = 0.49$
Low, Edelmann, & Sutton (1993)	81 F	EPQ	Endometriosis and other gynecological problems	VAS, McGill Pain Questionnaire	Higher I in patients with endometriosis	$p < 0.05$
Fan, Gu, & Zhou (1995)	64 F, 16 M	MMPI	Migraine	—	Higher I in migraine than normal controls	$p < 0.05$
Ziegler & Paolo (1995)	90 F, 14 M	MMPI-2	Headache	Structured interview	Headache patients seeking medical help more introverted than those not seeking help	$p < 0.04$
Morasso, Costantini, Baracco, Borreani, & Capelli (1996)	278 F, 156 M	EPQ	Cancer, variety of sites and degrees of severity	PDI	Negative correlation between psychological distress and E	$r = -0.34$

Note. — = not reported; E = extraversion; I = introversion; F = female; M = male; *NS* = not significant; EPI = Eysenck Personality Inventory; EPQ = Eysenck Personality Questionnaire; MMPI = Minnesota Multiphasic Personality Inventory; PAT = Pain Apperception Test; PDI = Psychological Distress Inventory; 16 PF = 16 Personality Factor Questionnaire (see page 193); TAS = Toronto Alexythymia Scale; VAS = Visual Analogue Scale.

proximately 80% of people in the United States will experience back pain at some point, and some of them will have chronic back pain. Love and Peck (1987) noted that people who report chronic lower back pain often report more pain and disability than appears to be warranted given their condition and that these individuals do not always respond to treatment. As a result, back pain often has been labeled "psychogenic," and premorbid personality characteristics were believed to contribute significantly to the condition. It should be noted, though, that the perspective that pain can be categorized as either psychogenic or functional is considered outdated and has been shown to have no empirical support (Baum et al., 1997).

Donham, Mikhail, and Meyers (1984) found significant relationships between ratings of pain by nurses and high scores on the Social Introversion scale of the MMPI, among others (Table 8.4). Nurses rated patients on whether they experienced "functional" or "organic" back pain, with functional pain being designated when clinical evidence is not sufficient to point to underlying organic pathology or when the symptoms reported contradict physical findings. When distributing patients on this functional–organic back pain dichotomy, significant differences were found on the Social Introversion, Depression, Psychasthenia, and Paranoia scales of the MMPI. Specifically, "functional" patients had significantly higher scores than did "organic" patients. Nurses described the "functional" group as more anxious, depressed, socially withdrawn, and suspicious. The authors noted that patients rated "organic" tend to have a more psychophysiological pain profile, whereas "functional" patients have a profile that is more somaticizing.

Headache is another common nonmalignant chronic pain condition that has been examined. Philips (1976) evaluated the difference in personality between people with headache and the general population, and between those with migraine and tension headache (Table 8.4). That study also examined whether headache sufferers who seek medical help are representative of all headache sufferers. Waters and O'Connor (1970) estimated that more than half of all headache sufferers seek no medical help. Bond and Pilowsky (1966) indicated that people who do seek help could tend to be more extraverted and more neurotic. Using the EPQ, Philips (1976) found no significant relationships between personality factors and headache sufferers. One explanation is that past findings might reflect only patients who complain of pain, whereas this study examined a sample of people independent of whether they had sought medical treatment or not.

Philips and Jahanshahi (1985) reported that chronic headache sufferers who complained more had higher levels of extraversion, neuroticism, and depression (Table 8.4). When these patients were compared with chronic back pain patients, the headache sufferers reported more pain behavior overall as measured by the McGill Pain Questionnaire and Pain Behavior checklist (Phillips & Hunter, 1982), in addition to more avoidance behavior, including avoiding social situations. They also had lower levels of help-seeking behavior compared with the back pain patients. Ziegler and Paolo (1995) studied the psychological characteristics of people who have headaches and who seek medical help, versus those who do not (Table 8.4). Headache sufferers seeking medical help were found to have significantly higher scores on the MMPI-2 on the Hypochondriasis, Depression, Hysteria, Psychasthenia, and Social Introversion scales. These results corroborate previous findings that these psychological factors are important in determining whether a person suffering from headaches will seek medical help. Finally, in a study of Chinese patients with migraine headaches, Fan,

Gu, and Zhou (1995) reported that the patients had elevated scores on the Hypochondriasis, Depression, Hysteria, Psychasthenia, Schizophrenia, and Social Introversion scales of the Chinese version of the MMPI (Table 8.4). Their results are similar to findings noted for patients seeking medical treatment for headache pain.

Summary and Conclusions

Research suggests that some individuals are more predisposed than others to experience symptoms of pain (Donham et al., 1984). Sternbach (1977) noted that many processes are involved in the complaint of pain, including physical and psychosocial processes, which are equally likely to play a part in the experience of pain. In addition to the physiological contribution, pain is affected by a person's ethnic background and by the levels of extraversion and neuroticism. Pain is clearly a biopsychosocial process, and all of these aspects are integral to the way a person experiences and reacts to pain. It is not likely that just one factor will account for all the variance or fully explain individual susceptibility or reactivity to pain conditions. Indeed, in the area of personality test interpretation in general, although a particular scale elevation serves to identify a specific trait or behavior, its utility is greatly enhanced when multiple scales are analyzed as a constellation, or profile, of scale scores (Baum et al., 1997).

This chapter examines research conducted over the past 40 years in the field of pain research, examining the personality factor of extraversion–introversion in the experience of pain. In general, this is a field that was most heavily researched in the 1960s and 1970s; interest has declined in more recent years. The earliest work used Eysenck's personality theory, which delineates two primary factors of personality—Extraversion–Introversion and Neuroticism–Stability. More recent research has primarily used the MMPI and other personality measures.

Most of the earliest research was done in the laboratory, using experimentally induced pain and extrapolating the results to explain clinical pain. With continued research suggesting that the results were not comparable to clinical situations, however, researchers began to turn away from laboratory studies. The clinical work has yielded varied results, but with the general finding that people who complain more about pain, who have higher tolerance for pain, and who have higher pain thresholds appear to be more extraverted. This has been demonstrated in clinical and experimental situations and across various pain conditions. In addition, it appears that as pain becomes more chronic in nature, higher introversion scores are seen.

It appears that extraversion–introversion is a factor that contributes to the pain phenomenon. However, it is just one of many factors that can affect how a person experiences and responds to pain. Baum et al. (1997), for example, identified mediators of stress to include social support, exercise, dispositional variables, and control. This idea can be applied to pain as well, with extraversion perhaps constituting one of several mediating variables that affect pain. It also appears that there are many factors related to extraversion–introversion that affect pain. Perhaps one way to explain the potential significance of this idea is to view extraversion as consisting of several covariates. In this way, it includes many factors that influence a person's reaction to pain, including reactive inhibition to pain, increased social support, increased expression of feelings, and social activity.

It has been noted that extraversion–introversion measures social tendencies: Extraverted individuals are more socially active, and introverts are more withdrawn. Therefore, it makes sense that where a person falls on this dimension could be related to the amount of social support he or she receives, thus making social support a covariate of extraversion. Extraverts could be more likely to have the resources to call on social support when they experience pain, whereas introverts might be more likely to remain isolated, failing to gather the social support they need. Indeed, social support has clearly been demonstrated to aid in decreasing stress, and stress has been shown to be a mediating variable in the experience of pain (Baum et al., 1997). It could be most heuristic, therefore, to view the relationship between extraversion–introversion and chronic pain as having several other important covariates, as depicted in Figure 8.1.

As Gatchel emphasizes in the final chapter of this volume, in the field of personality psychology, one *cannot* assume that a single assessment measure can be used as the sole conclusive, predictive, or descriptive variable for comprehensively elucidating a patient's reaction to pain or intervention methods. Such data should be

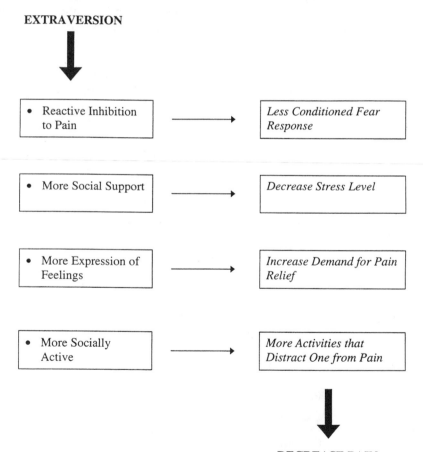

Figure 8.1. Relationship between extraversion–introversion and chronic pain and the major covariates.

viewed simply as one source of information to be used with other forms of assessment. This is certainly true for the personality variable of extraversion–introversion, and it is in keeping with the overall biopsychosocial perspective of chronic pain.

References

Barnes, G. E. (1975). Extraversion and pain. *British Journal of Social and Clinical Psychology, 14*, 303–308.

Bartol, C. R., & Costello, N. (1976). Extraversion as a function of temporal duration of electrical shock: An exploratory study. *Perceptual and Motor Skills, 42*, 1174.

Baum, A., Gatchel, R. J., & Krantz, D. S. (1997). *Introduction to health psychology* (3rd ed.). New York: McGraw-Hill.

Baumann, U., & Angst, J. (1972). Mark-Nyman Temperament Scale (MNT). *Zeitschrift fuer Klinische Psychologie, 3*, 189–212.

Beecher, H. K. (1956). Relationship of significance of wound to pain experienced. *Journal of the American Medical Association, 161*, 1609.

Beecher, H. K. (1959). *Measurement of subjective responses: Quantitative effects of drugs.* New York: Oxford University Press.

Bending, A. W. (1962). Pittsburgh scales of social extraversion–introversion and emotionality. *Journal of Psychology, 53*, 199–209.

Bond, M. R. (1971). Relation of pain to the Eysenck Personality Inventory, Cornell Medical Index and Whitely Index of Hypochondriasis. *British Journal of Psychiatry, 119*, 671–678.

Bond, M. R. (1973). Personality studies in patients with pain secondary to organic disease. *Journal of Psychosomatic Research, 17*, 257–263.

Bond, M. R., Glynn, J. P., & Thomas, D. G. (1976). Relation between pain and personality in patients receiving pentazocine (Fortral) after surgery. *Journal of Psychosomatic Research, 20*, 369–381.

Bond, M. R., & Pearson, I. B. (1969). Psychological aspects of pain in women with advanced cancer of the cervix. *Journal of Psychosomatic Research, 13*, 13–19.

Bond, M. R., & Pilowsky, I. (1966). Subjective assessment of pain and its relationship to the administration of analgesics in patients with advanced cancer. *Journal of Psychosomatic Research, 10*, 203.

Brown, R. A., Fader, K., & Barber, T. X. (1973). Responsiveness to pain: Stimulus-specificity versus generality. *Psychological Records, 23*, 1–7.

Butcher, J. N., Dahlstrom, W. G., Graham, J. R., Tellegen, A., & Kaemmer, B. (1989). *Minnesota Multiphasic Personality Inventory (MMPI-2): Manual for administration and scoring.* Minneapolis, MN: University of Minnesota Press.

Cattell, R. B. (1949). *Manual for forms A and B: Sixteen Personality Factors Questionnaire.* Champaign, IL: Institute for Personality and Ability Testing.

Claridge, G. S. (1967). Personality and arousal: A psychophysiological study of psychiatric disorders. In H. J. Eysenck (Ed.), *International series of monographs in experimental psychology* (Vol. 4, pp. 235–260). Oxford, England: Pergamon Press.

Cole. R. (1965). The problem of pain in persistent cancer. *Medical Journal of Australia, 52*, 682.

Costa, P. T., Jr., & McCrae, R. R. (1985). *NEO Personality Inventory (NEO PI): Professional manual.* Odessa, FL: Psychological Assessment Resources.

Costa, P. T., Jr., & McCrae, R. R. (1992). *Revised NEO Personality Inventory (NEO PI–R) and NEO Five-Factor Inventory (NEO–FFI): Professional manual.* Odessa, FL: Psychological Assessment Resources.

Dalrymple, D. G., Parbrook, G. D., & Steel, D. F. (1972). Effect of personality on postoperative pain and vital capacity impairment. *British Journal of Anaesthesia, 44,* 902.

Davidson, P. O., & McDougall, C. E. A. (1969a). Generality of pain tolerance. *Journal of Psychosomatic Research, 13,* 83–89.

Davidson, P. O., & McDougall, C. E. A. (1969b). Personality and pain tolerance measures. *Perceptual and Motor Skills, 28,* 787–790.

Digman, J. M. (1990). Personality structure: Emergence of the five-factor model. *Annual Review of Psychology, 41,* 417–440.

Donham, G. W., Mikhail, S. F., & Meyers, R. (1984). Value of consensual ratings in differentiating organic and functional low back pain. *Journal of Clinical Psychology, 40*(2), 432–439.

Drummond, R. (1985). Eysenck Personality Inventory. In D. J. Keyser & R. C. Sweetland (Eds.), *Test critiques* (Vol. II, pp. 258–262). Kansas City, MO: Test Corporation of America.

Exton-Smith, A. N. (1961). Terminal illness in the aged. *Lancet, 2,* 305.

Eysenck, H. J. (1959). *Maudsley Personality Inventory.* London: University of London Press. (Also published by Educational and Industrial Testing Service, Inc. [EDITS], San Diego, 1962.)

Eysenck, H. J. (1960). *Structure of human personality.* New York: Wiley.

Eysenck, H. J. (1967). Biological basis of personality. In S. Kugelmass (Ed.), *American lecture series no. 689: American lectures in living chemistry* (pp. 347–390). Springfield, IL: Charles C. Thomas.

Eysenck, H. J., & Eysenck, S. B. G. (1968). *Manual of the Eysenck Personality Inventory.* San Diego: Educational and Industrial Testing Service.

Eysenck, H. J., & Eysenck, S. B. G. (1975). *Eysenck Personality Questionnaire.* San Diego: Educational and Industrial Testing Service.

Fan, A. Y., Gu, R., & Zhou, A. (1995). MMPI control study: Chinese migraineurs during frequent headache attack intervals. *Headache, 35*(8), 475–478.

Fisher, R. A. (1938). *Statistical methods for research workers* (7th ed.) London: Oliver & Boyd.

Friedman, A. F. (1984). Eysenck Personality Questionnaire. In D. J. Keyser & R. C. Sweetland (Eds.), *Test critiques* (Vol. I, pp. 279–283). Kansas City, MO: Test Corporation of America.

Gil, K. M., Ginsberg, B., Muir, M., Sullivan, F., & Williams, D. A. (1992). Patient controlled analgesia: The relationship of psychological factors to pain and analgesic use in adolescents with postoperative pain. *Clinical Journal of Pain, 8,* 215–221.

Graham, J. R. (1990). *MMPI-2: Assessing personality and psychopathology.* New York: Oxford University Press.

Graham, J. R. (1993). *MMPI-2: Assessing personality and psychopathology* (2nd ed.). New York: Oxford University Press.

Haslam, D. R. (1967). Individual differences in pain threshold and level of arousal. *British Journal of Psychology, 58*(1–2), 139–142.

Huncke, B., & McCall, R. (1978). Chronic back pain. *Orthopedic Review, 7,* 12–19.

Huskisson, E. C. (1983). Visual analogue scales. In R. Melzack (Ed.), *Pain Measurement and Assessment* (pp. 33–37). New York: Raven Press.

Jess, P., & Bech, P. (1994). The validity of Eysenck's neuroticism dimension within the Minnesota Multiphasic Personality Inventory in patients with duodenal ulcer. *Psychotherapy and Psychosomatics, 62,* 168–175.

Kennard, M. (1952). Responses to painful stimuli of patients with severe chronic painful conditions. *Journal of Clinical Investigations, 31,* 245.

Lane, R. D., & Schwartz, G. E. (1987). Levels of emotional awareness: A cognitive–developmental theory and its application to psychopathology. *American Journal of Psychiatry, 144,* 133–143.

Levine, F. M., Tursky, B., & Nichols, D. C. (1966). Tolerance for pain, extraversion and neuroticism: Failure to replicate results. *Perceptual and Motor Skills, 23*, 847–850.

Love, A. W., & Peck, C. L. (1987). MMPI and psychological factors in chronic low back pain: A review. *Pain, 28*, 1–12.

Low, W. Y., Edelmann, R. J., & Sutton, C. (1993). Psychological profile of endometriosis patients in comparison to patients with pelvic pain of other origins. *Journal of Psychosomatic Research, 37*(2), 111–116.

Lynn, R., & Eysenck, H. J. (1961). Tolerance for pain, extraversion and neuroticism. *Perceptual and Motor Skills, 12*, 161–162.

Martin, J. E., & Inglis, J. (1965). Pain tolerance and narcotic addiction. *British Journal of Social and Clinical Psychology, 4*, 224–229.

Masson, A. H. B. (1966). Value and limitations of subjective assessments of pain and analgesia. *Proceedings of the Royal Society of Medicine* (Suppl. 81), 4.

Melzack, R. (1975). McGill Pain Questionnaire: Major properties and scoring methods. *Pain, 1*, 277–299.

Merskey, H., & Spear, F. G. (1967). *Pain, psychological and psychiatric aspects*. London: Balliére, Tindall & Cassell.

Millard, R. W., & Kinsler, B. L. (1992). Evaluation of constricted affect in chronic pain: An attempt using the Toronto Alexythymia Scale. *Pain, 50*, 287–292.

Millon, T., Green, C. J., & Meagher, R. B. (1982). *Millon Behavioral Health Inventory* (3rd ed.). Minneapolis, MN: National Computing Systems.

Morasso, G., Costantini, M., Baracco, G., Borreani, C., & Capelli, M. (1996). Assessing psychological distress in cancer patients: Validation of a self-administered questionnaire. *Oncology, 53*, 295–302.

Myers, I. B. (1977). *Myers/Briggs Type Indicator: Supplementary Manual*. Palo Alto, CA: Consulting Psychologists Press.

Petrie, A. (1960). Some psychological aspects of pain and the relief of suffering. *Annals of the New York Academy of Science, 85*, 13–37.

Petrie, A., Collins, W., & Solomon, P. (1960). Tolerance for pain and for sensory deprivation. *American Journal of Psychology, 73*, 80–90.

Petrovich, D. V. (1973). *Manual for the Pain Apperception Test*. Los Angeles: Western Psychological Services.

Philips, C. (1976). Headache and personality. *Journal of Psychosomatic Research, 20*, 535–542.

Philips, C., & Hunter, M. (1982). A psychophysiological investigation of tension headache. *Headache, 22*, 173–181.

Philips, H. C., & Jahanshahi, M. (1985). Effects of persistent pain: The chronic headache sufferer. *Pain, 21*, 163–176.

Poser, E. (1960). Figural aftereffect as a personality correlate. In *Proceedings of the 16th International Congress of Psychology*. Amsterdam: North Holland.

Robinson, H., Kirk, R. F., Jr., Frye, R. F., & Robertson, J. T. (1972). Psychological study of patients with rheumatoid arthritis and other painful diseases. *Journal of Psychosomatic Research, 16*, 53–56.

Schalling, D. (1970). Tolerance for experimentally induced pain as related to personality. *Reports from the Psychological Laboratories, University of Stockholm, 303*, 14.

Schalling, D., & Levander, S. (1964). Rating of anxiety-proneness and responses to electrical pain stimulation. *Scandinavian Journal of Psychology, 5*, 1–19.

Schalling, D., Rissler, A., & Edman, G. (1970). Pain tolerance, personality, and autonomic measures. *Reports from the Psychological Laboratories, University of Stockholm, 304*, 16.

Shagass, C., & Kerenyi, A. B. (1958). Neurophysiologic studies of personality. *Journal of Nervous and Mental Disorders, 126*, 141–147.

Snibbe, J. R., Peterson, P. J., & Sosner, B. (1980). Study of psychological characteristics of a workers' compensation sample using the MMPI and Millon Clinical Multiaxial Inventory. *Psychological Reports, 47*, 959–966.

Sternbach, R. A. (1975). Psychophysiology of pain. *International Journal of Psychiatry in Medicine, 6*(1–2), 63–73.

Sternbach, R. A. (1977). Psychological aspects of chronic pain. *Clinical Orthopedics and Related Research, 129*, 150–155.

Stone, M. (1985). Maudsley Personality Inventory. In D. J. Keyser & R. C. Sweetland (Eds.), *Test critiques* (Vol. I, pp. 279–283). Kansas City, MO: Test Corporation of America.

Taenzer, P., Melzack, R., & Jeans, M. E. (1986). Influence of psychological factors on postoperative pain, mood and analgesic requirements. *Pain, 24*, 331–342.

Tan, S.-Y. (1980). *Acute pain in a clinical setting: Effects of cognitive–behavioral skills training.* Unpublished doctoral dissertation, McGill University, Montreal, Quebec.

Taylor, G. J., Ryan, D., & Bagby, R. M. (1986). Toward the development of a new self-report alexythymia scale. *Psychotherapy & Psychosomatics, 44*(4), 191–199.

Turk, D. C. (1996). Biopsychosocial perspective on chronic pain. In R. J. Gatchel & D. C. Turk (Eds.), *Psychological approaches to pain management: A practitioner's handbook* (pp. 3–34). New York: Guilford Press.

Vando, A. (1969). *Personality dimension related to pain tolerance.* Unpublished doctoral dissertation, Columbia University, New York.

Wade, J. B., Dougherty, L. M., Hart, R. P., & Cook, D. B. (1992). Patterns of normal personality structure among chronic pain patients. *Pain, 48*(1), 37–43.

Wade, J. B., Dougherty, L. M., Hart, R. P., Rafii, A., & Price, D. D. (1992). Canonical correlation analysis of the influence of neuroticism and extraversion on chronic pain, suffering, and pain behavior. *Pain, 51*(1), 67–73.

Waters, W. E., & O'Connor, P. J. (1970). Clinical validation of a headache questionnaire. In A. L. Cochrane (Ed.), *Background to migraine.* London: Heinemann.

Williams, D. A. (1996). Acute pain management. In R. J. Gatchel & D. C. Turk (Eds.), *Psychological approaches to pain management: A practitioner's handbook* (pp. 55–77). New York: Guilford Press.

Woodforde, J. M., & Merskey, H. (1972). Personality traits of patients with chronic pain. *Journal of Psychosomatic Research, 16*, 167–172.

Ziegler, D. K., & Paolo, A. M. (1995). Headache symptoms and psychological profile of headache-prone individuals. *Archives of Neurology, 52*, 602–606.

Ziesat, H. A., Jr., & Gentry, W. D. (1978). Pain Apperception Test: An investigation of concurrent validity. *Journal of Clinical Psychology, 34*(3), 786–789.

Chapter 9
PERCEIVED OPTIMISM AND CHRONIC PAIN

John P. Garofalo

The personality dimension of optimism is one aspect of the broader study of pain and draws a great deal of attention as a significant mediator of stress in several psychological domains, including health and clinical psychology. Because of its health-promoting effects—observed across various physical conditions—there has been growing speculation that optimism could influence the course and experience of pain. This hypothesis coincides with a burgeoning body of literature that suggests not only that psychological factors are important in the experience of pain but that they represent a major influence in the response to treatment. To date, most pain research has focused primarily on the effects of stress, adversity, and other negative psychological variables on pain-related health outcomes. For example, high levels of stress and disturbed mood are generally believed to increase the likelihood of poorer health outcomes and to exacerbate pain severity and disability among pain patients (Jensen, Turner, Romano, & Karoly, 1991; Turk, 1996; Turk & Rudy, 1988). Additionally, the relatively high incidence of psychiatric morbidity (mood, anxiety, somatization, and personality disorders) among pain patients compared with the general population provides support for the idea that psychological factors influence the pain experience, and possibly its pathogenesis (Dworkin & Gitlin, 1991; Gatchel, 1996; Gatchel, Garofalo, Ellis, & Holt, 1996; Katon, Egan, & Miller, 1985; Polatin, Kinney, Gatchel, Lillo, & Mayer, 1993).

Despite the growing interest in the effects of psychological variables on pain, the relationship between optimism and pain has never been systematically examined. This chapter addresses this poorly understood relationship by reviewing and summarizing the limited research to date on the effects of optimism on pain. Because of the paucity of research conducted in this area, the studies reviewed here will be collapsed so that pain conditions are treated as a homogeneous group. In doing so, this approach might neglect the heterogeneity of these conditions and the unique properties that distinguish one pain condition from another.

This chapter is probably the first attempt at exploring the relationship between optimism and pain. Before beginning, it is appropriate to present a review of optimism and its apparent health-promoting effects. This should offer insight into the possible application to assessment and treatment of pain. One primary aim of this chapter is to determine whether the effects of optimism are applicable to pain conditions. This information could be particularly useful for developing a tentative model to account for the role of optimism in pain, its mechanisms, any ensuing health benefits pain patients might experience, and perhaps ways to inform treatment strategies.

Optimism

Optimism is the tendency to hold positive expectations about the future—a tendency that has been associated with psychological well-being and an overall positive outlook on life. The belief that positive expectations represent a potential mediator of stress is not a novel one, as evidenced by the work of Bandura (1977) and Rotter (1954), both of whom viewed optimism as highly influenced by a sense of self-efficacy. These authors speculated that the anticipation of positive outcomes will sustain, and possibly reenergize, one's goal-directed efforts in situations with undetermined outcomes. On the other hand, the anticipation of negative outcomes can attenuate or end efforts toward an intended goal (Scheier, Weintraub, & Carver, 1986). Thus, the anticipation of success or failure is believed to influence behavior and outcomes.

Before continuing with the review on optimism, it is important to note several related constructs that have been explored. Depending on the variable being measured, optimism is alternatively described as a disposition, a world view, a defense, a coping style, a situation-specific construct, a cognitive bias, or a combination of these. Despite the numerous ways researchers have described optimism, it is generally agreed that maintaining distinction is important, particularly when each construct carries different implications. Schwarzer (1994) reviewed the different operational definitions of optimism, noting that framing one's expectations in a positive light can lead to two different purposes: a functional one and a defensive one.

Functional optimism refers to adaptive effects that have been attributed to optimism. Two examples of this construct are the optimistic explanatory style and dispositional optimism (Peterson & Seligman, 1987; Scheier & Carver, 1985, 1987, 1992; Seligman 1991). The optimistic explanatory style, sometimes called *learned optimism*, is best understood as the opposite of the "depressive attributional style" (Abramson, Seligman, & Teasdale, 1978). Seligman (1991) posited that, whereas a depressed individual interprets a negative event in terms of internal, stable, and global attributions, the optimist will make external, variable, and specific attributions to explain the same event. The optimist's attributions appear more self-serving in the face of a good event; such an event is believed to reflect internal, stable, and global attributes. It should be noted that the construct of the optimistic explanatory style is only recently developed; therefore, this construct and its interaction with stress require further scrutiny.

Dispositional optimism is defined as generalized positive expectations for the future. Longitudinal follow-up has demonstrated that this tendency to anticipate positive outcomes appears relatively stable over time and across situations (Scheier & Carver, 1985, 1992). Dispositional optimism is frequently explained as a model of self-regulation, by which optimism's effectiveness depends on the degree to which one's expectations are congruent with the likelihood of realistic, favorable outcomes. That is, optimistic expectations, coupled with a realistic appraisal of a future event, might prompt one to behave in a manner that increases the likelihood of success. Based on this premise, an optimist stranded on a deserted island would be inclined to make a fire to signal for help; a pessimist's "why bother" outlook could lead to no action whatsoever. Thus, an optimistic outlook appears to serve as an important source of motivation to engage in behaviors that will directly influence outcome. During the past 15 years, dispositional optimism has received a great deal of support for its positive effects on both psychological and physical well-being.

Schwarzer's (1994) concept of defensive optimism refers to the tendency to unrealistically underestimate one's vulnerability to threat. Findings suggest that such an outlook can result in either positive or negative consequences. Optimism, even when unrealistic or inaccurate, nevertheless appears to be a good indicator of psychological well-being. Three mechanisms by which "positive illusions" (Taylor, 1983) exert positive benefits are self-aggrandizement, an increased sense of personal control, and an overly optimistic outlook (Taylor & Armor, 1996). In terms of self-aggrandizement, patients often wish to think of themselves more favorably than others, particularly with respect to health domains. That is, many patients see themselves as less vulnerable than other people are to the threat of disease, as evidenced by the attitude "it could never happen to me" (Helgeson & Taylor, 1993). Consequently, a tendency to self-aggrandize can result in more effective coping.

Second, there are data that support Taylor and Armor's (1996) contention that the perception of having increased control over events frequently results in successful adjustment to adverse experiences, including life-threatening traumas and disease (Bulman & Wortman, 1977; Taylor & Armor, 1996; Taylor & Brown, 1988). Bulman and Wortman reported that the tendency to blame oneself for a trauma predicted good coping, whereas blaming others predicted poor coping.

Perhaps even more striking are findings relating to the third mechanism, unrealistic optimism, which has been related to lengthened survival for AIDS and cancer patients (Greer, Morris, Pettingale, & Haybittle, 1990; Reed, Kemeny, Taylor, Wang, & Visscher, 1994). According to Taylor and Armor (1996), unrealistic optimists had less difficulty adjusting to disease and were more likely to return to their prior level of functioning. One possible explanation is that being overly optimistic could allow one to confront a negative situation that normally would be avoided. For example, Taylor et al. (1992) observed an increased rate of health-promoting behavior among gay men who tested positive for HIV or who had been diagnosed with AIDS.

On the other hand, several contexts have been identified for which unrealistic optimism can lead to negative consequences. One example includes the development of appraisals that markedly underestimate the likelihood of a realistic outcome. These "positive illusions" can compromise the capacity to take appropriate action by instilling a false sense of invulnerability to a threat, such as illness (Janoff-Bulman & Frieze, 1983; Tennen & Affleck, 1987). For example, a woman with a family history of breast cancer might neglect to do breast self-examination or obtain mammograms, maintaining the "it-could-never-happen" belief. The false sense of invulnerability can lead to inappropriate action. A driver who speeds excessively is probably ignoring the increased danger associated with speeding. While defensive optimism does not account for all risk behaviors, Schwarzer (1994) asserted that it is significant in a person's perception of risk and vulnerability.

Measures of Optimism

The literature describes several psychosocial instruments that measure optimism. The Minnesota Multiphasic Personality Inventory (MMPI; Hathaway & McKinley, 1943), a frequently used clinical and research assessment measure of personality, has been described as capable of measuring positive outlook in several ways. The Optimism–Pessimism Scale (PSM) for the MMPI consists of 298 items that have been used to measure this construct as a relatively stable personality trait (Colligan, Offord, Malinchoc, Schulman, & Seligman, 1994). The total score is based on a continuum in which a high score reflects an optimistic explanatory style, and a low score reflects a pessimistic explanatory style. Costello, Schoenfeld, Ramamurthy, and Hobbs-Hardee (1989) reported that optimism–pessimism can be measured by taking the sum of the basic scale of depression and the social introversion scale and subtracting the basic scale of mania. More recently, Malinchoc, Offord, and Colligan (1998) compared the PSM to regression equations that convert noncorrected K raw scores on the MMPI, traditionally a measure of defensiveness, to an estimated optimism–pessimism score. Their findings revealed that the optimism–pessimism score represents a reliable measure. Because of its length, however, researchers often use shorter measures of optimism to decrease the amount of time participants spend filling out paperwork.

The gold standard measure of dispositional optimism is the Life Orientation Test (LOT), a brief, psychometrically reliable, and valid self-report scale developed by Scheier and Carver (1985). The original version consisted of eight items (e.g., "In uncertain times, I usually expect the best."). Respondents endorse the degree to which they agree with each item. The LOT measures generalized outcome expectancies, precluding any measure of attribution, morale, mood, psychological well-being, locus of control, or any other construct associated with optimism. Internal reliability has been reported to be good ($\alpha = .76$); the LOT has also demonstrated good test–retest reliability ($\alpha = .71$). The test does not attempt to delineate situation-specific expectations, but instead conceptualizes optimism as a world view that good things are going to happen for the individual. Most studies described in this chapter used the LOT as the primary measure.

There are several other noteworthy psychosocial instruments. For example, Seligman's (1991) optimistic explanatory style is measured with the Attributional Style Questionnaire, an instrument whose subscales demonstrate good efficiency, reliability, and validity. The Generalized Expectancy for Success Scale (Fibel & Hale, 1978) measures expectations across different life domains instead of taking a global perspective. The Hopelessness Scale (Beck, Weissman, Lester, & Trexler, 1974) differs from the LOT in its focus on tendencies rather than expectations. This scale also distinguishes itself from other measures of optimism by assessing a wide range of affective experiences. Another measure of optimism includes the Optimism–Pessimism Prescreening Questionnaire (Norem & Cantor, 1986), which was developed to identify individuals who use optimistic and pessimistic defense strategies when dealing with issues surrounding academics. Despite the adequate reliability and validity demonstrated by these instruments, their selection as a means to measure optimism over the LOT should depend on how the investigator conceptualizes optimism and the particular domain being targeted.

In contrast to the LOT's assessment of dispositional optimism, the Health Optimism Scale (Estlander, 1991) assesses expectations of positive health outcomes. The scale demonstrates good internal reliability and consistency ($\alpha =. 72$). Aside from its health-specific focus, this measure does not approach optimism as a dispositional construct. Instead, the origin of expectations is traced to past health experiences. For example, negative health experiences appear to foster pessimistic expectations, whereas positive experiences foster more positive expectations. Because they relate directly to external experiences, the strength of these expectations is seen to be particularly malleable.

Optimism and Health

There is a growing body of research that supports the positive effects of optimism on physical health as well as psychological well-being (Affleck & Tennen, 1996; Carver et al., 1993, 1994; Fitzgerald, Tennen, Affleck, & Pransky, 1993; Jenkins, 1996; Nelson, Karr, & Coleman, 1995; Scheier & Carver, 1987; 1992; Scheier et al., 1989). In a landmark study, Scheier and Carver (1985) found an inverse association between dispositional optimism and physical symptoms. College undergraduates with high levels of optimism reported fewer physical symptoms; those with low optimism reported more physical symptoms. Another study showed that, in a sample of college undergraduates, optimism was associated with fewer physical symptoms and fewer daily hassles (Nelson et al., 1995). Nelson and colleagues found a positive relationship between levels of outside emotional support and dispositional optimism. Other studies have found optimism to relate to improved treatment outcomes and faster rates of postsurgical recovery among heart and cancer patients (Carver et al., 1993; 1994; Chamberlain, Petrie, & Azariah, 1992; Kiyak, Vitaliano, & Crinean, 1988). Although all of these studies suggest that optimism positively influences health, the promotion mechanisms are not well understood.

Much of the research on the relationship between optimism and health has drawn its conclusions by contrasting optimists to their counterparts—pessimists. Based on these comparisons, several mechanisms have been proposed to explain the beneficial effects of optimism on physical and mental well-being. One is that optimism serves as a buffer to the effects of stress on health, whereas pessimism does not (Adler, Horowitz, Garcia, & Moyer, 1998; Haerkaepaeae, Jaervikoski, & Estlander, 1996). That is, positive expectations might shield a recently diagnosed patient from the onset of the negative psychological sequelae that generally accompany disease. This protection results in overall improved psychological adjustment (Carver et al., 1993, 1994; Taylor, 1983). Better psychosocial adjustment could result in improved treatment outcomes as well as overall improvement in quality of life during the course of the disease. For example, in a prospective study on breast cancer patients, optimism was inversely related to levels of distress at each time point during a 12-month follow-up, and higher levels of dispositional optimism reliably predicted adjustment and recovery (Carver et al., 1993, 1994). In contrast, cancer patients with higher levels of pessimism experienced poorer adjustment at each time point.

Another possible mechanism involves the optimist's use of coping strategies that are more effective than those used by pessimists when confronted by threat or challenge. Optimists appear to demonstrate superior adaptation when dealing with the onset and course of some medical conditions (Fitzgerald et al., 1993; Scheier et al., 1989). These differences do not identify the more effective "copers" per se, but instead suggest that some coping strategies mediate the health-promoting effects of optimism by increasing the likelihood of improved adjustment.

Carver, Scheier, and Weintraub (1989) argued that optimists rely more on problem-focused coping strategies than do pessimists, who rely more on emotion-focused coping strategies. Carver et al. (1993) monitored a group of breast cancer patients, revealing that optimists were more likely to refrain from behavioral disengagement. That is, patients with higher levels of positive expectations worked toward remaining active, thereby engaging in behaviors that retain a high level of structure and order within their lives. Breast cancer patients with greater levels of optimism seemed less likely to yield a helpless response to their diagnosis and treatment; instead, they presented themselves as more ready to accept the reality of the situation. This style coincides with findings that suggest optimists take an active, head-on approach to emerging obstacles and challenges. It is noteworthy that, although such coping strategies seem to mediate the effects of optimism, they do not fully account for its health-promoting effects (Scheier & Carver, 1992). Nevertheless, the pessimist's failure to use these coping styles creates a portrait of a patient who avoids confronting the reality of a situation, who disengages behaviorally and socially, and in turn who can experience distress and poorer overall adjustment to the demands that accompany a decline in health.

A growing body of literature contends that optimists are healthier than pessimists and that they engage in more health-promoting behaviors (Peterson & Bossio, 1991; Scheier & Carver, 1992; Seligman, 1991). Supporters of this hypothesis argue that a positive outlook instills a sense of control over the future and an improved sense of self-regulation. When comparing healthy individuals to acutely ill college students, Kulik and Mahler (1987) observed that the latter group reported feeling more susceptible to future health problems. The investigators concluded that this increased sense of vulnerability would reduce the likelihood that ill patients would take preventive action against factors that lead to the onset of new problems or that will aggravate continuing problems.

Some research suggests that personality factors influence physical health directly rather than indirectly through health behaviors. Kamen-Siegel, Rodin, Seligman, and Dwyer (1991) found that a pessimistic explanatory style was associated with poorer immune system functioning. Segerstrom, Taylor, Kemeny, and Fahey (1998) reported that optimism was associated with higher numbers of helper T-cells and higher natural killer-cell cytotoxicity. However, mood and perceived stress partially accounted for the relationship.

Another difference between optimists and pessimists could reside in the way people anticipate the future, as suggested by proponents of the optimistic explanatory style. Ascribing negative events to external, unstable, and specific causes is associated not only with positive mood and perceived reduction of risk for disease, but it appears to instill the belief that one can prevent future health problems (Peterson & Bossio, 1991; Peterson & DeAvila, 1995; Schwarzer, 1994; Seligman, 1991). In contrast, a pessimistic explanatory style is associated with depressed mood and is characterized by assessing negative events as internal, stable, and global. This cognitive bias might compromise or delay coping efforts with stress, thereby augmenting the likelihood of negative consequences (Jenkins, 1996).

Optimism and Pain

As evidence grows to suggest that optimism is an important mediator of stress and health, many now hypothesize that optimism could have significant effects on pain. Indeed, some research indicates that an optimistic disposition could lead to successful treatment of patients with pain (Gruen, 1972; Haerkaepaeae et al., 1996; Jamison, Taft, O'Hara, & Ferrante, 1993; Novy, Nelson, Hetzel, Squitieri, & Kennington, 1998). For an estimated 50 million Americans pain conditions are a major source of life stress (Turk, 1996). Pain is complex, and it is characterized by negative sensory, affective, and cognitive changes. Many patients report depressed mood, poor adjustment, and a compromised quality of life as pain interferes with social and occupational functioning (Anderson, Bradley, Young, McDaniel, & Wise, 1985; Dworkin & Gitlin, 1991; Turk, 1996). These accompanying features are significant in the course of pain and in the entire experience of the patient. The shift from a biomedical paradigm to a biopsychosocial approach clearly underscores the growing awareness among researchers of the importance of psychological and environmental factors in pain.

Despite the extensive influence psychological factors demonstrate, few researchers have examined the role of optimism in the pain experience. There are several reasons such sparse attention has been given to this relationship. First, most mind–body research has focused on the influence of negative psychological factors, neglecting the effects of positive factors on health. For example, a common treatment goal set for patients involves reducing the use of catastrophizing as a coping style. With training, patients can learn alternative ways to cope with pain. This leads to a reduction in catastrophizing, which results in reduced pain intensity and disability (Turner & Clancy, 1986). Second, optimism is not observed often among pain patients; many patients report significant pessimism. Despite advances in treatment, many chronic pain patients report continuous, intense, disabling pain that is psychologically taxing. That is, frustrated with the perceived limited success of treatment, many patients report despair and feelings of hopelessness for the future (Turk & Holzman, 1986).

Although there has been no systematic investigation of the influence of unrealistic optimism on pain, other related constructs have been examined (see Love & Peck, 1987, for a review). Costello and colleagues (1989) used the MMPI to identify four types of pain patients demonstrating different elevations on the basic clinical scales: the psychpathological-looking patient, the Conversion V patient, the infirmary-type patient, and the normal-appearing patient. Optimism and pessimism differentiated two of the subgroups. That is, Conversion V patients were particularly more optimistic than were infirmary-type patients, whose label was coined because of the long history of multiple surgeries and hospitalizations observed in this subgroup. Patients with a Conversion V profile rarely report significant distress. Instead, they generally present themselves as overly optimistic, marked by a Pollyannaish view of the world and the future, and with a decreased concern with physical symptoms (Graham, 1990). Taylor (1983) alluded to possible benefits from unrealistic optimism. Positive expectations can provide patients exhibiting this profile with a sense of psychological well-being, but findings from other research suggest that unrealistic optimism does not yield pain relief (Love & Peck, 1987; Sherman, Camfield, & Arena, 1995). Instead, patients with Conversion V profiles generally report greater pain intensity and increased resistance to treatment. This appears to coincide with the view that such patients prefer to focus on somatic complaints and to ignore or avoid the possibility that psychological factors influence pain.

In the limited number of studies conducted, optimism has indeed demonstrated positive effects on the course and experience of pain. Haerkaepaeae et al. (1996) evaluated psychological factors' capacity to predict treatment outcomes in a multimodal back treatment program. The study followed 175 patients with chronic or recurrent back pain who had completed an intensive, 12-month treatment program. The investigation revealed that health-related optimism and control beliefs predicted treatment outcome. Patients who held more optimistic views on their health and the course of their back pain, coupled with greater perceived control, appeared to have longer term improvement after treatment. Further analysis also revealed a significant association between health optimism and work status. Patients who had more optimistic expectations about their health were more likely to return to work than were patients with pessimistic expectations. The authors noted that dispositional optimism, as measured by the LOT, does not relate to their findings. Instead, they used the Health Optimism Scale (Estlander, 1991). This measure does not share the stability of dispositional optimism, but instead posits that health optimism is derived from past and current experiences and is therefore susceptible to change.

Research has found that coping style and appraisal are two important factors in adaptation to pain (Rosenstiel & Keefe, 1983; Turk, 1996). It is generally established that active-coping strategies are associated with improved outcomes. Physically active pain patients adjust better to their pain when they use more active coping strategies and avoid catastrophizing (Hill, Niven, & Knussen, 1995; Turk, 1996; Turk & Rudy, 1992). Passive pain management strategies, in which the patient focuses on nociceptive stimulation or catastrophizing—expecting the worst possible outcome —are seen frequently in pain patients (Keefe, Brown, Wallston, & Caldwell, 1989; Smith & Wallston, 1992; Van Lankveld, Van't Pad Bosch, Van de Putte, Naring, & Van der Staak, 1994; Zautra & Manne, 1992).

Long and Sangster (1993) expanded this area of study by including the role of dispositional optimism in their comparison of coping strategies exhibited by rheumatoid arthritis and osteoarthritis patients. The investigators observed differential psychological adjustment among the two groups that were not fully accounted for by the influence of optimism and pessimism on coping style, but that they attributed to the nature of the pain condition. More optimistic patients in both groups primarily used problem-solving coping strategies; more pessimistic patients primarily used wishful thinking. Although the findings did not reveal an association between successful adjustment to a pain condition and problem-solving coping, an optimistic disposition was associated with improved psychological adjustment for both groups, and dispositional pessimism was directly related to poorer adjustment in the rheumatoid arthritis group. Only an indirect relationship was found between pessimism and membership in the osteoarthritis group: Poorer psychological adjustment was more likely when wishful thinking and physical disability accompanied pessimistic expectations. One possible explanation for the difference could relate to the disease course of osteoarthritis, which is less ambiguous and more predictable than is rheumatoid arthritis. Specifically, increased uncertainty and ambiguity are associated with rheumatoid arthritis, which result in poorer coping.

Long and Sangster's (1993) work reported an association between the use of wishful thinking—accompanied by physical disability—and poor adjustment. These findings are consistent with other reports that suggest wishful thinking is relatively ineffective in helping patients deal with stress (Felton & Revenson, 1984; Scheier & Carver, 1985). Despite its apparent relationship with optimism, the use of problem solving did not significantly influence psychological adjustment for either group of patients in the Long and Sangster study. Instead, dispositional optimism alone had an overall positive effect on adjustment toward illness. The investigators hypothesized that—in contrast to pessimism, for which wishful thinking has a mediating effect—coping strategies might not be the mechanism by which optimism exerts its health-promoting effects.

Novy et al. (1998) observed two patterns of coping strategies among 90 chronic pain patients, most of whom had reported low back pain. The investigators found that a higher level of optimism was related to active-coping strategies. These strategies, in turn, were associated with the perception of an ability to control pain. The second pattern of optimistic coping differed from the first in the notable absence of a perceived ability to regulate one's pain. Instead, the strategy was characterized by the presence of hoping and praying as primary means for dealing with stress. Both patterns were negatively associated with the tendency to catastrophize.

In terms of appraisal, many pain patients perceive situations as more stressful than other people might, and because they view their resources as inadequate, they report feelings of helplessness and hopelessness (Smith, Peck, & Ward, 1990; Smith & Wallston, 1992). The sense of helplessness often reflects the way patients perceive their pain and their inability to control it (Rosenstiel & Keefe, 1983). Tennen, Affleck, Urrows, Higgins, and Mendola (1992) examined the influence of perceived pain control and pain benefit appraisals among a group of rheumatoid arthritis patients. Two questions the investigators addressed involved whether dispositional optimism accounted for the level of control a patient perceives as well as the tendency to appraise benefits from the pain. Their findings reveal that individuals with greater perceived control experienced less daily pain. Although optimism was unrelated to perceived pain control and pain benefit appraisals, it did predict emotional well-being.

Brenner, Melamed, and Panush (1994) explored and identified several determinants of psychosocial adjustment to rheumatoid arthritis. In a sample of 66 patients, greater dispositional optimism, perceived support, and less disability were related to better psychosocial adjustment. However, only dispositional optimism predicted improved psychosocial adjustment over time, regardless of disability. In addition, optimism assessed at baseline predicted the use of problem-focused coping 16 months later. Consistent with the literature, a positive relationship was observed between this style of coping and psychosocial adjustment, and wishful thinking was related to negative adjustment. The authors hypothesized that, because optimism related to psychosocial adjustment at each time point, it was likely that the perception of being able to cope with future stressors accrued over time.

Recent research suggests that it is not necessarily only the patient who needs to demonstrate a high level of dispositional optimism to experience improved health. Members of a patient's support system must as well (Beckham, Burker, Rice, & Talton, 1995; Block & Boyer, 1984). Beckham and colleagues (1995) reported that optimism appears to have positive effects on pain when a caregiver frames expectations in a positive light. This investigation observed a positive relationship between rheumatoid arthritis patients' pain, expectations about control over symptoms, and caregiver optimism. A relatively strong relationship was found between physical status and caregiver pessimism. Patients with poorer physical and mental health had caretakers who were less optimistic, and patients with more optimistic caretakers reported better physical and mental health. Because the design of the study was correlational, it is impossible to determine the direction of the relationship. For example, one might hypothesize that patients who have experienced a recent improvement in health status would reduce the caretaker's burden, which could account for the increased optimism scores of the caretakers. Alternatively, optimistic caretakers could differ from pessimistic caretakers in coping style, which in turn could lead to improved interactions with and better overall care of patients. This could represent a more tenable hypothesis in light of recent evidence suggesting that patients' perceptions of their spouses' responsive behavior will predict pain behavior (Williamson, Robinson, & Melamed, 1997).

Optimism Model in Pain

The biopsychosocial model perhaps best accounts for the wide range of expression of pain by examining the dynamic interplay of biological, psychological, and environmental factors. Despite numerous studies that support an association between optimism and beneficial outcomes for a variety of medical conditions, including pain disorders, the biopsychosocial model has neglected the role of optimism as an influential psychological factor on pain. No model currently accounts for optimism's positive effects on the course and experience of pain or for how optimists might differ from their pessimistic counterparts in treatment response.

According to Turk and Holzman (1986), pain patients resemble patients from other medical populations in their response to the onset of symptoms. That is, when they experience a symptom, they seek to understand it by attempting to match the symptom to experiences that can account for changes in health status. However, when symptoms do not coincide with their experience, patients rely on attitudes and beliefs that influence future appraising, coping strategies, and response to subsequent treatment. Optimism and pessimism often typify the patient's general world view and perhaps reflect the underlying attitudes to which Turk and Holzman (1986) alluded. According to Carver and Scheier (1994), several factors influence behavior; ultimately, however, behavior will be determined by whether one anticipates success or failure. If so, dispositional optimism would serve as a point of reference for the patient who cannot match pain symptoms to experience. That is, the optimistic patient will maintain the belief that "everything will be okay," whereas the pessimistic patient will anticipate the worst.

Optimism and pessimism appear to influence pain patients' use of coping strategies in dealing with adversity. These strategies, problem-focused and emotion-focused coping, in turn, differentially relate to psychosocial adjustment (Figure 9.1). As noted by Scheier and Carver (1992), greater optimism leads patients to use more active, problem-focused coping for positive outlook and instills in a patient the belief that goals are attainable. This type of coping has been related to more adaptive functioning, reduced psychological sequelae, and improved treatment outcome (Brown & Nicassio, 1987; Fernandez & Turk, 1989; Turk, 1996).

Fernandez and Turk (1989) observed a reduction in pain intensity when patients were instructed to use more adaptive coping measures. Alternatively, emotion-focused coping, including catastrophizing and wishful thinking, related to negative adjustment. Patients who catastrophize generally demonstrate greater pain intensity and disability (Heyneman, Fremouw, Gano, Kirkland, & Heiden, 1990; Turk, 1996). Greater pessimism among pain patients has been linked to a perceived lack of control over pain. Perceptions of being incapable of controlling symptoms can result in feelings of demoralization (Turk, 1996). Moreover, patients who have a pessimistic

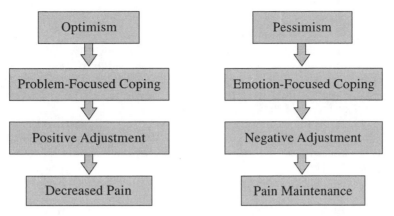

Figure 9.1. Optimism and pain.

outlook might have less interest or see little value in taking preventive measures to reduce pain (Kulik & Mahler, 1987). Although the model presented in Figure 9.1 is overly simplistic and excludes several factors associated with the pain experience, it provides a rudimentary view of how optimism can influence pain.

Conclusion

Optimism is clearly a complex construct whose health-promoting effects warrant greater exploration. There have been two primary approaches in examining the relationship between optimism and health: (a) studying healthy individuals or those who are at risk for illness, and (b) studying patients' adjustment to a medical condition. There are several reliable and valid instruments for measuring optimism and related constructs. Despite the paucity of research on its relationship with pain, preliminary evidence suggests that optimism has positive effects on the pain experience. Although the preponderance of research is based on observations of other medical populations, the mechanisms by which optimism exerts its health-promoting effects are hypothesized to be analogous to pain. And although problem-focused coping has been identified as a style generally used by optimists, emotion-focused coping (catastrophizing) has been identified as a factor that could account for increased pain reporting by pessimists. The use of these coping strategies mediates the quality of psychosocial adjustment that, in turn, will likely influence the course of pain. These findings substantiate the belief, held by researchers and clinicians alike, that a patient's overall outlook on life will influence treatment response. Further exploration of the relationship between optimism and pain, and its role as a protective factor in the experience of pain, is needed.

References

Abramson, L. Y., Seligman, M. P. E., & Teasdale, J. (1978). Learned helplessness in humans: Critique and reformulation. *Journal of Abnormal Psychology, 87,* 49–74.

Adler, N., Horowitz, M., Garcia, A., & Moyer, A. (1998). Additional validation of a scale to assess positive states of mind. *Psychosomatic Medicine, 60,* 26–32.

Affleck, G., & Tennen, H. (1996). Construing benefits from adversity: Adaptational significance and dispositional underpinnings. *Journal of Personality, 64,* 899–922.

Anderson, K. O., Bradley, L. A., Young, L. D., McDaniel, L. K., & Wise, C. M. (1985). Rheumatoid arthritis: Review of psychological factors related to etiology, effects and treatment. *Psychological Bulletin, 98,* 358–387.

Bandura, A. (1977). *Social-learning theory.* Englewood Cliffs, NJ: Prentice-Hall.

Beck, A. T., Weissman, A., Lester, D., & Trexler, L. (1974). Measurement of pessimism: The Hopelessness Scale. *Journal of Consulting and Clinical Psychology, 42,* 861–865.

Beckham, J. C., Burker, E. J., Rice, J. R., & Talton, S. L. (1995). Patient predictors of caregiver burden, optimism, and pessimism in rheumatoid arthritis. *Behavioral Medicine, 20,* 171–178.

Block, A. R., & Boyer, S. L. (1984). Spouse's adjustment to chronic pain: Cognitive and emotional factors. *Social Science and Medicine, 19,* 1313–1317.

Brenner, G. F., Melamed, B. G., & Panush, R. S. (1994). Optimism and coping as determinants of psychosocial adjustment to rheumatoid arthritis. *Journal of Clinical Psychology in Medical Settings, 2,* 115–134.

Brown, G., & Nicassio, P. (1987). Development of a questionnaire for the assessment of active and passive coping strategies in chronic pain patients. *Pain, 31,* 53–62.

Bulman, R. J., & Wortman, C. B. (1977). Ambitions of blame and coping in the "real world." Severe accident victims react to their lot. *Journal of Personality and Social Psychology, 35,* 351–363.

Carver, C. S., Pozo, C., Harris, S. D., Noriega, V., Scheier, M. F., Robinson, D. S., Ketcham, A. S., Moffat, F. L., & Clark, K. C. (1993). How coping mediates the effect of optimism on distress: A study of women with early stage breast cancer. *Journal of Personality and Social Psychology, 65,* 375–390.

Carver, C. S., Pozo, C., Harris, S. D., Noriega, V., Scheier, M. F., Robinson, D. S., Ketcham, A. S., Moffat, F. L., & Clark, K. C. (1994). Optimism versus pessimism predicts the quality of women's adjustment to early stage breast cancer. *Cancer, 73,* 1213–1320.

Carver, C. S., & Scheier, M. F. (1994). Optimism and health-related cognition. What variables actually matter? *Psychology and Health, 9,* 191–195.

Carver, C. S., Scheier, M. F., & Weintraub, J. K. (1989). Assessing coping strategies: A theoretically based approach. *Journal of Personality and Social Psychology, 56,* 267–283.

Chamberlain, K., Petrie, K., & Azariah, R. (1992). Role of optimism and sense of coherence in predicting recovery following surgery. *Psychology and Health, 7,* 301–310.

Colligan, R., Offord, K., Malinchoc, M., Schulman, P., & Seligman, M. E. (1994). CAVEing the MMPI for an Optimism–Pessimism Scale: Seligman's attributional model and the assessment of explanatory style. *Journal of Clinical Psychology, 50,* 71–95.

Costello, R. M., Schoenfeld, L. S., Ramamurthy, S., & Hobbs-Hardee, B. (1989). Sociodemographic and clinical correlates of P-A-I-N. *Journal of Psychosomatic Research, 33,* 315–321.

Dworkin, R. H., & Gitlin, M. J. (1991). Clinical aspects of depression in chronic pain. *Clinical Journal of Pain, 7,* 79–94.

Estlander, A. (1991). Assessment and treatment of chronic low back pain patients. Some cognitive behavioural aspects. In *Research reports 25.* Helsinki, Finland: Rehabilitation Foundation.

Felton, B. J., & Revenson, T. A. (1984). Coping with chronic illness: A study of illness controllability and the influence of coping strategies on psychological adjustment. *Journal of Consulting and Clinical Psychology, 52,* 343–353.

Fernandez, E., & Turk, D. C. (1989). Utility of cognitive coping strategies for altering perceptions of pain: A meta-analysis. *Pain, 38,* 123–135.

Fibel, B., & Hale, W. D. (1978). Generalized Expectancy for Success Scale—A new measure. *Journal of Consulting and Clinical Psychology, 46*, 924–931.

Fitzgerald, T., Tennen, H., Affleck, G., & Pransky, G. (1993). Relative importance of dispositional optimism and control appraisals in quality of life after coronary artery bypass surgery. *Journal of Behavioral Medicine, 16*, 25–43.

Gatchel, R. J. (1996). Psychological disorders and chronic pain. In R. J. Gatchel & D. C. Turk (Eds.), *Psychological approaches to pain management* (pp. 33–52). New York: Guilford Press.

Gatchel, R. J., Garofalo, J. P., Ellis, E., & Holt, C. (1996). Major psychological disorders in acute and chronic TMD pain: An initial examination. *Journal of the American Dental Association, 127*, 1365–1374.

Graham, J. R. (1990). *MMPI-2: Assessing personality and psychopathology.* New York: Oxford University Press.

Greer, S., Morris, T., Pettingale, K. W., & Haybittle, J. L. (1990). Psychological response to breast cancer and 15-year outcome. *Lancet, 335*, 49–50.

Gruen, W. (1972). Successful application of systematic self-relaxation and self-suggestions about postoperative reactions in a case of cardiac surgery. *International Journal of Clinical and Experimental Hypnosis, 20*, 143–151.

Haerkaepaeae, K., Jaervikoski, A., & Estlander, A. M. (1996). Health optimism and control beliefs as predictors for treatment outcome of a multimodal back treatment program. *Psychology and Health, 12*, 123–134.

Hathaway, S. R., & McKinley, J. (1943). *Minnesota multiphasic personality inventory.* Minneapolis: University of Minnesota Press.

Helgeson, V. S., & Taylor, S. E. (1993). Social comparisons and adjustment among cardiac patients. *Journal of Applied Social Psychology, 23*, 1171–1195.

Heyneman, N. E., Fremouw, W. J., Gano, D., Kirkland, F., & Heiden, L. (1990). Individual differences in the effectiveness of different coping strategies. *Cognitive Therapy and Research, 14*, 63–77.

Hill, A., Niven, C. A., & Knussen, C. (1995). Role of coping in adjustment to phantom limb pain. *Pain, 62*, 79–86.

Jamison, R. N., Taft, K., O'Hara, J. P., & Ferrante, F. M. (1993). Psychosocial and pharmacologic predictors of satisfaction with intravenous patient-controlled analgesia. *Anesthesia Analgesia, 77*, 121–125.

Janoff-Bulman, R., & Frieze, I. H. (1983). Theoretical perspective for understanding reactions to victimization. *Journal of Social Issues, 39*, 1–17.

Jenkins, C. D. (1996). While there's hope, there's life. *Psychosomatic Medicine, 58*, 122–124.

Jensen, M. P., Turner, J. A., Romano, J. M., & Karoly, P. (1991). Coping with chronic pain: A critical review of the literature. *Pain, 47*, 249–283.

Kamen-Siegel, L., Rodin, J., Seligman, M. P. E., & Dwyer, J. (1991). Explanatory style and cell-mediated immunity in elderly men and women. *Health Psychology, 10*, 229–235.

Katon, W., Egan, K., & Miller, D. (1985). Chronic pain: Lifetime psychiatric diagnoses and family history. *American Journal of Psychiatry, 142*, 1156–1160.

Keefe, F. J., Brown, G. K., Wallston, K. A., & Caldwell, D. S. (1989). Coping with rheumatoid arthritis pain: Catastrophizing as a maladaptive strategy. *Pain, 37*, 51–56.

Kiyak, H. A., Vitaliano, P. P., & Crinean, J. (1988). Patient's expectations as predictors of orthognathic surgery outcomes. *Health Psychology, 7*, 251–268.

Kulik, J. A., & Mahler, H. I. (1987). Health status, perceptions of risk, and prevention interest for health and nonhealth problems. *Health Psychology, 6*, 15–27.

Long, B. C., & Sangster, J. I. (1993). Dispositional optimism/pessimism and coping strategies: Predictors of psychosocial adjustment of rheumatoid and osteoarthritis patients. *Journal of Applied and Social Psychology, 23*, 1069–1091.

Love, A. W., & Peck, C. L. (1987). MMPI and psychological factors in chronic low back pain: A review. *Pain, 28*, 1–12.

Malinchoc, M., Offord, K. P., & Colligan, R. (1998). Pessimism in the profile. *Journal of Clinical Psychology, 54*, 169–173.

Nelson, E. S., Karr, K. M., & Coleman, P. K. (1995). Relationships among daily hassles, optimism and reported physical symptoms. *Journal of College Student Psychotherapy, 10*, 11–26.

Norem, J. K., & Cantor, N. (1986). Defensive pessimism: Harnessing anxiety as motivation. *Journal of Personality and Social Psychology, 51*, 1208–1217.

Novy, D. M., Nelson, D. V., Hetzel, R. D., Squitieri, P., & Kennington, M. (1998). Coping with chronic pain: Sources of intrinsic and contextual variability. *Journal of Behavioral Medicine, 21*, 19–34.

Peterson, C., & Bossio, L. M. (1991). *Health and optimism*. New York: Free Press.

Peterson, C., & DeAvila, M. (1995). Optimistic explanatory style and the perception of health problems. *Journal of Clinical Psychology, 51*, 128–132.

Peterson, C., & Seligman, M. E. P. (1987). Explanatory style and illness. *Journal of Personality, 55*, 237–265.

Polatin, P. B., Kinney, R. K., Gatchel, R. J., Lillo, E., & Mayer, T. G. (1993). Psychiatric illness and chronic low back pain. *Spine, 18*, 66–71.

Reed, G. M., Kemeny, M. E., Taylor, S. E., Wang, H. Y. J., & Visscher, B. R. (1994). Realistic acceptance as a predictor of decreased survival time in gay men with AIDS. *Health Psychology, 13*, 299–307.

Rosenstiel, A. K., & Keefe, F. J. (1983). Use of coping strategies in chronic low back pain patients: Relationship to patient characteristics and current adjustment. *Pain, 17*, 33–44.

Rotter, J. B. (1954). *Social learning and clinical psychology*. New York: Prentice-Hall.

Scheier, M. F., & Carver, C. S. (1985). Optimism, coping and health: Assessment and implication of generalized outcome expectancies. *Health Psychology, 4*, 219–247.

Scheier, M. F., & Carver, C. S. (1987). Dispositional optimism and physical well-being: The influence of generalized outcome expectancies on health. *Journal of Personality, 55*, 169–210.

Scheier, M. F., & Carver, C. S. (1992). Effects of optimism on psychological and physical well-being: Theoretical overview and empirical update. *Cognitive Therapy and Research, 16*, 201–228.

Scheier, M., Matthews, K., Owens, J., Magovern, G., Lefebvre, R., Abbot, R., & Carver, C. (1989). Dispositional optimism and recovery from coronary artery bypass surgery: The beneficial effects on physical and psychological well-being. *Journal of Personality and Social Psychology, 57*, 1024–1040.

Scheier, M., Weintraub, J. K., & Carver, C. S. (1986). Coping with stress: Divergent strategies of optimists and pessimists. *Journal of Personality and Social Psychology, 51*, 1257–1264.

Schwarzer, R. (1994). Optimism, vulnerability, and self-beliefs as health-related cognitions: A systemic overview. *Psychology and Health, 9*, 161–180.

Segerstrom, S. C., Taylor, S. E., Kemeny, M. E., & Fahey, J. L. (1998). Optimism is associated with mood, coping and immune change in response to stress. *Journal of Personality and Social Psychology, 74*, 1646–1655.

Seligman, M. E. P. (1991). *Learned optimism*. New York: Knopf.

Sherman, R. A., Camfield, M. R., & Arena, J. G. (1995). Effect of presence or absence of low back pain on the MMPI's Conversion V. *Military Psychology, 7*, 29–38.

Smith, C. A., & Wallston, K. A. (1992). Adaptation in patients with chronic rheumatoid arthritis: Application of a general model. *Health Psychology, 11*, 151–162.

Smith, T. W., Peck, J. R., & Ward, J. R. (1990). Helplessness and depression in rheumatoid arthritis. *Health Psychology, 9*, 377–389.

Taylor, S. E. (1983). Adjustment to threatening events: A theory of cognitive adaptation. *American Psychologist, 38,* 1161–1173.

Taylor, S. E., & Armor, D. A. (1996). Positive illusions and coping with adversity. *Journal of Personality, 64*(4), 873–898.

Taylor, S. E., & Brown, J. D. (1988). Illusion and well-being: A social psychological perspective on mental health. *Psychology Bulletin, 103,* 193–210.

Taylor, S. E., Kemeny, M. E., Aspinwall, L. G., Schneider, S. C., Rodriguez, R., & Herbert, M. (1992). Optimism, coping, psychological distress, and high-risk, sexual behavior among men at risk for AIDS. *Journal of Personality and Social Psychology, 63,* 460–473.

Tennen, H., & Affleck, G. (1987). Costs and benefits of optimistic explanations and dispositional optimism. *Journal of Personality, 55*(2), 377–393.

Tennen, H., Affleck, F., Urrows, S., Higgins, P., & Mendola R. (1992). Perceived control, construing benefits, and daily processes in rheumatoid arthritis. *Canadian Journal of Behavioural Science, 24*(2), 186–203.

Turk, D. C. (1996). Biopsychosocial perspective on chronic pain. In R. J. Gatchel & D. C. Turk (Eds.), *Psychological approaches to pain management* (pp. 3–32). New York: Guilford Press.

Turk, D. C., & Holzman, A. D. (1986). Commonalities among psychological approaches in the treatment of chronic pain: Specifying the meta-constructs. In A. D. Holzman & D. C. Turk (Eds.), *Pain management: A handbook of psychological treatment approaches* (General Psychology Series 136, pp. 257–267). Elmsford, NY: Pergamon.

Turk, D. C., & Rudy, T. E. (1988). Toward an empirically derived taxonomy of chronic pain patients: Integration of psychological assessment. *Journal of Consulting and Clinical Psychology, 56,* 233–238.

Turk, D. C., & Rudy, T. E. (1992). Cognitive factors in persistent pain: A glimpse into Pandora's Box. *Cognitive Therapy and Research, 16,* 99–122.

Turner, J. A., & Clancy, S. (1986). Strategies for coping with chronic low back pain: Relationship to pain and disability. *Pain, 24,* 355–363.

Van Lankveld, W., Van't Pad Bosch, P., Van de Putte, L., Naring, G., & Van der Staak, C. (1994). Disease-specific stressors in rheumatoid arthritis: Coping and well-being. *British Journal of Rheumatology, 33,* 1067–1073.

Williamson, D., Robinson, M. E., & Melamed, B. (1997). Pain behavior, spouse responsiveness, and marital satisfaction in patients with rheumatoid arthritis. *Behavior Modification, 21,* 97–118.

Zautra, A. J., & Manne, S. L. (1992). Coping with rheumatoid arthritis: A review of a decade of research. *Annals of Behavioral Medicine, 14,* 31–39.

Part IV

Personality Disorders and Chronic Pain

Chapter 10
STUDIES INVESTIGATING THE PREVALENCE OF PERSONALITY DISORDERS IN PATIENTS WITH CHRONIC PAIN

James N. Weisberg

Although numerous clinicians and researchers have studied the various personality characteristics and traits of patients with chronic pain, few have examined specific personality disorders, their prevalence, and their significance in the chronic pain population. Many of the chapters in this text, in fact, are dedicated to a review of findings on personality traits and characteristics of pain patients. Clinicians often incorrectly refer to chronic pain patients as a homogenous group having specific personality disorders without empirical evidence to support their assertions. This chapter reviews the relatively sparse data examining the epidemiology of personality disorders in patients with chronic pain. Unfortunately, this has been a much-overlooked area. However, there is a relative amount of consistency between the findings of these studies. Although there does appear to be a higher proportion of patients with personality disorders in the chronic pain population than in the general population, there does not appear to be one "pain personality"; a variety of disorders are represented. This chapter also presents a rationale for early and accurate diagnosis of personality disorders in chronic pain patients.

The chapter introduces the reader to common epidemiological terms, discusses methods that have been used to diagnose personality disorders, reviews the few studies that have diagnosed such disorders in chronic pain patients, and discusses the future of personality disorder diagnosis and the clinical application of working with pain patients.

Issues in Methodology

Much of the difficulty in diagnosing personality disorders arises from problems with their conceptualization and from the methodological and psychometric properties of the measures typically used to assess them (Holdwick, Hilsenroth, Castlebury, & Blais, 1998). Specifically, poor reliability between clinicians, fair stability of diagnosis over time, comorbidity with Axis I disorders, and overlap between Axis II personality disorder are some of the major issues that have been and need to be further addressed. In addition, a significant amount of time is involved in diagnosis.

Although there are several criteria one must meet to diagnose a personality disorder, according to the construct of the *Diagnostic and Statistical Manual of Mental Disorders*, Third Edition, Revised (*DSM-III-R*, American Psychiatric Association [APA], 1987), there is no "gold standard" of what constitutes specific disorders. Studies of personality disorders have demonstrated that patients may receive different Axis II diagnoses from different clinicians. Some diagnoses, such as antisocial personality disorder, appear to have better interrater reliability than others. In the case of borderline personality disorder, for example, many constructs have been used to explain the underlying pathology and provide a diagnosis. These constructs range from psychodynamic formulations (i.e., Kernberg, 1975) to biological bases for the disorder. Therefore, despite the diagnostic criteria listed in the *DSM*, depending on the diagnosing clinician's underlying paradigm, the patient might be considered to have or to not have the disorder in question.

It is well documented that clinical (Axis I) disorders cloud personality disorder diagnosis, and that they simultaneously often coexist and overlap with personality disorders (Holdwick et al., 1998; Links, Heslegrave, & Villella, 1998; Siever & Davis, 1991). Furthermore, the particular Axis I disorder and the immediate state of the patient being interviewed for personality disorders affects his or her reporting of Axis II symptomatology (Joffe, 1988, cited in Links et al., 1998; Weisberg, 1992). For example, the individual with borderline personality disorder may appear stable and emotionally unreactive on a relatively "good" day and, therefore, could under-report lifetime symptomatology. That same individual, under extreme emotional stress, might acknowledge all criteria for borderline personality disorder. This issue speaks both to overlap and to stability of diagnosis over time, as the *DSM* considers personality disorders, by definition, "stable over time." In addition to overlap between Axis I and Axis II disorders, diagnostic overlap is a problem among the personality disorders. Therefore, studies have proposed that they be viewed on a continuum, or as a spectrum of disorders, with groupings according to their commonalties (Widiger, Trull, Hurt, Clarkin, & Frances, 1987).

Following the introduction of the *Diagnostic and Statistical Manual of Mental Disorders, Third Edition (DSM-III*, APA, 1980), Reich, Rosenblatt, and Tupin (1983) attempted to clarify *DSM-III* nomenclature as it applies to chronic pain patients. These authors attempted to provide a research rationale for diagnosing both Axis I (clinical) and Axis II (personality) disorders, based on the assumption that treatment plans and expected outcomes differ greatly between the groups. Because of the structure of the *DSM-III*, these authors believed that chronic pain patients are potentially more accurately diagnosable, thereby increasing the knowledge about chronic pain and therapeutic practices with chronic pain syndromes. In their paper, Reich, Rosenblatt, and Tupin discussed the advances made by *DSM-III* in increasing diagnostic reliability among personality disorders despite the relatively low test–retest reliability ($\kappa = .54$) of personality diagnosis. The authors further note the integration of psychiatric and medical diagnoses in the *DSM-III*. This last point is particularly salient for the diagnosis of persons with chronic pain, as it allows for the recognition of an underlying physiological disorder concurrent with psychiatric diagnosis.

Rationale for Diagnosing Personality Disorders

Personality disorders, as opposed to personality traits or patterns, suggest a pathological function; the characteristics are present to such a degree that they interfere with the individual's ability to function on a daily basis, to interact with others, and, at times, to maintain reality testing. Furthermore, these characteristics are believed to develop early in life and are believed to be pervasive and relatively stable throughout life (APA, 1980). The methods used to diagnose personality disorders, and the subsequent treatment provided to persons suffering from these disorders, has greatly improved since the advent of the *DSM-III* (APA, 1980). In an effort to increase the reliability of psychiatric diagnosis, the association has published a series of manuals delineating specific criteria that must be met before an individual can be given a particular diagnosis. The most recent versions of the *DSM* (APA, 1980, 1987, 1994) allow for diagnosis on five axes, each corresponding to a different class of disorder.

An Axis I diagnosis corresponds to clinical disorders, such as depression, anxiety, or schizophrenia. The individual usually experiences symptoms of these disorders as troubling and seeks treatment as a result of the symptomatology. Treatment usually focuses on the reduction or amelioration of symptoms through the use of psychotropic medications, various forms of psychotherapy, or both. Axis II diagnoses consist of the personality disorders. In the *DSM-IV* these are: (a) paranoid personality disorder, (b) schizoid personality disorder, (c) schizotypal personality disorder, (d) antisocial personality disorder, (e) borderline personality disorder, (f) histrionic personality disorder, (g) narcissistic personality disorder, (h) avoidant personality disorder, (i) dependent personality disorder, (j) obsessive–compulsive personality disorder, and (k) personality disorder not otherwise specified (used when an individual displays features of more than one disorder, but does not meet the full criteria for any of them). This class of disorders might or might not be directly psychologically troubling for the individual, but it can contribute to deficits in interpersonal functioning, reality testing, defenses, and ego (Table 10.1; Weisberg & Keefe, 1997). Axis III allows for the diagnosis of a physical disorder such as diabetes, cardiac condition, or an intervertebral disc herniation. Axis IV is used to note the individual's psychosocial stressors. Axis V rates the patient's overall level of functioning in the past year on a scale from zero to 100. By using a common nomenclature, or nosology, it is believed that many of the difficulties in obtaining consistent diagnoses and treatment plans can be achieved among the clinicians who make the diagnosis.

In addition to the above, there have been few factors, whether physiological, psychological, or social, that appear to consistently help clinicians guide treatment or predict its outcome. As recently as 1996, Gatchel noted that prospective studies are needed to "substantiate these retrospective recall results more clearly" (p. 36) because it is unknown whether many of the psychopathological features observed in chronic pain patients are the consequences of the chronic pain and its related difficulties, or whether preexisting psychopathology predisposes some individuals to develop chronic pain.

Epidemiological Factors

There are many ways to quantify the rates of medical and psychiatric disorders in the population. The most basic of these, *point prevalence*, measures the number of individuals in a population who have a disorder at a given time, calculated as the number of new cases divided by the total population at a specific time. The number of existing cases is obtained with this method, but there is no assessment of the likelihood of new cases developing. *Incidence* is the number of new cases diagnosed with the condition over a specific period. This is obtained by dividing the new cases of the condition by the at-risk population and multiplying it by a period of time. *Period prevalence* refers to the number of cases over a given period, and it is ob-

Table 10.1—*DSM-IV Personality Disorders*

Personality Disorder	Intrapsychic Function–Affect	Interpersonal Function	Defense Mechanism	Cognition–Reality Testing
Paranoid	Unable to accept responsibility, tense, restricted affect	Suspicious, mistrustful, hypersensitive	Projection, occasional ideas of reference	Concrete, suspicious, distorted
Schizoid	Restricted affect	Withdrawn, aloof	Intellectualization, splitting	Abstract, intact reality testing
Schizotypal	Constricted affect, unaware of own affect, anhedonia	Poor, inappropriate interpersonal relations	Paranoia, suspiciousness	Magical thoughts, perceptual aberrations, may have breaks with reality under stress
Antisocial	Seemingly unaware of affect	Unable to conform to social norms, superficially charming, manipulative	Impulsivity, externalization	Good reality testing, sometimes heightened
Borderline	Unstable affect, poor self-image, free-floating anxiety	Tumultuous relations, overvalue–undervalue others	Projection, splitting, devaluation, impulsivity	Poor reality testing at times, may be psychotic under extreme stress

Histrionic	Poorly modulated affect, insecurity	Attention-seeking, dramatic	Repression, conversion, dissociation	Impaired when under stress, vague, global, impressionistic
Narcissistic	Grandiose sense of self, fragile self-esteem	Exploitative of others, manipulative	Entitlement	Fantasies of success, beauty, brilliance, no psychotic thinking
Avoidant	Insecurity	Desires relations but shy, withdrawal at fear of rejection	Vigilance	Good reality testing, occasional cognitive interference
Dependent	Self-doubt, insecurity	Subverts own needs to those of others, needs excessive advice and reassurance	Submissiveness	Intact reality testing, difficulty with decision making
Obsessive–Compulsive	Emotional constriction	Unable to compromise, eager to please authority figures	Repetitive acts, intellectualization	Inflexible thought pattern, ruminative, over-control, detail-oriented

From "Personality disorders in the chronic pain population: Basic concepts, empirical findings and clinical implications," by J. N. Weisberg, & F. J. Keefe, 1997, *Pain Forum, 6*(1), Table 2, p. 3. Copyright 1997, Saunders. Reprinted with permission.

tained by dividing the number of existing cases by the average population over a given period (Mausner & Kramer, 1985).

Each of these definitions is important to understand, both because the epidemiology of personality disorders and chronic pain disorders has been studied using the various methods and because of the implications for primary prevention (preventing the occurrence of chronic pain), secondary prevention (preventing the consequences of chronic pain, such as psychological and physiological dysfunction), and tertiary prevention (multimodal treatment). Without going into detail about the point-prevalence rates of various pain syndromes, a more appropriate concern is that the pattern of prevalence varies between studies and, therefore, there appears to be no consistent pattern other than that the prevalence of back pain increases in men up to age 50 (LeResche & Korff, 1999). Women appear to have higher rates of joint pain than men do, with point-prevalence rates increasing with age, presumably because of hormonal changes. Headaches appear more common in women of all ages, including both migraine and tension-type headache. The highest period prevalence for both genders appears between 35 and 45 years of age (Stewart, Lipton, Celentano, & Reed, 1992, cited in LeResche & Korff, 1999). In contrast to the data on prevalence, LeResche and Korff note the paucity of incidence data or studies that assess risk factors associated with pain onset. The studies that do exist focus on measures such as the Minnesota Multiphasic Personality Inventory (Hathaway & McKinley, 1943) or on Axis I (clinical) diagnoses, such as depression, but are methodologically flawed.

Methods of Personality Disorder Diagnosis

Traditionally, diagnosis of personality disorders has been accomplished through the use of a clinical interview by a mental health clinician. Unfortunately, this method often results in diagnostic discrepancies between clinicians. Recent advances in diagnostic techniques and the increasingly sophisticated nosology of the *DSM* (APA, 1980, 1987, 1994) have led to the proliferation of structured (each question predetermined) and semistructured (some variation in follow-up questions) interviews to obtain a more reliable clinical diagnosis than was previously available for Axis I diagnoses (SADS; Spitzer & Endicott, 1979; SCID; Spitzer, Williams, Gibbon, & First, 1988) and for Axis II diagnoses (PDE; Loranger, Lehman-Susman, Oldman, & Russakof, 1985; SIDP-III-R; Pfohl, Blum, Zimmerman, & Stangl, 1989; SIDP-IV; Pfohl, Blum, Zimmerman, & Stangl, 1995; SCID-II; Spitzer et al., 1988). Although semistructured interviews have been used to provide research diagnoses of the general psychiatric population (Coccaro et al., 1989; Coccaro, Silverman, Klar, Horvath, & Siever, 1994; Oldham et al., 1992; Siever et al., 1986; Silverman et al., 1993), they have not been widely used with chronic pain patients. One reason is the length of time required to administer, score, and interpret a semistructured interview, which is costly in the clinical setting of a pain service, and can range from 3 to 5 hours. However, diagnostic techniques that have been used in research with other populations should, and could, be used in the chronic pain population to establish the most accurate epidemiological information regarding personality disorders and chronic pain. With the increasing sophistication of psychiatric and medical techniques and investigation, the need has arisen for more reliable and valid personality diagnosis of pain patients in order either to confirm or to refute the clinical observations that often presume psychopathology in this population.

Semistructured instruments have been used to yield diagnoses in studies of thought disorder in personality disorders (Weisberg, 1992), biological markers of personality disorders (Siever et al., 1986), family history studies of schizophrenia-related disorders (Siever et al., 1990), personality disorders (Coccaro et al., 1994), and family history studies of schizophrenia and personality disorders (Silverman et al., 1993). Studies using the SIDP (Structured Interview for DSM Personality Disorders) with pain patients have not yet been published, although my colleagues and I are currently conducting such a study. Structured interviews, such as the Structured Clinical Interview for *DSM-III-R* (SCID I and SCID II; Spitzer et al., 1988), have been used with the pain population (Polatin, Kinney, Gatchel, Lillo, & Mayer, 1993). Before reviewing these findings, it is important to explain the methodological rigor that has been applied in biological psychiatry. Because there is no gold standard for personality disorder diagnosis, these studies take unique steps to ensure the accuracy, reliability, and validity of diagnosis. In addition, the methodology demonstrates the effort put into making the diagnosis, and it demonstrates the time and financial commitment one must make when using semistructured instruments.

Silverman et al. (1993) used the SIDP–R (Pfohl, Blum, Zimmerman, & Stangl, 1989) to diagnose 67 psychiatric patients according to *DSM-III* personality disorder criteria. They were examining the psychiatric morbidity of probands (close relatives) of people with schizophrenia and individuals with schizotypal personality disorder. Axis I disorders were first ruled out, because of the above-mentioned difficulties with overlap and confounding of the diagnosis, by administering the Schedule for Affective Disorders and Schizophrenia (Spitzer & Endicott, 1979). Therefore, the personality disorder, rather than any clinical syndrome, was the primary diagnosis. Both the patient and a "knowledgeable informant" (due to the connotation, the term *informant* has been replaced with *historian*; R. L. Trestman, personal communication, August 1995) were interviewed with the SIDP–R. The purpose of the historian (usually a spouse, relative, or close friend) in semistructured interviews is to provide information that either confirms or refutes information obtained from the patient. After both interviews, which were obtained independently by different interviewers, information was pooled by the interviewers, and a consensus was reached for each of the criteria for every Axis II diagnosis. This information was then presented for final diagnosis by an expert diagnostician who was blind to the case. The total time involved in such an undertaking varies, but often exceeds 5 hours, including time for interviews, scoring of the diagnostic criteria, and the consensus conferences.

High interrater reliabilities of schizotypal ($\kappa = .73$) and borderline ($\kappa = .81$) diagnosis were reported (Silverman et al., 1993). Without a rigorous, highly reliable diagnostic instrument, the investigators would have had less credibility in their results because of the decreased reliability of clinical Axis II diagnosis. Thus, the semistructured interview format led to increased reliability, validity, and assurance of a correct diagnosis. One can see that a significant amount of time and effort are put into the process of achieving these diagnoses. In the context of a clinical service, time translates to cost. In addition, patients who are evaluated for back pain are typically resistant to any psychological or psychiatric assessment. The use of a semistructured interview is likely to be perceived by patients as intrusive or inappropriate. However, in the context of clinical research, my experience has demonstrated that patients are generally cooperative, and in many cases, they find that interviews help provide them with some insight about their personality function, as feedback is often given during a "debriefing."

Personality Diagnosis in Chronic Pain

Who Needs it?

Although many pain clinicians and researchers have described, and at times "labeled," chronic pain patients according to *DSM* Axis II terminology, the methods used to obtain these personality diagnoses have been questionable at best, and perhaps inconsistent and inappropriate in some cases. The pain clinician reading this chapter will, undoubtedly, recall case conferences, presentations, and team meetings in which chronic pain patients have been loosely referred to as "dependent" or "borderline," for example. Although this practice might be helpful for explaining difficult or disturbed behavior in a patient or serve as an outlet for the team members to vent their frustrations, it can be inaccurate and lead to incorrect and stigmatizing labeling of the patient. In fact, in most cases, these individuals, like the population in general, likely might have traits or tendencies of many personality disorders, but they do not meet the full criteria for any specific personality disorder diagnosis. The recently developed research interviews used in diagnostic psychiatry research can be used to provide evidence that either supports or refutes such clinical hunches.

Understanding premorbid personality (including psychopathology) in the patient before the onset of chronic pain has several advantages that can lead to better outcome. First, it provides both a frame and a vantage point to help the treating clinicians conceptualize the case. The clinicians can understand the patient's earlier level of functioning and tailor treatment accordingly, rather than either overestimate or underestimate premorbid personality functioning. Second, the conceptual advantage can translate into improved management planning and treatment. Traditionally, accurate diagnosis and a conceptual formulation helped physicians and clinicians to develop the most appropriate techniques for successfully matching treatment modalities (medication, behavior therapy, biofeedback) to an individual case. By knowing, a priori, an individual's personality structure, one can develop the most effective treatment plan. Finally, personality disorder diagnosis aids in the epidemiological study of disorders and diseases.

Categorical or Dimensional Diagnosis?

After the introduction of the *DSM-III* it was proposed that personality disorders be considered as dimensions rather than as discrete entities because of the overlap between personality disorders and the difficulty with operationalizing each specific diagnosis. In addition, individuals often have many traits of various personality disorders but rarely exhibit all the traits of one (Widiger et al., 1987). That is, patients might be subthreshold for a particular diagnosis if they exhibit most or all of the necessary criteria. This phenomenon would result in an individual being diagnosed with traits of the personality disorder, but not the disorder itself. It has been suggested that a subthreshold might change, to reach threshold under the physical, mental, and emotional stress of pain (Weisberg & Keefe, 1997).

Because most people will have more or less of any given diagnosis, based on factor-analytic studies, Widiger and colleagues (1987) described three personality clusters: (a) social personality disorders, consisting of the paranoid, schizoid, and schizotypal personality disorders; (b) flamboyant personality disorders, consisting of the borderline, histrionic, and narcissistic personality disorders; and (c) anxious personality disorders, containing the avoidant, dependent, obsessive–compulsive, and passive–aggressive personality disorders. These clusters were first formally introduced in the *DSM-III-R* and are maintained in the *DSM-IV*. The terminology has been changed, such that the asocial cluster is called the odd–eccentric cluster, the flamboyant cluster consists of the dramatic–emotional styles, and the anxious cluster includes the term *fearful* in its definition.

The dimensional approach also has been advocated to explain the developmental differences between children and the patterns of behavior they exhibit in adulthood (Siever & Davis, 1991). Viewing major categories (dimensions) of behavior, such as impulsivity–aggression, affective instability, cognitive organization, and anxiety–inhibition, these authors make the case that viewing personality and personality disorders along the above dimensions has several advantages. First, although each dimension bisects various disorders (aggression bisects antisocial and borderline personality disorders, depending on developmental diatheses), they are more easily validated externally than are categorical diagnoses. The dimensional approach also provides a link between the overlap previously mentioned between Axis I and Axis II disorders. That is, on one continuum of function (for example, cognitive–perceptual organization) lie both schizophrenia (Axis I) and schizoid personality disorder (Axis II). Similarly, the same continuum is hypothesized to exist in the other developmental dimensions discussed by Siever and Davis (1991).

Studies Using Clinical Interviews of Personality Diagnosis in Chronic Pain Patients

Semistructured-Interview Studies

Reich, Tupin, and Abramowitz used a semistructured interview to diagnose personality disorders in 43 individuals experiencing chronic pain. The 2-hour-long interview was based on flow sheets derived from the *DSM-III* listing of personality disorders. Results indicated that 20 of the 43 patients (47%) met criteria for Axis II disorders. The most frequent diagnoses were histrionic ($n = 6$) and dependent ($n = 5$). One interesting finding was the wide range of disorders identified in the sample—7 of the 12 possible disorders were represented, thereby supporting the heterogenity of the peer population. The authors suggested that further studies on other samples might cross-validate their findings (see Table 10.2).

Reich and Thompson conducted a study of *DSM-III* personality disorder clusters of patients with chronic pain. They used odds ratios to compare the prevalence of personality disorders in three groups of patients: (a) patients with chronic pain, (b) psychiatric patients applying for disability benefits, and (c) psychiatric patients undergoing mental competency hearings. All patients were given a semistructured in-

Table 10.2—*Personality Diagnosis of Chronic Pain Patients*

	Reich, Tupin, & Abramowitz (1983)	Large (1986)	Fishbain et al. (1986)	Polatin et al. (1993)	Gatchel et al. (1996)[a]	Weisberg et al. (1996)	Monti et al. (1998)[b]
Participants	n = 43	n = 50	n = 283	n = 200	n = 50	n = 55	CPRS = 25[c] DRR = 25[d]
Diagnostic measure	Flow sheet interview	Maudsley-style	2-hr semi-structured	SCID-II[e]	SCID-II	Longitudinal	SCID-II
Reliability	None reported	κ = .46	None reported	κ = .63 (n = 20)	None reported	κ = .52 (n = 10)	None reported
Axis II disorders	47%	40%	59%	51%		31%	60% CRPS 64% DRR
Paranoid		2% (traits)	3%	33%	18%	2%	
Schizoid	2%		2%	4%		2%	
Schizotypal	5%			4%	2%	4%	
Histrionic	14%	6%	12%	4%	8%		
Antisocial				5%			
Narcissistic	2%	2% (traits)	2%	5%		2%	
Borderline	7%	2% (traits)	1%	15%	10%	13%	
Avoidant				14%	4%		
Dependent	12%	10%	17%	3%		11%	

Obsessive–compulsive	8% (traits)	7%	6%	10%		28% CRPS 12% DRR
Passive–aggressive[f]	6% (traits)	15%	12%	6%	2%	
Self-defeating[g]			10%	4%	7%	20% CRPS 12% DRR 4% CRPS 20% DRR
Mixed[h]	22%					
	5%					
PD NOS (DSM-IV)			2%	2%	27%	

[a] Based on patients with chronic temporomandibular joint disorder.
[b] $n = 50$.
[c] CRPS = Complex Regional Pain Syndrome.
[d] DRR = disk-related radiculopathy.
[e] SCID = Structured Clinical Interview for *DSM-III-R* (Spitzer et al., 1988).
[f] *DSM-III-R* passive-aggressive category.
[g] *DSM-III-R* self-defeating category.
[h] *DSM-III-R* mixed personality disorder category.

PD = not otherwise specified, used when the individual has features of more than one personality disorder, but does not meet full criteria for any one personality disorder (*DSM-IV*; APA, 1994). From J. N. Weisberg & F. J. Keefe, 1997, "Personality disorders in the chronic pain population: Basic concepts, empirical findings, and clinical implications," 1997, *Pain Forum*, 6(1), Table 3, p. 5. Copyright 1997, Saunders. Reprinted with permission.

terview (not cited) to elicit both Axis I and Axis II *DSM-III* diagnoses. Based on the personality diagnosis, patients were placed in one of the three personality disorder clusters. In instances in which a patient had personality diagnoses in more than one cluster, the patient was placed in the cluster that best reflected the most severe symptom. Results indicated that, on average, patients with chronic pain were more likely to have a diagnosable personality disorder than were individuals in the group undergoing mental competency hearings. Thirty-seven percent of the chronic pain patients met diagnostic criteria for a personality disorder, compared with 11.8% of patients undergoing mental competency hearings. Patients with chronic pain were more likely to have personality disorders in the *DSM-III-R* anxious cluster (Cluster C) than were individuals either in the group undergoing mental competency hearings or in the group applying for disability. Patients with chronic pain also were more likely to have personality disorders in the flamboyant cluster (Cluster B) than were patients in the group undergoing mental competency hearings. Taken together, the results suggest a relatively high level of personality disorder in chronic pain patients, the most frequent of which are those in a cluster containing anxiety-spectrum disorders (Cluster C).

Fishbain, Goldberg, Meagher, Steele, and Rosomoff (1986) reported on an extensive study of 283 chronic pain patients admitted to the University of Miami's Comprehensive Pain and Rehabilitation Center. They conducted a 2-hour semistructured interview to elicit *DSM-III* Axis II diagnoses. The interviews were consistent with *DSM-III* guidelines and structured in the manner recommended for interviewing patients (D. Fishbain, personal communication, November 1994). The authors cite two primary rationales for their study: the knowledge that chronic pain patients often suffer from concomitant psychiatric illness and the fact that only one previous study had used operational criteria for reaching diagnostic decisions. This was the first rigorous attempt at *DSM-III* Axis I and Axis II diagnosis using operational criteria. The authors also collected lifetime occupational and social history in determining Axis II diagnosis. They present detailed demographic information on their sample and thoroughly discuss all of the diagnoses. The patients exhibited a higher incidence (59% vs. 47%) of at least one Axis II diagnosis than found by Reich, Tupin, and Abramowitz (1983). The diagnoses found most frequently by Fishbain et al. (1986) were dependent (17%), passive–aggressive (15%), histrionic (12%), and compulsive personality disorders (7%). More men met the criteria for paranoid and narcissistic personality disorders; women were more likely diagnosed as histrionic. Agreeing with Reich, Rosenblatt, and Tubin (1983), the authors concluded that the *DSM-III* classification system is useful for chronic pain patients but that, because of site differences and difficulties with *DSM-III* criteria, it is difficult to compare their diagnoses with those obtained in other studies. The major difficulty with the study of Fishbain et al., which was a major advance from earlier studies, is the use of a nonstandardized diagnostic interview without multiple-site testing and demonstrated reliability and validity. The authors acknowledged this problem and believe that comparison with other studies might be somewhat mitigated by the use of a structured interview with demonstrated reliability and validity in various populations.

Large (1986) undertook a study to examine the *DSM-III* nosology as it applies to chronic pain patients. Fifty patients at the Auckland (New Zealand) Pain Center were psychiatrically evaluated using a semistructured interview, which led to *DSM-III* diagnoses. Reliability was established by presenting case histories on six randomly selected patients. The Axis II diagnosis (κ = .27 to κ = .46) depended on the clinician. Results indicated that, in addition to patients meeting criteria for an Axis I disorder, 20 met the criteria for a personality disorder, with the mixed category (mixed personality disorder) being most prevalent (n = 11), followed by histronic personality disorder (6%) and dependent personality disorder (10%). Dependency traits were most common in the mixed category; compulsive and dependency traits were most common in those patients who did not fulfill criteria for the mixed (meeting partial criteria for more than one diagnosis) personality disorder. The author acknowledged the difficulties of single-clinician studies and of obtaining accurate, reliable data from pain patients using a semistructured interview. Given the prevalence of Axis II pathology (40%), Large proposed the use of a multiaxial system to diagnose chronic pain patients, with the belief that such a system recognizes differences between patients. Furthermore, the multiaxial system acknowledges physical and mental disease, as well as levels of function, and it encourages individualized treatment on all five axes.

Weisberg, Gallagher, and Gorin (1996) presented data on 55 chronic pain patients evaluated and treated at a comprehensive pain and rehabilitation center. Their study used retrospective, longitudinal data that included a clinical interview and treatment outcome measures, clinic notes, and family and self-report data to diagnose personality disorders. Interrater reliability (n = 10) was consistent with reliabilities found in other studies (κ = .52). The results of this study found slightly lower rates of Axis II disorders than previously reported. Thirty-one percent of the patients met the criteria for a personality disorder. The most frequent diagnosis was personality disorder not otherwise specified (27%; used when an individual meets incomplete criteria for two or more disorders). The next most common diagnoses were borderline personality disorder (13%) and dependent personality disorder (11%; see Table 10.2). The authors are conducting further research that uses a semistructured interview with the same individuals to compare diagnoses obtained through longitudinal chart review with a valid, reliable interview schedule (Pfohl et al., 1997). Although longitudinal diagnosis could provide the most accurate method for obtaining a personality disorder diagnosis, it is by definition impossible to do so during an intake evaluation. The authors believed that a brief, reliable screening instrument given at intake is likely to guide treatment decisions earlier in the course of treatment, thereby decreasing cost and improving outcome (Weisberg et al., 1996; Weisberg & Keefe, 1997).

Structured-Interview Studies

Polatin et al. (1993) conducted a methodologically sophisticated study of personality disorders in chronic pain. The participants were 200 patients with chronic low back pain who were interviewed at the time of entry into a comprehensive pain and rehabilitation program. This was the first study to apply the same type of semistructured interviews that had been used in psychiatric studies previously mentioned. Diagnostic interviews used the SCID and SCID-II (Spitzer et al., 1988), which evaluate Axis I and Axis II disorders, respectively. The SCID-II is based on the patient's self-report of 120 items derived from *DSM-III-R* personality disorder criteria. Although diagnostic reliability for the personality disorder diagnoses (κ = .632) was lower than that for Axis I (κ = .905–1.00), it was still in the acceptable range. Fifty-one percent of patients met criteria for one personality disorder; 30% met criteria for more than one personality disorder. The most common diagnoses were paranoid (33%), borderline (15%), avoidant (14%), and passive–aggressive (12%). Polatin et al. (1993) also found a high prevalence of lifetime Axis I disorder (98%) and current major depressive disorder (45%), which could have affected their Axis II findings. As discussed earlier, in the biological psychiatry literature on personality disorders, primary Axis I disorders are a rule-out for personality diagnosis because of the overlap between Axis I and Axis II disorders and because a patient's immediate emotional state can significantly affect the self-report of interpersonal and intrapsychic functioning needed for an Axis II diagnosis.

In another study, Gatchel, Garofalo, Ellis, and Holt (1996) used the SCID and SCID-II to diagnose *DSM-III-R* Axis I and Axis II disorders in 51 acute and 50 chronic patients with temporomandibular joint disorder. Results of the SCID-II demonstrated a higher prevalence of personality disorders in chronic than in acute patients, although this difference was statistically insignificant. The most common Axis II disorders in the chronic patients were paranoid personality disorder (18%), followed by both obsessive–compulsive personality disorder (10%) and borderline personality disorder (10%).

Personality disorders and clinical syndromes were assessed in patients suffering from Complex Regional Pain Syndrome (CRPS) Type I (Monti, Herring, Schwartzman, & Marchese, 1998), a painful condition that usually develops following trauma to the affected area. The pain appears disproportionate to tissue damage and does not always follow dermatomal distribution (Monti et al., 1998). It is usually described as burning, dysasthetic pain, and is often accompanied by edema, temperature changes, and trophic changes. Within the pain population, patients with the syndrome often are noted to be among the more difficult to treat, both medically and psychologically. As with other pain syndromes, recent research has attempted to discern whether specific personality traits and temperaments predispose individuals to developing the syndrome or are a response to their medical condition. Monti et al. attempted to answer the chicken–egg question by comparing CRPS I patients with patients who had chronic low back pain due to disk-related radiculopathy (DRR) on the SCID and SCID-II. They chose the structured interview because it offers more objectivity than do clinical interviews. Patients with primary Axis I disorders, as assessed by the SCID, were not included in the study.

Psychiatrists trained and experienced in the SCID and SCID-II conducted all interviews (Monti et al., 1998). Demographic results indicated a much higher percentage (point prevalence) of women with CRPS I (80%). In addition, the CRPS patients were less likely to be working following diagnosis than were back pain patients. Axis I diagnoses, mostly depression, were evident in 24% of the CRPS I group and in 20% of the back pain group, a prevalence rate lower than found in previous studies, presumably because of the methodological rigor of the SCID. Depression followed diagnosis (rather than preexisting) in 80% of the CRPS I patients with depression. Of patients without Axis I pathology, 60% of the CRPS I patients had Axis II disorders compared with 64% of back pain patients. The most common *DSM III-R* Axis II diagnoses were obsessive–compulsive personality disorder (CRPS I = 28%; DRR = 12%) and self-defeating personality disorder (CRPS I = 20%; DRR = 12%). The authors commented on the high percentage of self-defeating patients and believe learned helplessness, guilt, and self-blame may account for it. Unfortunately, they did not cite the prevalence of other personality disorders in either group. The authors cited the *diathesis–stress model* of personality disorders in chronic pain (Weisberg & Keefe, 1997) by acknowledging that a "sustained state of pain and disability would intensify this coping mechanism, perhaps to the point of what would appear to be an (obsessive–compulsive) personality disorder" (Monti et al., 1998, p. 301). In brief, the application of the diathesis-stress model to personality disorders in chronic pain posits that underlying personality traits (diathesis) are exacerbated under the stress of pain and disability, and the individual's coping techniques and defense mechanisms fail, leading to a personality disorder (see chapter 12). They suggested that future research might focus on personality-disorder-specific treatment approaches to increase the use of adaptive-coping techniques and decrease the possibility of these traits becoming expressed as personality disorders.

The above studies suggest a high prevalence of personality disorders in patients with chronic pain. All studies found the prevalence of personality disorders to be considerably higher than that found in the general population (Gatchel et al., 1996). The findings underscore the scope of the problem of personality disorders in clinical samples of chronic pain patients. They do not, however, address the causal nature of the relationship or provide support for or refute the diathesis–stress model of personality disorders in this population. Without truly prospective studies of personality disorders at the pain onset—and longitudinal follow-up of these individuals—the causality will remain enigmatic.

Clinical Application of Personality Disorder in Chronic Pain

As discussed earlier, in addition to the epidemiological benefits of accurate diagnosis, and the ethical advantages of prudently diagnosing individuals rather than haphazardly "sticking on a label," personality diagnosis serves many useful clinical functions. First, after an assessment of both premorbid and current personality, changes attributable to the onset of pain might be determined, and treatment could be aimed at returning the individual to his or her previous style of interaction. Second, in cases in which a severe personality disturbance is evident, such as a borderline patient, clinicians can modify their reactions to the patient accordingly. Third, the treatment modality can be fitted to the individual more successfully, optimizing the likelihood of a successful outcome. This point is most crucial, as the treatment success (defined by decreased pain perception, increased function, and decreased health care use) with patients with personality disorders is low, and any way to maximize compliance, independence, decreased emotionality, and other features of personality disorders are likely to result in improved outcomes.

Turk and Okifuji (1998) discussed the "myth" cited by Gallagher et al. (1989) that all chronic pain patients are similar and thus benefit from the same treatment. Based on previous findings of 3 subgroups (Turk & Rudy, 1988) on the MPI (Kerns, Turk, & Rudy, 1985), Turk, Zaki, and Rudy (1993) designed a "dysfunctional" group and found significantly greater changes in behavioral, psychosocial, and physical measures with treatment that targeted the unique characteristics of those patients. Turk and Okifuji (1998) suggested that, although all patients might receive a standard program of physical therapy and psychological interventions, individuals might need additional specific interventions based on their unique characteristics. They also suggested research to assess the differential effects of customizing treatment to patients' psychological and personality characteristics.

Conclusions

Appropriate Axis II diagnosis can aid in the treatment of chronic pain patients by tailoring the treatment to the individual's personality style, common defense mechanisms, and ways of coping. In the medical field, diagnosis leads to treatment. Those of us in the mental health field traditionally have been less concerned with the diagnosis as it relates to treatment. However, for appropriate treatment to occur, accurate, reliable, and valid personality diagnosis must first occur. Semistructured personality disorder interview techniques have been introduced in the psychiatric literature since the advent of *DSM-III* that have been used for several purposes in diagnostic and biologic psychiatry. Although there exists no gold standard for Axis II diagnoses, more reliable and valid diagnoses are now possible with the recent advances of these interview diagnostic techniques. Several studies cited here approximate the advocated goal. In addition to the immediate benefit to the patient who is appropriately diagnosed, the research benefits to be gained from a rigorous diagnostic protocol should either validate or nullify the common belief that some patterns of personality are associated with the chronic pain population. It is time that we incorporate diagnostic technologies introduced by biological psychiatry and put them to use in advancing the field of diagnosis and treatment of chronic pain patients, many of whom are believed to have serious personality deficits.

In the meantime, how should we best assess and treat the chronic pain patient with a personality disorder? We must remember the following: First, diagnosis is of little value if it does not guide treatment decisions. Therefore, rather than haphazardly labeling individuals according to "one size fits all," the use of a personality disorder diagnosis should be made only in cases in which it will provide structure and substance to the treatment team. As an alternative to personality disorder diagnosis, Kahana and Bibring (1964) proposed diagnostic categories that they clearly stated do not represent personality disorders. Their system of delineating personality types has, as its goal, helping the medical physician understand the needs, meanings of illness, and coping styles of the patient. This system of classification has been used in medical settings to assist physicians in assessment and treatment, and the reader is encouraged to review their classic chapter for further information. In addition to the nonpathological method of understanding personality function, newer assessment instruments, such as the NEO–PI (Neuroticism, Extroversion, Openness-Personality Inventory; Costa & McCrae, 1985) and the Millon Behavioral Health Inventory (Millon, Green, & Meagher, 1983), have been investigated extensively in the pain population.

Second, inappropriate or overdiagnosis can be detrimental to an individual both within and beyond the treatment setting, and we must be reminded to "first do no harm." Although there are brief screening measures for *DSM-IV* personality disorders used in research (SIDP–IV; personal communication, B. Pfohl, April 7, 1995; Schedule for Nonadaptive and Adaptive Personality; Clark, 1993), until there is a timely, reliable, and valid instrument to make personality disorder diagnosis in the chronic pain population, diagnosis should be made only after careful evaluation, observation, and consensus between treating clinicians. In addition, obtaining historical information about the patient from family or close friends is necessary to establish that behavior predates onset of chronic pain. In most instances, the stress of the pain and disability will exacerbate premorbid character pathology.

References

American Psychiatric Association. (1980). *Diagnostic and statistical manual of mental disorders* (3rd ed.). Washington, DC: Author.

American Psychiatric Association. (1987). *Diagnostic and statistical manual of mental disorders* (3rd ed., rev.). Washington, DC: Author.

American Psychiatric Association. (1994). *Diagnostic and statistical manual of mental disorders* (4th ed.). Washington, DC: Author.

Clark, L. (1993). *Schedule for Nonadaptive and Adaptive Personality (SNAP)*. Minneapolis: University of Minneapolis Press.

Coccaro, E., Siever, L., Klar, H., Maurer, G., Cochrane, K., Cooper, T., Mohs, R., & Davis, K. (1989). Serotonergic studies in patients with affective and personality disorders: Correlates with suicidal and impulsive aggressive behavior. *Archives of General Psychiatry, 46*, 587–599.

Coccaro, E. F., Silverman, J. M., Klar, H. M., Horvath, T. B., & Siever, L. J. (1994). Familial correlates of reduced central serotonergic system function in patients with personality disorders. *Archives of General Psychiatry, 51*, 318–324.

Costa, P. T., & McCrae, R. R. (1985). *The NEO Personality Inventory Manual*. Orlando, FL: Psychological Assessment Resources.

Fishbain, D. A., Goldberg, M., Meagher, B. R., Steele, R., & Rosomoff, H. (1986). Male and female chronic pain patients categorized by the DSM-III psychiatric diagnostic criteria. *Pain, 26*, 181–197.

Gallagher, R. M., Raugh, V., Haugh, L. D., Milhous, R., Callas, P. W., Langelier, R., McClallen, J. M., & Frymoyer, J. (1989). Determinants of return-to-work among low back pain patients. *Pain, 39*, 55–67.

Gatchel, R. (1996). Psychological disorders and chronic pain: Cause and effect relationships. In R. Gatchel & D. C. Turk (Eds.), *Psychological approaches to pain management* (pp. 33–52). New York: Guilford Press.

Gatchel, R. J., Garofalo, J. P., Ellis, E., & Holt, C. (1996). Major psychological disorders in acute and chronic TMD: An initial examination. *Journal of the American Dental Association, 127*, 1365–1374.

Hathaway, S. R., & McKinley, J. C. (1943). Minnesota Multiphasic Personality Inventory. Minneapolis: University of Minnesota Press.

Holdwick, D. J., Hilsenroth, M., Castlebury, R., & Blais, M. (1998). Identifying the unique and common characteristics among the DSM-IV Antisocial, Borderline, and Narcissistic personality disorders. *Comprehensive Psychiatry, 39*(5), 277–286.

Kahana, R., & Bibring, G. (1964). Personality types in medical management. In N. Zinberg (Ed.), *Psychiatry and medical practice in a general hospital* (pp. 108–123). New York: International Universities Press.

Kernberg, O. (1975). Borderline conditions and pathological narcissism. New York: Aronson.

Kerns, R. D., Turk, D. C., & Rudy, T. E. (1985). The West Haven-Yale multidimensional pain inventory (WHYMPI). *Pain, 23*, 345–356.

Large, R. G. (1986). DSM-III diagnoses in chronic pain: Confusion or clarity? *Journal of Nervous and Mental Disease, 174*(5), 295–303.

LeResche, L., & Korff, M. V. (1999). Epidemiology of chronic pain. In A. Block, E. Kremer, & E. Fernandez (Eds.), *Handbook of pain syndromes: Biopsychological perspectives* (pp. 3–22). Mahwah, NJ: Earlbaum.

Links, P., Heslegrave, R., & Villella, J. (1998). Psychopharmacological management of personality disorders: An outcome-focused model. In K. Silk (Ed.), *Biology of personality disorders* (pp. 93–127). Washington, DC: American Psychiatric Association.

Loranger, A., Lehman-Susman, V., Oldman, J., & Russakof, L. (1985). *Personality Disorders Examination (PDE): A structured interview for DSM-III-R personality disorders.* White Plains, NY: New York Hospital—Cornell Medical Center, Westchester Division.

Mausner, J., & Kramer, S. (1985). *Epidemiology—An introductory text.* Philadelphia: W. B. Saunders.

Millon, T., Green, C., & Meagher, R. (1983). *Millon Behavioral Health Inventory* (3rd ed.). Minneapolis: National Computer Systems.

Monti, D., Herring, C., Schwartzman, R., & Marchese, M. (1998). Personality assessment of patients with Complex Regional Pain Syndrome Type I. *Clinical Journal of Pain, 14*(4), 295–302.

Oldham, J., Skodol, A., Kellman, H., Hyler, S., Rosnick, L., & Davies, M. (1992). Diagnosis of DSM-III-R personality disorders by two structured interviews: Patterns of comorbidity. *American Journal of Psychiatry, 149*(2), 213–220.

Pfohl, B., Blum, N., Zimmerman, M., & Stangl, D. (1989). *Structured interview for DSM-III-R personality disorders.* University of Iowa.

Pfohl, B., Blum, N., & Zimmerman, M. (1997). *Structured interview for DSM-IV personality disorders.* Washington, DC: American Psychiatric Press.

Polatin, P. B., Kinney, R. K., Gatchel, R. J., Lillo, E., & Mayer, T. G. (1993). Psychiatric illness and chronic low-back pain. The mind and the spine—Which goes first? *Spine, 18*(1), 66–71.

Reich, J., Rosenblatt, R., & Tupin, J. (1983). DSM-III: A new nomenclature for classifying patients with chronic pain. *Pain, 16*, 201–206.

Reich, J., & Thompson, D. (1987). DSM-III personality disorder clusters in three populations. *British Journal of Psychiatry, 150*, 471–475.

Reich, J., Tupin, J. P., & Abramowitz, S. I. (1983). Psychiatric diagnosis of chronic pain patients. *American Journal of Psychiatry, 140*(11), 1495–1498.

Siever, L. J., Coccaro, E. P., Klar, H., Losonczy, M. P., Silverman, J. P., & Davis, K. L. (1986). *Biologic markers in borderline and related personality disorders.* In proceedings of the World Congress of Biologic Psychiatry, 566–568.

Siever, L. J., & Davis, K. L. (1991). Psychobiological perspective on the personality disorders. *American Journal of Psychiatry, 148*(12), 1647–1658.

Siever, L. J., Silverman, J. M., Horvath, T. B., Klar, H., Coccaro, E., Keefe, R. S. E., Pinkham, L., Rinaldi, P., Mohs, R. C., & Davis, K. L. (1990). Increased morbid risk for schizophrenia-related disorders in relatives of schizotypal personality disorder. *Archives of General Psychiatry, 47*, 634–640.

Silverman, J. M., Siever, L. J., Horvath, T. B., Coccaro, E. F., Klar, H., Davidson, M., Pinkman, L., Apter, S. H., Mohs, R. C., & Davis, K. L. (1993). Schizophrenia-related and affective personality disorder traits in relatives of probands with schizophrenia and personality disorders. *American Journal of Psychiatry, 150*(3), 435–442.

Spitzer, R., & Endicott, J. (1979). *Schedule for Affective Disorders and Schizophrenia— Lifetime version.* New York: New York State Institute, Biometrics Research.

Spitzer, R. L., Williams, J. B., Gibbon, M., & First, M. B. (1988). *Structured Clinical Interview for DSM-III-R.* New York: New York State Psychiatric Institute.

Stewart, W. F., Lipton, R. B., Celentano, D. D., & Reed, M. L. (1992). Prevalence of migraine headache in the United States: Relation to age, income, race and other sociodemographic factors. *Journal of the American Medical Association, 267*, 64–69.

Turk, D., & Okifuji, A. (1998). Directions in prescriptive chronic pain management based on diagnostic characteristics of the patient. *APS Bulletin, 8*, 5–11.

Turk, D. C., & Rudy, T. E. (1988). Toward an empirically derived taxonomy of chronic pain patients: Integration of psychological assessment data. *Journal of Consulting and Clinical Psychology, 56*, 233–238.

Turk, D. C., Zaki, H. S., & Rudy, T. E. (1993). Effects of intraoral appliance and biofeedback/stress management alone and in combination in treating pain and depression in TMD patients. *Journal of Prosthetic Dentistry, 70*, 158–160.

Weisberg, J. (1992). Assessment of formal thought disorder in personality disorders. *Dissertation Abstracts International, 54*(5).

Weisberg, J. N., Gallagher, R. M., & Gorin, A. (1996, November). *Personality disorder in chronic pain: A longitudinal approach to validation of diagnosis.* Paper presented at the 15th Annual Scientific Meeting of the American Pain Society, Washington, DC.

Weisberg, J. N., & Keefe, F. J. (1997). Personality disorders in the chronic pain population: Basic concepts, empirical findings, and clinical implications. *Pain Forum, 6*(1), 1–9.

Widiger, T. A., Trull, T. J., Hurt, S. W., Clarkin, J., & Frances, A. (1987). A multidimensional scaling of the DSM-III personality disorders. *Archives of General Psychiatry, 44*, 557–563.

Chapter 11
HOW PRACTITIONERS SHOULD EVALUATE PERSONALITY TO HELP MANAGE PATIENTS WITH CHRONIC PAIN

Robert J. Gatchel

The search for specific personality or psychosocial factors that predispose individuals to develop chronic pain problems has always been a major focus in the field of psychosomatic medicine. Investigators have attempted to identify specific disorder personality types, such as a "migraine personality," as well as a more general "pain-prone personality" (Blumer & Heilbronn, 1982). By and large, these efforts have received little empirical support and in fact have been challenged (Turk & Salovey, 1984). Although there is no research to consistently demonstrate a link between a *specific* personality type and the development of chronic pain disability, there can be no doubt that, based on their experiences, people develop unique ways of interpreting information and coping with stress. These patterns affect pain perceptions and responses to the presence of pain, and if they are maladaptive, then one would expect more difficulty in coping.

Individuals with a personality disorder *in general* would be expected to display an inability to cope with a major stressor such as chronic pain. Millon (1981) suggested that there are three major characteristics of individuals with personality disorders: (a) Their style of perceiving and relating to challenges tends to perpetuate or intensify preexisting difficulties. (b) Their coping style leaves them extremely vulnerable under conditions of subjective stress. (c) Their actual coping strategies are few and appear to be protected rigidly. As discussed in this chapter, a major contention is that the presence of a personality disorder or cluster, in general—and not necessarily a specific type of personality disorder—impairs coping ability and could be related to problems with chronic pain disability. This, in turn, has major clinical implications for how to best manage chronic pain patients.

Base Rates of Psychopathology

If we review the results from the National Institute of Mental Health (NIMH) epidemiologic study on 1-month prevalence of various mental disorders in the general population (Regier et al., 1988) we should not be surprised to find that there are chronic pain patients who often experience psychiatric problems because the base rates for such problems in the general population are quite high. For example, the statistics show a 7.3% prevalence rate for anxiety disorders and a rate of 5.1% for affective disorders in the general population. The rate for symptoms of schizophrenia is 0.7%, and the rate for drug and alcohol abuse is about 3.8%. Therefore, 15.4% of

The writing of this chapter was supported in part by grants DE10713-05 and MH46452-05 from the National Institutes of Health.

the noninstitutionalized population has some significant mental health disorder. An earlier study of *lifetime* prevalence of those disorders assessed across three sites showed rates that were even higher (Robins et al., 1984). One can easily argue that these disorders will become greatly exacerbated under the stress of a chronic pain disability.

The NIMH prevalence statistics do not account for the equally prevalent personality disorders, such as antisocial, borderline, and paranoid personalities, estimated at between 10% and 18% in the general population (Weissman, 1993; Zimmerman & Coryell, 1989). There are also data to suggest that patients with codiagnoses on Axis I and Axis II (*Diagnostic and Statistical Manual of Mental Disorders DSM-IV*; American Psychiatric Association [APA], 1994) have a poor prognosis and higher relapse rate than do comparable patients who do not have an Axis II diagnosis (e.g., Fyer, Frances, Sullivan, Hurt, & Clarkin, 1988; Joffe & Regan, 1988). Thus, a personality disorder, together with a major psychiatric illness, can be an especially poor prognostic sign and perhaps an index of greater vulnerability to major stressors, such as chronic pain and disability. Pain management specialists must be aware of such psychological characteristics to manage their patients' pain effectively.

Indeed, the demonstration of the presence of personality disorders in a chronic pain population was the result of the first large-scale study of this association by Fishbain, Goldberg, Meagher, Steel, and Rosomoff (1986). These investigators evaluated chronic pain patients who were administered a semistructured interview that yielded *DSM* personality disorder diagnoses. They found that 59% of chronic pain patients met criteria for a personality disorder diagnosis. In a more methodologically rigorous study, by Polatin, Kinney, Gatchel, Lillo, and Mayer (1993), 200 chronic pain patients underwent a structured interview—the Structured Clinical Interview for *DSM-III-R* (SCID and SCID II; Spitzer, Williams, Gibbon, & First, 1988)—at the time of entry into a comprehensive pain rehabilitation program. The SCID evaluates current and lifetime incidence of Axis I and II disorders. The SCID II was used to diagnose personality disorders. Interview questions on this measure are based on a patient's self-report of 120 items. Results revealed that 51% of the patients met the criteria for one personality disorder, and 30% met criteria for more than one.

In another study, Gatchel, Garofalo, Ellis, and Holt (1996) used the SCID and SCID II for the diagnosis of 51 acute and 50 chronic patients with temporomandibular joint disorders (TMD). Results revealed that chronic TMD patients had higher rates of Axis II personality disorders than did acute TMD patients (although the difference was not statistically significant). The most common Axis II disorders in the chronic TMD patients were paranoid personality disorder (18%), obsessive–compulsive personality disorder (10%), and borderline personality disorder (10%).

In yet another study, Gatchel, Polatin, Mayer, and Garcy (1994) evaluated whether the success of a comprehensive functional restoration program for patients with chronic low back pain would be adversely affected by the psychopathology of the patients. The SCID and SCID II were administered to 152 patients before they entered a functional restoration program. Consistent with other studies, 58% met criteria for an Axis II personality disorder. At a 1-year posttreatment evaluation of important socioeconomic outcomes, such as return to work and health care use rates, 85% of the patients, regardless of personality characteristics, demonstrated successful outcomes. The findings are interpreted as a clear example of the fact that, when a rehabilitation program is planned to help manage clinical psychiatric symptoms and personality issues (as functional restoration does), the psychopathology of patients need not interfere with successful program completion and such socioeconomic outcomes as return to work.

Personality Factors and Chronic Pain

Weisberg and Keefe (1999) noted that "one of the most challenging tasks for pain clinicians is dealing with personality factors in the patients they treat" (p. 56). These authors provide common examples of this phenomenon: Patients with neurotic personalities persist in worrying about even minor pain or physical complaints even after the initial pathology that produced the pain is long since resolved. Patients with borderline personality disorder make more demands on clinical staff for immediate attention and specialized treatment, becoming angry and passive–aggressive if their demands are not met. Patients with depressive personalities present themselves as hopeless about the future prospect of pain relief and as helpless when asked to assume an active role in their own treatment program. To deal effectively with such patient characteristics, which can create significant barriers to recovery, pain management professionals need to have assessment approaches to better identify and explain the characteristics of personality.

The introduction of the multiaxial diagnostic system in the *DSM-III* (APA, 1980) reflected the view that temperament and trait factors are important in the development of psychiatric symptoms and disorders. It was seen as essential to conceptualize patients' clinical symptoms or major psychopathology (Axis I, clinical disorders) within the broader context of lifelong styles of coping and relating to the world (Axis II, personality disorders). This generated considerable research on the more precise definition and assessment of personality disorders. There were important distinctions made among the various disorders as described in the *DSM-III-R* (APA, 1987), as well as the subsequent *DSM-IV* (APA, 1994). To differentiate among these disorders, the Axis II criteria of the *DSM-III-R* and DSM-IV follow a *categorical* taxonomic system. As described by Gorton and Akhtar (1990), the criteria are based almost exclusively on qualitative behavioral, cognitive, and interpersonal indicators rather than on quantitative indicators. The distinctions between normal and abnormal personality proposed in the *DSM* categorical format were not derived empirically; they were originally determined on the basis of clinical judgment. Although significant efforts, based on recent empirical evidence, have gone into the revision of the Axis II personality disorders based on more recent empirical evidence, the basic criticisms of the *DSM-III-R* continue to hold true for the *DSM-IV*.

Indeed, the investigation of chronic pain patients, such as those with low back pain, using the *DSM-III* criteria revealed great inconsistency in which personality disorders were reported to be more prevalent. One reason most likely was the low reliability of the *DSM-III* personality disorders (Frances, 1980; Zimmerman, 1994). Thus, although there is evidence to support the high rates of personality pathology in the population with chronic low back pain, the interpretation of the exact nature of this pathology varies greatly. Some investigators suggest that the presence of virtually *any* type of personality disorder could be a more significant characteristic of the chronic pain syndrome than is any *specific* array of disorders. Indeed, in our own research, we have not yet found any specific array of personality disorders to be more associated than another. Moreover, we have found that many patients do not meet all the criteria needed for diagnosis. However, when we did a preliminary analysis of the data to include patients who met all of the criteria but one (sub-threshold), the predictive relationship was much stronger and more statistically significant (Gatchel, 1996).

In addition to the lack of empirical evidence to support differentiation among the personality diagnostic categories in normal and patient groups, there are several other significant criticisms that question the use of a categorical approach (as opposed to a dimensional approach) to personality disorder assessment: (a) the difficulty inherent in classifying patients who fall at the boundaries of a category; (b) the loss of information when patients fall just below threshold for a disorder (as we found in our research; Gatchel, 1996); (c) the high degree of heterogeneity often found within diagnostic groups; (d) the high degree of overlap among diagnostic groups; and (e) the need for wastebasket categories, such as "mixed" or "atypical" (Frances & Widiger, 1986; Widiger, Frances, & Spitzer, 1988; Widiger, Trull, & Hurt, 1987). Such shortcomings lead many investigators to suggest that a dimensional approach to personality disorder assessment is much more sensitive than is a categorical system (Clark, 1993c; Cloninger, 1987; Eysenck, 1987; Widiger, 1992; Widiger et al., 1987). Eysenck (1987), in fact, has argued that practically all of the behaviors used to describe the various categories of personality disorders in the *DSM-III* were conceptualized in terms of "more or less" rather than "either or," thus making it an implicit dimensional assumption rather than a categorical one. Indeed, the *DSM-IV* embraces three underlying dimensions in its cluster organization of disorders: degree of oddness or eccentricity (Cluster A: schizoid, schizotypal, paranoid), degree of dramatic affect or emotionality (Cluster B: histrionic, borderline, narcissistic, antisocial), and degree of anxiety or fear (Cluster C: passive–aggressive, avoidant, dependent, compulsive).

The debate continues about whether a categorical or dimensional approach is more appropriate. Traditionally, personality researchers have assumed a dimensional approach and an emphasis on a range from normal–adaptive to abnormal–maladaptive. However, it is important to acknowledge that the two systems are not mutually exclusive. Clark (1992) argued that a dimensional approach is a necessary precursor to the investigation of categorical entities. That is to say, it allows for the investigation of whether and how personality traits combine to form discrete categories, thus having the potential to provide a much-needed empirical basis for the description of personality disorders. Another advantage of a dimensional approach is that the boundaries between normal and abnormal personality function can be established empirically.

Assessment Instruments

There are several instruments to assess personality and its disorders. Most approaches provide scores for the *DSM* Axis II diagnoses (they follow a categorical approach). These include semistructured clinical interviews, such as the Structured Interview for *DSM-III* Personality Disorders (Pfohl, Stangl, & Zimmerman, 1983); the Personality Disorder Examination (Loranger, Susman, Oldham, & Russakoff, 1985); and the SCID-II (Spitzer et al., 1988), which we have used in our research (Gatchel, 1996). Although these instruments are significant improvements over earlier, unstructured approaches to personality assessment, they are still susceptible to many of the limitations associated with the categorical system. Moreover, investigators often cite multiple personality diagnoses for the same patient when assessment is based on structured instruments. Clark (1993b) summarized various studies that revealed that, on average, 85% of patients diagnosed with a personality disorder received multiple Axis II diagnoses. He also stated that the average degree of overlap between any two specific pairs of personality disorders was 10% (ranging from 0% to 45%). These data raise questions about the distinct boundaries assumed to exist between specific Axis II diagnostic categories.

Dimensions

Several instruments assess personality disorders from a dimensional approach. These include semistructured interviews, such as the Personality Assessment Schedule (Tyrer & Alexander, 1979); the *Personality Interview Questionnaire* (Widiger & Frances, 1985); and self-report measures, such as the Millon Clinical Multiaxial Inventory (MCMI; Millon, 1983) and the Minnesota Multiphasic Personality Inventory scales (MMPI-2) that assess traits (Morey, 1985). Unfortunately, most measures that assess personality from a dimensional or trait perspective also have psychometric limitations (Widiger, 1992). The MCMI, which is probably the most widely used to assess personality disorders clinically, was constructed and validated to measure the personality typology developed by Millon (1981), and it also is associated with significant psychometric difficulties (Widiger & Sanderson, 1987) as is the MCMI–II (Streiner & Miller, 1989). There is now also the MCMI–III.

One instrument used to assess personality traits and disorders from a dimensional approach that has addressed many of the limitations found in earlier tests is the Schedule for Nonadaptive and Adaptive Personality (SNAP; Clark, 1993b). The SNAP, which is discussed in greater detail in chapter 12 of this text, is a factor-analysis-derived, self-report instrument that assesses Axis II pathology in terms of trait dimensions. The SNAP has 15 scales—12 are considered "trait" scales that assess primary traits important in the domain of personality disorders, and 3 are considered "temperament" scales that measure general affective traits. It also has 5 validity scales and an overall validity index. The scale scores derived from the SNAP are designed to reflect personality trait variation, ranging from nonpathological to severely disordered. All of the scales are internally consistent and have acceptable retest reliability. The primary trait scales are all relatively independent. The SNAP contains items to assess the Axis II personality disorder criteria of the *DSM-IV*, and the dimensions evaluated relate well to the five-factor model of personality proposed by Costa and McCrae (1989). In fact, Clark (1993a) reported that a greater portion of variance for several personality disorders is accounted for in the SNAP than in the five-factor model. One reason is that the five-factor model was developed primarily on the normal range of personality, whereas the SNAP was developed to capture a wider range of the normal and the abnormal.

Preliminary research using the SNAP is quite promising. In an initial study by Clark, McEwen, Collard, and Hickok (1993), three groups of individuals varying in

personality pathology were assessed using the SNAP (college students, college students seeking outpatient counseling, and inpatients from a substance abuse unit and
a personality disorders unit at a state hospital). Results demonstrated systematic
patterns of scale-level differences emerging from the SNAP profiles of the three
groups, suggesting its validity.

Personality Disorders and Coping

One hallmark of individuals with personality disorders is a failure of, or inadequate,
coping skills. Indeed, the *DSM-IV* explicitly defined personality disorders in terms
of traits or styles that "are inflexible and maladaptive and cause either significant
functional impairment or subjective distress" (APA, 1994, p. 630). As such, one
would expect independent evaluation of coping skills to further document these deficits in individuals with personality disorders. There is growing demonstration of a
relationship between ineffective pain-coping strategies and chronic pain (e.g.,
Kleinke, 1994; Turk & Rudy, 1986). Jayson (1997) noted the potential importance
of coping strategies in affecting outcomes for treatment of low back pain. Much of
the research has been correlational, although there is evidence that patients who are
taught effective pain-coping strategies deal more effectively with their pain (e.g.,
Keefe et al., 1990). There has been very little research directly evaluating the relationship between personality disorder and coping style.

One instrument that accounts for the issue of personality and coping is the
Multidimensional Pain Inventory (MPI), also known as the West Haven–Yale Multidimensional Pain Inventory (Kerns, Turk, & Rudy, 1985), which was developed to
measure three psychosocial dimensions of pain: (a) patient self-reported pain and the
effect of pain, (b) responses of significant others to the communications of pain
patients, and (c) level of daily living activities. Kerns et al. demonstrated in developing this instrument that the MPI has good psychometric properties. Turk and Rudy
(1988) subsequently developed a classification system, using the MPI, which categorized patients according to three subgroups that predicted response to treatment:
dysfunctional, interpersonally distressed, and adaptive copers. According to their system, dysfunctional subgroup patients are hypothesized not to respond as well to
intervention as would patients in the other two subgroups. A study by Asmundson,
Norton, and Alterdings (1997) reported that patients with chronic low back pain who
were classified as dysfunctional on the MPI reported more pain-specific fear and
avoidance than did patients in the other two subgroups. Such characteristics were,
in turn, related to poorer coping ability in these dysfunctional chronic pain patients.
Turk and Okifuji (1998) reviewed the research demonstrating the utility of the MPI
with other chronic pain conditions.

Which Personality Assessment Tools Should We Use?

As noted in the past (Gatchel, 1991), no single psychological device can be used
reliably in all personality assessments; one cannot assume that one instrument can
be used as a sole conclusive predictive or descriptive variable. Such data should be
viewed as just one source of information to be considered along with other types of

information. One also must know about a patient's history of social relationships, the presence or absence of social support networks, job and life satisfaction and success, the history of coping with stressors, and so on, to make a probability statement concerning the prediction of some behavior such as response to pain (e.g., a person with a history of coping well with stressors has an 80% probability of not displaying a great deal of pain behaviors). It is extremely rare to be able to make a completely accurate prediction of some behavior based on a single psychological or personality assessment instrument. Multiple sources of data should be used to provide a comprehensive evaluation of a chronic pain patient. This section reviews various assessment procedures that can be used to elucidate pain patients' personality characteristics. These should not be viewed as a Holy Grail of personality assessment, but as important pieces of the personality puzzle that have helped pain management professionals treat chronic pain patients. Many of these procedures are also discussed in other chapters of this text.

Beck Depression Inventory–II

The Beck Depression Inventory–II (BDI–II) consists of 21 items with a cumulative scoring system focusing on physical manifestations, such as sleep disturbance, sexual dysfunction, and weight change, and psychological symptoms, such as anhedonia. The original BDI was developed by Beck (1967) as a means of assessing the cognitive components of depression. Depression, like anxiety, is a frequent concomitant of chronic pain and, therefore, is an important psychosocial variable to evaluate. Although it is unclear whether depression precedes or follows the onset of pain symptoms in most cases, knowledge of its presence can be helpful. For example, offering depressed patients pharmacologic treatment can encourage greater patient motivation and compliance with therapy. Indeed, the adjunctive use of antidepressant medication has become increasingly popular in the treatment of chronic pain.

The simplicity of the BDI–II also makes it attractive. Patients complete the form in about 5 minutes, and scoring takes less than 1 minute. The BDI–II also can be repeated to gauge progression of the patient's depressive symptoms and the effects of treatment programs. When the BDI–II is used in conjunction with a psychosocial interview, grossly exaggerated or underplayed scores on this instrument can provide significant insight to the clinician concerning a patient's defense mechanisms and approach to pain, and they can suggest the need for more psychiatric or psychological counseling in a comprehensive treatment program. For example, patients who deny the existence of depressive symptoms but who have considerable pain and functional impairment are often defensive about acknowledging any psychological aspect of their illness. Patients who have excessively high scores often are quite fragile psychologically. Those with high BDI–II scores, but with low functional impairment, generally are dependent and feel overwhelmed by all stressors.

Finally, the BDI–II primarily measures cognitive factors in depression. For a more careful evaluation of vegetative signs of depression, such as loss of appetite or sleep, the Hamilton Rating Scale for Depression (Hamilton, 1960) can be used. The major drawback of this scale is that an interviewer must be trained to administer it orally.

Minnesota Multiphasic Personality Inventory-2

Ever since Hanvik (1951) first used MMPI scale descriptors with a chronic pain population, an abundance of research has expanded this form of evaluation of the 10 primary clinical scales by which MMPI-2 responses are classified. The hysteria, depression, and hypochondriasis scales are the most important for assessing chronic pain patients. MMPI profiles are reviewed in Part I of this text. Numerous other scales have been developed for the MMPI-2 that could be useful with a chronic pain population. The McAndrew scale was initially standardized on an outpatient group of alcoholics. It helps a clinician to recognize a patient with an alcoholic or drug-dependent personality type. Therefore, it can often help determine which patients could be at risk for drug abuse, before habituation occurs. Patients who have positive scores on the McAndrew scale need not be active drug users, and even former substance abusers often score high. This scale can be useful for evaluating patients with acute low back pain to identify those who might be particularly susceptible to long periods of hospitalization for bed rest and to excessive analgesic use. Patients with high scores tend to be prolonged users of oral opiate analgesics and tranquilizing muscle relaxants as their pain becomes more chronic. Because the personality profile of the dependent drug abuser bears some resemblance to that of many chronic pain patients, abnormalities on this scale can raise a red flag to help clinicians be aware of early adverse behavioral changes.

Another scale of the MMPI-2—the ego-strength scale—can help identify patients who have limited emotional resources. Patients who exhibit particularly low ego-strength scores, concurrent with other psychological problems, usually are less likely to benefit from treatment regimens that demand motivation and personal responsibility than are patients who score higher. This scale can help the clinician determine whether patients need more or less motivation or training in acquiring personal control and accepting responsibility for their behaviors.

Another MMPI-2 profile that can provide important information concerning personality characteristics is the Conversion V profile. When this profile is found in women, in combination with a V pattern on the Psychopathic Deviate, Masculinity–Femininity, and Paranoia scales, there is often a great deal of anger, acting-out and paranoia that accompany the high somatization. The V pattern is elevation of the sociopathy and paranoia scales and a low masculinity–femininity scale. Patients who exhibit this pattern usually are extremely difficult to work with in treatment. The staff therefore usually will be required to make additional efforts in managing such patients.

As an alternative to the MMPI-2, the System Check List 90–Revised (SCL-90–R; Derogatis, Lipman, & Covi, 1973) can be administered. This test was developed to measure psychopathology in psychiatric and medical outpatients, and it has a high degree of convergence with the MMPI-2. It takes only about 20 minutes to complete, and it provides an alternative to the much longer MMPI-2. Unlike the MMPI-2, though, specific profile patterns that can be useful in a population of chronic pain patients have not been developed. The SCL-90–R is a general red flag of emotional distress clinically when there are significant elevations on major scales such as depression, anxiety, fear, somatic distress, and as a measure of overall symptomatology when there is an elevation of the global symptom reporting summary scale (Kinney, Gatchel, & Mayer, 1991).

Multidimensional Pain Inventory

Earlier in this chapter, it was pointed out that the MPI (Kerns et al., 1985) can serve as a useful measure of coping displayed by pain patients. The MPI consists of a set of empirically derived scales to assess chronic pain. Its benefits include its brevity, its empirical derivation, and its connection to a normative data base of chronic pain patients. The MPI has 13 scales: pain severity, interference, life control, affective distress, support, punishing responses, solicitous responses, distracting responses, household chores, outdoor work, activities away from home, social activities, and general activity level. The factor structure and psychometric properties have been replicated in numerous studies in the United States, Germany, Sweden, and the Netherlands. On the basis of cluster analyses on a heterogeneous sample of chronic pain patients' responses, Turk and Rudy (1988) identified three distinct profiles to differentiate between pain patients in various areas such as observed physical functioning, self-reported pain, depressive moods, quality of interpersonal relationships, and perceived functional limitation. Such behaviors obviously would be extremely important for pain management specialists to consider.

1. *Dysfunctional profile* patients tend to perceive the severity of their pain to be high and to report that pain interferes with much of their lives. They also report a higher degree of psychological distress because of their pain and, as a consequence, usually report low levels of activity.
2. *Interpersonally distressed* patients are similar to dysfunctional profile patients, but they also perceive that their significant others are not very understanding about their conditions. Thus, they think they have no good social support to help them with their pain behavior problems.
3. *Adaptive coper* patients report a high level of social support and relatively low levels of pain and perceived interference with their lives. They also report relatively high levels of activity despite their pain, and they usually respond well to pain management procedures.

Turk and Okifuji (1998) noted that the clinical robustness of this profile taxonomy has been shown across several pain syndromes, including chronic low back pain, headache pain, TMD pain, and fibromyalgia. The authors state that assessment of MPI profiles will lead to important "tailoring" of needs or treatment strategies to account for the different personality characteristics of patients. For example, patients with the interpersonally distressed profile might need additional clinical attention addressing interpersonal skills to perform effectively in a group-oriented treatment program. Pain patients with dysfunctional and interpersonally distressed profiles demonstrate more indications of acute and chronic personality differences than do adaptive coper profile patients, and they would therefore require more clinical management (e.g., Etscheidt, Steiger, & Braverman, 1995). Such additional attention, though, would not be essential for patients with the adaptive coper profile.

Millon Behavioral Health Inventory

Millon, Green, and Meagher (1982) developed the Millon Behavioral Health Inventory (MBHI), a 150-question true–false test based on 20 clinical scales that reflect medically related concerns, such as compliance with treatment regimens and reaction to treatment personnel. Although it is usually not perceived as a personality assessment test, it was intended as an alternative to the MMPI-2 for use with an actual medical population, including pain patients. One advantage of the MBHI over the MMPI-2 is that it requires only about 20 minutes to complete. Moreover, most patients find it less threatening than the MMPI-2 because it includes questions related to medical care.

The MBHI's clinical scales include those that rate introversive style, cooperative style, sociable style, premorbid pessimism, pain treatment responsivity, and emotional vulnerability. Several of these scales are clinically meaningful in assessment of chronic pain patients. For example, in our treatment programs for patients with chronic low back pain disability, we often find that people who score low on the cooperative style scale and high on the sensitive style scale demonstrate poor treatment outcome (Gatchel, Mayer, Capra, Diamond, & Barnett, 1986). These patients usually tend not to follow advice and can be unpredictable and moody. Obviously, such personality characteristics can be detrimental to any group-oriented treatment process. In marked contrast, patients scoring high on the cooperative and sociable scales demonstrate excellent outcome. We also have found that patients who score high on the emotional vulnerability scale usually require additional psychological treatment in dealing with their pain and disability, as we found in treating chronic headache patients (Gatchel, Deckel, Weinberg, & Smith, 1985). The MBHI scales can be useful for helping treatment personnel to better understand important personality characteristics that are directly related to response to a medical treatment environment, such as an interdisciplinary pain management program.

Structured Clinical Interview for the DSM-IV

Reich, Rosenblatt, and Tupin (1983) were the first to argue that a uniform diagnostic nomenclature should be used to develop a more accurate means for classifying patients with chronic pain. They suggest that the construct of the *DSM-III* (APA, 1980) —and now the *DSM-IV* (APA, 1994)—would be a useful way to categorize chronic pain patients. However, one problem encountered in using the *DSM* for nomenclature is the semistructured clinical interview. A semistructured or unstructured format can present a problem if one is interested in comparing the content and material gathered from the same patients by different interviewers. The different experiences and clinical skills of interviewers can render comparisons of data difficult—if not impossible. To overcome this problem, the use of a structured clinical interview was advocated. One of the most widely used such interviews is the SCID (Spitzer et al., 1988), which requires the interviewer to ask the same set of questions to all patients, either to rule in or to rule out various *DSM* diagnoses. It ensures that all patients are asked the same questions. It allows a structured means of making more precise statements concerning the presence of any major psychiatric or personality disorder that can affect the course of treatment. In addition, the SCID has a further advantage in that it has good reliability and promising validity. Moreover, as noted earlier, there have been several studies using the SCID for making personality diagnoses. Continued clinical use of the SCID will ensure commonality of personality diagnosis nomenclature across various clinical sites, which offers the added advantage of providing a consistent way to communicate personality diagnoses to third-party carriers.

Schedule for Nonadaptive and Adaptive Personality

The SNAP (Clark, 1993b, 1993c) is a 375-item, multiple-choice instrument that assesses three temperament dimensions and 12 personality dimensions. Vittengl, Clark, Owen-Salters, and Gatchel (1999) used this test to evaluate a sample of 125 patients with chronic low back pain and reported that it reveals, consistent with the existing literature, that patients who seek treatment for chronic low back pain can demonstrate a broad range of psychopathology. More important, in terms of personality characteristics, as measured by the SNAP, patients with chronic low back pain differed significantly from a normal comparison group on three of the six validity indices. Specifically, the two groups did not differ on the content-balanced inconsistency scales of variable, true, and desirable responding; however, the patient sample endorsed more rare virtues and greater deviance, and the group scored higher on the overall invalidity index than did the "normal" control patients. The two groups also differed on 12 of the 15 trait scales. The only trait scales that were *not* different were eccentric perceptions, dependency, and propriety. Thus, not at all surprisingly, the patients described themselves as higher on negative temperament and on a range of traits related to this factor (mistrust, aggression, and self-harm) and lower on positive temperament and related scales (lower exhibitionism and entitlement; higher detachment). The patients also described themselves as less disinhibited, impulsive, and manipulative and as more workaholic than the normal comparison group. The results of this study clearly indicate that personality pathology, as measured by the SNAP, was quite evident. The SNAP appears to be useful for assessing personality characteristics that will direct management of chronic pain patients.

Short Form Health Survey

The Short Form Health Survey (SF-36; Ware & Sherbourne, 1992) was developed for various uses, including clinical practice and research. It has good psychometric properties and is becoming a favorite of third-party payers for outcome monitoring of patients who have chronic medical conditions. The SF-36 has eight scales that measure health concepts, such as physical functioning, bodily pain, social functioning, and mental health. There are two global summary or component scales: a physical component summary scale and a mental component summary scale. Elevated scores on the mental component scale are usually a good index of potential emotional distress in patients. The absolute clinical utility of the SF-36 with individual patients is not well-established because of the test's psychometric limitations (Gatchel, Polatin, Mayer, Robinson, & Dersh, 1998), but its advantages are that it is brief (taking approximately 10–20 minutes to complete) and it does divide health into distinct physical, social, and mental health components. Thus, as a global index of emotional distress, it can be useful for those patients who are not resistant to acknowledging such problems.

Stepwise Approach

Most clinicians are under various time constraints, as well as billing constraints imposed by third-party payers, when considering the best method of evaluating possible personality pathology in their patients with chronic pain. Therefore, a frequently asked question is, "If I were to choose the most time- and cost-efficient assessment method, which one should I select?" Unfortunately, one must not make the assumption that there is a single instrument that can serve as the best assessment. For many patients, several assessments will be needed. Rather than asking which instrument should be used, a better question is, "What sequence of testing should I consider to develop the best understanding of potential personality problems that might be encountered with chronic pain patients?"

Psychosocial personality assessment should be viewed as a stepwise process, proceeding from global indices of emotional distress and disturbance to more detailed evaluations of specific diagnoses of Axis I clinical and Axis II personality disorders. Figure 11.1 is a flow chart for such a process. It should be noted that specific assessment tools have been developed for many types of chronic pain disorders, including the Roland and Morris Disability Questionnaire for Chronic Low Back Pain (Roland & Morris, 1983) and the Research Diagnostic Criteria for Temporomandibular Disorders (Dworkin & LeResche, 1992). Turk and Melzack (1992) have provided a detailed source book of various specific assessment instruments. These tools, which address particular issues associated with specific conditions, would be used in addition to the diagnostic process delineated in Figure 11.1.

An initial screening process to flag obvious psychological distress, which can be done efficiently, might consist of the administration of the BDI–II, the SCL-90–R, and the SF-36. Pronounced scale elevations on these instruments would alert clinical staff to the degree of emotional distress or dysfunction in a chronic pain patient and indicate the need for a more thorough evaluation. This would include the administration of the MMPI-2, as well as the SCID or the SNAP (the SCID could be administered only if trained personnel were available; the SNAP is a self-report instrument).

If no pronounced elevations were displayed on the BDI–II, SCL-90–R, and SF-36, the MMPI-2 would still be administered, because third-party payers are accustomed to having this widely accepted test as part of a chronic pain evaluation. If there were no meaningful profile elevations on the MMPI-2, then one could proceed directly to a clinical interview. If elevations on the MMPI-2 were exhibited, the SCID or the SNAP would be administered. Administration of either one supports an official *DSM-IV*–based diagnosis of an Axis I or Axis II disorder.

The next step is administration of a psychosocial clinical interview, which is indeed a powerful assessment tool of the clinician. In addition to the traditional areas explored in a clinical history, there are other areas that should be explored with chronic pain patients. The clinician will be sensitized to which need attention as a result of the structured psychosocial–personality test results. Some issues that are important to cover in a clinical interview consist of potential barriers to recovery that could affect response to treatment:

- patient and family history of mental health, such as depression and substance abuse
- history of head injury, convulsions, or impairment of function
- any stressful changes in lifestyle or marital status before or since the injury that precipitated the pain

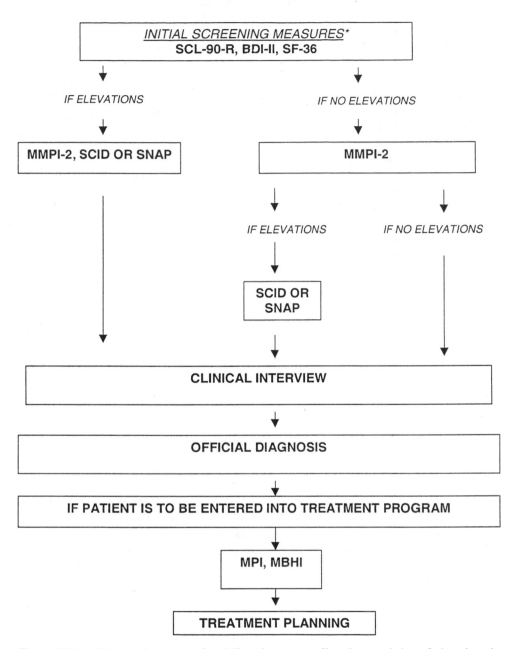

Figure 11.1. Diagnostic process for delineating personality characteristics of chronic-pain patients. For some disorders, there also could be a specific assessment tool developed that would be administered at this time.

- work history, including explanation of job losses, changes, and dissatisfaction
- financial history, contrasting current income with past, and comparing these with current cost-of-living requirements
- Any litigation pending for the patient's current medical and pain problem.

In addition, the determination of the patient's motivation for change is another important, if unstated, purpose of the interview process. Many chronic pain patients restrict their lives by avoiding any risk of experiencing pain, through immobilization and use of analgesics. Patients who are not candidates for surgical intervention (for any reason) and who refuse to work toward active rehabilitation clearly have suspect motivation for change. Jensen (1996) has provided an excellent review of methods for enhancing patient motivation in pain treatment programs.

The clinical interview allows the clinician to contrast the patient's current psychosocial functioning with past functioning, and to compare the testing data with the interview data. The clinician can then estimate the potential for getting the patient to change behavior and work toward rehabilitation. Finally, with this clinical assessment material in hand, if it is decided that the patient is a suitable candidate to enter a comprehensive pain management program, an additional set of assessment instruments should be administered—the MPI and the MBHI. These instruments are beneficial for treatment personnel, who can use the results to identify the best approach for pain management and to anticipate potential problems in the pain management program.

Conclusions

The major premise of this chapter is that the presence of a personality disorder or cluster *in general*—and not necessarily a specific personality disorder—can impair the coping ability of a chronic pain patient and could be related to problems with chronic pain disability. Obviously, this has major clinical implications for the effective management of patients. The high prevalence of personality disorders in the general population, and in the chronic pain population specifically, demands that such disorders be carefully evaluated to develop the effective pain treatment programs. Several assessment instruments were reviewed: the Beck Depression Inventory–II, the Minnesota Multiphasic Personality Inventory-2, the Multidimensional Pain Inventory, the Millon Behavioral Health Inventory, the Structured Clinical Interview for *DSM*, the Schedule for Nonadaptive and Adaptive Personality, the Short Form Health Survey, and the clinical interview. Finally, a stepwise approach to personality assessment is advocated, proceeding from global indices of emotional distress and disturbance to more detailed evaluations of specific Axis I clinical and Axis II personality disorders.

References

American Psychiatric Association. (1980). *Diagnostic and statistical manual of mental disorders* (3rd ed.). Washington, DC: Author.

American Psychological Association. (1987). *Diagnostic and statistical manual of mental disorders* (3rd ed., rev.). Washington, DC: Author.

American Psychiatric Association. (1994). *Diagnostic and statistical manual of mental disorders* (4th ed.). Washington, DC: Author.

Asmundson, G. J. G., Norton, G. R., & Alterdings, M. D. (1997). Fear and avoidance in dysfunctional chronic back pain patients. *Pain, 69,* 231–236.

Beck, A. (1967). *Depression: Clinical, experimental, and theoretical aspects.* New York: Harper & Row.

Blumer, D., & Heilbronn, M. (1982). Chronic pain as a variant of depressive disease: The pain-prone disorder. *Journal of Nervous and Mental Disease, 170,* 381–406.

Clark, L. A. (1992). Resolving taxonomic issues in personality disorders: The value of large scale analyses of symptom data. *Journal of Personality Disorders, 6,* 360–376.

Clark, L. A. (1993a). Personality disorder diagnosis: Limitations of the five-factor model. *Psychological Inquiry, 4,* 100–104.

Clark, L. A. (1993b). *Schedule for Nonadaptive and Adaptive Personality and Its Disorders.* Dallas: Author.

Clark, L. A. (1993c). *SNAP: Manual for administration, scoring, and interpretation.* Minneapolis: University of Minnesota Press.

Clark, L. A., McEwen, J., Collard, L., & Hickok, L. (1993). Symptoms and traits of personality disorder: Two new methods for their assessment. *Psychological Assessment, 5*(1), 81–91.

Cloninger, R. (1987). A systematic method for clinical description and classification of personality variance. *Archives of General Psychiatry, 44,* 473–588.

Costa, P. T., & McCrae, R. R. (1989). *NEO Personality Inventory/NEO Five-Factor Inventory manual supplement.* Odessa, FL: Psychological Assessment Resources.

Derogatis, L. R., Lipman, R. S., & Covi, L. (1973). SCL-90: An outpatient psychiatric rating scale. *Psychopharmacology Bulletin, 9,* 13–28.

Dworkin, S. F., & Le Resche, L. (1992). Research diagnostic criteria for temporomandibular disorders: Review, criteria, examinations and specifications, critique. *Journal of Craniomandibular Disorders, 6,* 301–355.

Etscheidt, M. A., Steiger, H. G., & Braverman, B. (1995). Multidimensional Pain Inventory profile classifications and psychopathology. *Journal of Consulting and Clinical Psychology, 51,* 29–36.

Eysenck, H. J. (1987). The definition of personality disorders and the criteria for their description. *Journal of Personality Disorders, 1*(3), 211–219.

Fishbain, D. A., Goldberg, M., Meagher, B. R., Steele, R., & Rosomoff, H. (1986). Male and female chronic pain patients categorized by DSM-III psychiatric diagnostic criteria. *Pain, 26,* 181–197.

Frances, A. (1980). The DSM-III personality disorders section: A commentary. *American Journal of Psychiatry, 137,* 1050–1054.

Frances, A., & Widiger, T. (1986). Methodological issues in personality disorder diagnosis. In T. Millon & G. Klerman (Eds.), *Contemporary directions in psychopathology: Toward the DSM-IV* (pp. 381–400). New York: Guilford Press.

Fyer, M. R., Frances, A. J., Sullivan, T., Hurt, S. W., & Clarkin, J. (1988). Comorbidity of borderline personality disorder. *Archives of General Psychiatry, 45,* 348–352.

Gatchel, R. J. (1991). Early development of physical and mental deconditioning in painful spinal disorders. In T. G. Mayer, V. Mooney, & R. J. Gatchel (Eds.), *Contemporary conservative care for painful spinal disorders* (pp. 278–289). Philadelphia: Lea & Febiger.

Gatchel, R. J. (1996). Psychological disorders and chronic pain: Cause-and-effect relationships. In R. J. Gatchel & D. C. Turks (Eds.), *Psychological approaches to pain management: A practitioner's handbook* (pp. 33–52). New York: Guilford Press.

Gatchel, R. J., Deckel, A. W., Weinberg, N., & Smith, J. E. (1985). The utility of the Millon Behavioral Health Inventory in the study of chronic headache. *Headache, 25,* 49–54.

Gatchel, R. J., Garofalo, J. P., Ellis, E., & Holt, C. (1996). Major psychological disorders in acute and chronic TMD patients: An initial evaluation of the "chicken or egg" question. *Journal of the American Dental Association, 127,* 1365–1374.

Gatchel, R. J., Mayer, T. G., Capra, P., Diamond, P., & Barnett, J. (1986). Millon Behavioral Health Inventory: Its utility in predicting physical function in patients with low back pain. *Archives of Physical Medicine and Rehabilitation, 67,* 878–882.

Gatchel, R. J., Polatin, P. B., Mayer, T. G., & Garcy, P. D. (1994). Psychopathology and the rehabilitation of patients with low back pain disability. *Archives of Physical Medicine and Rehabilitation, 75,* 666–670.

Gatchel, R. J., Polatin, P. B., Mayer, T. G., Robinson, R., & Dersh, J. (1998). Use of the SF-36 Health Status Survey with a chronically disabled back pain population: Strengths and limitations. *Journal of Occupational Rehabilitation, 8,* 237–246.

Gorton, G., & Akhtar, S. (1990). The literature on personality disorders, 1985–1988: Trends, issues, and controversies. *Hospital and Community Psychiatry, 41*(1), 39–51.

Hamilton, M. (1960). A rating scale for depression. *Journal of Neurology, Neurosurgery and Psychiatry, 23,* 56–62.

Hanvik, L. J. (1951). MMPI profiles in patients with low back pain. *Journal of Consulting Psychology, 15,* 350–353.

Jayson, M. I. V. (1997). Presidential address: Why does acute back pain become chronic? *Spine, 22,* 1053–1056.

Jensen, M. P. (1996). Enhancing motivation to change in pain treatment. In R. J. Gatchel & D. C. Turk (Eds.), *Psychological approaches to pain management: A practitioner's handbook* (pp. 78–111). New York: Guilford Press.

Joffe, R. T., & Regan, J. J. (1988). Personality and depression. *Journal of Psychiatric Research, 22,* 279–286.

Keefe, F. J., Caldwell, D. S., Williams, D. A., Gil, K. M., Mitchell, D., Robertson, C., Martinez, S., Nunley, J., Beckham, J. C., Crissom, J. E., & Helms, M. (1990). Pain coping skills training in the management of osteoarthritic knee pain: A comparative study. *Behavior Therapy, 21,* 49–62.

Kerns, R. D., Turk, D. C., & Rudy, T. E. (1985). The West Haven–Yale Multidimensional Pain Inventory (WHYMPI). *Pain, 23,* 345–356.

Kinney, R., Gatchel, R. J., & Mayer, T. G. (1991). SCL-90-R: Evaluated as an alternative to the MMPI for psychological screening of chronic low back pain patients. *Spine, 16,* 940–942.

Kleinke, C. L. (1994). MMPI scales as predictors of pain-coping strategies preferred by patients with chronic pain. *Rehabilitation Psychology, 39,* 123–128.

Loranger, A. W., Susman, V. L., Oldham, J. M., & Russakoff, M. (1985). *Personality Disorder Examination (PDE): A structured interview for DSM-III-R personality disorders.* White Plains, NY: New York Hospital—Cornell Medical Center, Westchester Division.

Millon, T. (1981). The nature of personality. In T. Millon (Ed.), *Disorders of personality* (pp. 1–44). New York: Wiley.

Millon, T. (1983). *Millon Clinical Multiaxial Inventory.* Minneapolis: National Computer Services.

Millon, T., Green, C. J., & Meagher, R. B. (1982). *Millon Behavioral Health Inventory* (3rd ed.). Minneapolis: Interpretive Scoring System.

Morey, L. C. (1985). A comparison of three personality disorder assessment approaches. *Journal of Psychopathology and Behavioral Assessment, 8*(1), 25–30.

Pfohl, B., Stangl, D., & Zimmerman, M. (1983). *Structured Interview for DSM-III Personality Disorders (SIDP*; 2nd ed.). Unpublished manual. University of Iowa, College of Medicine, Iowa City.

Polatin, P. B., Kinney, R. K., Gatchel, R. J., Lillo, E., & Mayer, T. G. (1993). Psychiatric illness and chronic low back pain. *Spine, 18,* 66–71.

Regier, D. A., Boyd, J. H., Burke, J. D., Rae, D. S., Myers, J. K., Kramer, M., Robins, L. N., George, L. K., Karno, M., & Locke, B. Z. (1988). One-month prevalence of mental disorders in the United States. *Archives of General Psychiatry, 45,* 977–986.

Reich, J., Rosenblatt, R. M., & Tupin, J. (1983). DSM-III: A new nomenclature for classifying patients with chronic pain. *Pain, 16,* 201–206.

Robins, L. N., Helzer, J. E., Weissman, M. M., Orvaschel, D. A., Gruenberg, E., Burke, J. D., & Regier, D. A. (1984). Lifetime prevalence of specific psychiatric disorders in three sites. *Archives of General Psychiatry, 41,* 949–958.

Roland, M., & Morris, R. (1983). A study of the natural history of back pain. Part I. Development of a reliable and sensitive measure of disability in low back pain. *Spine, 8,* 141–144.

Spitzer, R. L., Williams, J. B. W., Gibbon, M., & First, M. (1988). *Structured clinical interview for the DSM-III-R.* New York: New York State Psychiatric Institute.

Streiner, D. L., & Miller, H. R. (1989). The MCMI–II: How much better than the MCMI? *Journal of Personality Assessment, 53*(1), 81–84.

Turk, D. C., & Melzack, R. (1992). *Handbook of pain assessment.* New York: Guilford Press.

Turk, D. C., & Okifuji, A. (1998). Directions in prescriptive chronic pain management based on diagnostic characteristics of the patient. *APS Bulletin, 8,* 5–11.

Turk, D. C., & Rudy, T. E. (1986). Assessment of cognitive factors in chronic pain: A worthwhile enterprise? *Journal of Consulting and Clinical Psychology, 54,* 760–768.

Turk, D. C., & Rudy, T. E. (1988). Toward an empirically derived taxonomy of chronic pain patients: Integration of psychological assessment data. *Journal of Consulting and Clinical Psychology, 56,* 233–238.

Turk, D. C., & Salovey, P. (1984). Chronic pain as a variant of depressive disease: A critical reappraisal. *Journal of Nervous and Mental Disease, 172,* 398–404.

Tyrer, P., & Alexander, J. (1979). Classification of personality disorder. *British Journal of Psychiatry, 135,* 163–167.

Vittengl, J. R., Clark, L. A., Owen-Salters, E., & Gatchel, R. J. (1999). Diagnostic change and personality stability following functional restoration treatment in a chronic low back pain patient sample. *Assessment, 6,* 79–91.

Ware, J. E., & Sherbourne, C. D. (1992). The MOS 36-Item Short Form Health Survey (SF-36). *Medical Care, 30,* 473–483.

Weisberg, J. N., Gallagher, R. M., & Gorin, A. (1996, October). *Personality disorder in chronic pain: A longitudinal approach to validation of diagnosis.* Poster presented at the 12th Annual Scientific Meeting of the American Pain Society, Washington, DC.

Weisberg, J. N., & Keefe, F. J. (1999). Personality, individual differences and psychopathology in chronic pain. In R. J. Gatchel & D. C. Turk (Eds.), *Psychological factors in pain: Critical perspectives* (pp. 56–73). New York: Guilford Press.

Weissman, M. M. (1993). The epidemiology of personality disorders. *Journal of Personality Disorders* (Suppl. 1), 44–62.

Widiger, T. A. (1992). Categorical versus dimensional classification: Implications from and for research. *Journal of Personality Disorders, 6,* 287–300.

Widiger, T. A., & Frances, A. (1985). The DSM-III personality disorders. Perspectives from psychology. *Archives of General Psychiatry, 42,* 615–623.

Widiger, T., Frances, A., & Spitzer, R. (1988). The DSM-III-R personality disorders: An overview. *American Journal of Psychiatry, 145,* 786–795.

Widiger, T. A., & Sanderson, C. (1987). The convergent and discriminant validity of the MCMI as a measure of the DSM-III personality disorders. *Journal of Personality Assessment, 51*(2), 228–242.

Widiger, T. A., Trull, T., & Hurt, S. (1987). A multidimensional scaling of the DSM-III personality disorders. *Archives of General Psychiatry, 44,* 557–563.

Zimmerman, M. (1994). Diagnosing personality disorders: A review of issues and research methods. *Archives of General Psychiatry, 51,* 225–245.

Zimmerman, M., & Coryell, W. (1989). DSM-III personality disorder diagnoses in a nonpatient sample: Demographic correlates and comorbidity. *Archives of General Psychiatry, 46,* 682–689.

Chapter 12
PERSONALITY AND PAIN:
Summary and Future Perspectives

James N. Weisberg, Jeffrey R. Vittengl, Lee Anna Clark,
Robert J. Gatchel, and Amy A. Gorin

The preceding chapters of this text review the history of personality investigation in chronic pain; personality measures currently in use in the chronic pain population; and promising new instruments to help guide clinicians toward early, accurate diagnosis of personality traits and disorders. A major goal of early, accurate diagnosis is providing clinicians with increased knowledge about how patients' personality function is or is not related to their pain, thereby helping to optimize treatment outcomes. Ultimately, understanding an individual's personality characteristics or disorders should increase early detection of those at risk for developing chronic, debilitating pain, allowing intervention on as many dimensions as possible during the acute and subacute phases of pain as a way to prevent the progression to chronicity.

In this chapter, we summarize the advantages of personality assessment and some of the best instruments to use, including a recently developed method of assessing personality pathology from a trait dimensional perspective—the Schedule for Nonadaptive and Adaptive Personality (SNAP). We also present a model of personality disorders in chronic pain recently introduced in the literature—the diathesis–stress model (Weisberg & Keefe, 1997). This model provides a testable hypothesis for the observation that many chronic pain patients have comorbid personality disorders, the presence of which they, their families, and their friends deny before the onset of pain.

The Diathesis–Stress Model

A diathesis–stress model of personality disorders in chronic pain has been proposed (Weisberg & Keefe, 1997) to explain the discrepancy between the rates of those disorders in the general population and in the chronic pain population. The model posits that personality disorders develop as an interaction between underlying personality predispositions (or *diatheses*) and the extreme stress of pain and its physical, psychological, and social consequences. In this model, disorder is a consequence of acute and subacute pain, and it also can perpetuate chronic, disabling pain. The summary here provides a theoretical rationale for such a model to be tested for its heuristic and predictive value, and it provides information to help clinicians assess personality function in the context of long-standing traits and current stressors.

It is well-established that personality disorders are highly prevalent in patients with chronic pain (Gatchel, Garofalo, Ellis, & Holt, 1996; Livengood & Johnson, 1998; Weisberg & Keefe, 1997). Comparisons with other psychiatric and medical populations support the observation that chronic pain patients demonstrate high levels of personality psychopathology (Gatchel, Polatin, Mayer, & Garcy, 1994; Reich & Thompson, 1987). The rate in the general population ranges from 0.5% to 3%, according to the fourth edition of the *Diagnostic and Statistical Manual of Mental Disorders* (*DSM-IV*; American Psychiatric Association [APA], 1994). In outpatient psychiatric clinical populations, the prevalence rate varies greatly. One study of more than 18,000 individuals reported a prevalence rate of 12.9% (Fabrega, Ulrich, Pilkonis, & Mezzich, 1993). Rates vary widely in other outpatient clinical samples, depending on sample demographics and assessment methods. One study found that 54% of clinic outpatients presenting with anxiety and depressive disorders also met criteria for at least one personality disorder as assessed by a structured interview (Flick, Roy-Byrne, Cowley, Shores, & Dunner, 1993). This appears consistent with studies by Sanderson, Wetzler, Beck, and Betz (as cited in Zuckerman, 1999), which found 35% of individuals with anxiety disorders and 53% of individuals with depressive disorders also met criteria for a personality disorder. In comparison, prevalence rates in the chronic pain population range between 31% and 59%. When disorders in that population are subdivided into *DSM-IV* clusters, Cluster B (antisocial, borderline, histrionic, and narcissistic personality disorders) appears to contain the highest percentage of individuals, followed closely by Cluster C (avoidant, dependent, passive–aggressive) and Cluster A (paranoid, schizoid, and schizotypal personality disorders). The reader is referred to Weisberg and Keefe (1997) for a review.

Pain and Personality Disorders

Although it seems clear that the prevalence rate of personality disorders in people who experience chronic pain is both significant and similar to that found in other psychiatric populations, the causal relationship between personality and pain is enigmatic and controversial. The diathesis–stress model challenges traditional understanding of the genesis of personality disorders, and we suggest that the *DSM* definitions might not be applicable in the chronic pain population. Personality is often viewed along a spectrum from healthy attributes to pathological characteristics. When defining personality, one refers to the constellation of attributes that makes each person unique. It is the differences between individuals that lead to the particular expression of emotions, thoughts, and behaviors. Personality disorders, however, indicate a pathological expression of these thoughts, emotions, and behaviors (APA, 1994) that are inconsistent with social norms.

The term *personality disorder* refers to a long-standing pattern—as opposed to a few instances of maladaptive response—of disordered behavior and emotions, usually evident by adolescence or early adulthood, with symptoms severe enough to interfere with an individual's ability to function, interact with others and, in some cases, maintain reality testing. This is a double-edged sword in chronic pain. Patients with pain, and their significant others, often present a very different description of the patient's premorbid (before pain onset) personality function from that observed after the onset of pain. According to *DSM-IV* (APA, 1994) criteria, in these cases, a personality disorder cannot be diagnosed because these individuals do not exhibit the "long-standing" criterion of the necessary characteristics. Despite the discrepancy, such a diagnosis often is provided in the treatment setting, perhaps as a means of attributing a patient's presenting behavior to something other than pain. By viewing the personality disorder according to a diathesis–stress model, the discrepancy between premorbid and postmorbid personality function becomes better accounted for, and it could provide a testable model for the heuristic understanding of what happens to pain patients after the acute onset of pain.

History of the Model

As pointed out in the Introduction of this text, biological predispositions have been assigned a primary role in the etiology of physical illness at least as far back as the time of Hippocrates (Monroe & Simmons, 1991). Focusing on physical characteristics and "imbalances," Hippocrates identified four basic body fluids, the humors, associated with specific behavior patterns and health consequences. An individual with a diathesis for black bile was believed to be at increased risk for developing depressive symptoms; a preponderance of blood was thought to be associated with a cheerful disposition (Hunt, 1993). The relationship between chronic pain and a variety of personality characteristics also has been a topic of inquiry since antiquity. Hippocrates believed that pain arose when one humor was in excess or depleted (Bonica, 1990). Plato believed that pain occurred not only from peripheral stimulation but also from emotions in the soul and the heart (Bonica, 1990). In *DeAnima*, Aristotle echoed the belief of his mentor, Plato, that pain was a quality of the soul. In the mid-19th century, Griesinger (1867/1965) cited his belief in the connection between pain and personality when he described a case in which a patient with "very severe pain may also call forth an attack of insanity in an individual who is predisposed" (p. 179). He described this insanity as "hysteria" that moves rapidly from one area of the nervous system to another. Over the past century, these observations have led to an effort to assess, measure, and quantify individual differences in pain.

More modern studies of diatheses have focused on genetic vulnerabilities that predispose individuals to disease (Falconer, 1965). The discoveries of genetic markers for some types of breast cancer (Newman & Liu, 1998), Parkinson's disease (Gasser et al., 1998) and for Huntington's disease and neurofibromatosis (Rosenberg & Iannaccone, 1995) are examples of this trend. The presence of a genetic marker does not necessarily mean there is an underlying biological predisposition, but it is one of the closest measurements, other than specific gene typing, currently available for assessing genetic predisposition. Genetic markers have been identified in psychiatric illness, such as schizophrenia (Pickar et al., 1986; Siever et al., 1991) and depression (Buchsbaum, Goodwin, & Muscettola, 1981; Silverman et al., 1993). Psychological or social diatheses also have been proposed as the medical model has evolved into a more biopsychosocial approach (Engel, 1977). Uhl, Sora, and Wang (1999) apparently have isolated a gene that controls pain sensitivity. Thus, there might be a genetic predisposition for the degree to which people experience pain.

The stress component of the model is just as important. Although many definitions of *stress* have been advanced, perhaps one of the best is given by Lazarus and Folkman (1984): Stress is the physiological, psychological, or mental influences that exert pressure on the organism, taxing or exceeding its capacity to respond. Recognition of the influence of stress on health is a relatively recent advance in our conceptualization of health and illness. Indeed, Selye's *general adaptation syndrome* (Selye, 1956) has had a tremendous influence on the study of illness and on behavioral interventions to change the maladaptive response to stress. Along with other influences (e.g., biopsychosocial factors), the general adaptation syndrome has resulted in the exploration of the operation of environmental factors on disease. A relatively new field of study—psychoneuroimmunology—also has increased our understanding of the complex connection between stress and illness. This area of research has shown that, during times of stress, immune functions weaken (e.g., Ader, Felton, & Cohen, 1990), leaving one more susceptible to minor illnesses, such as the common cold or flu, or to severe diseases, such as Crohn's disease and coronary artery disease. Psychosocial stressors that tax immune systems include negative life events, such as marital discord (Kiecolt-Glaser & Glaser, 1987), bereavement (Schleifer, Keller, Camerino, Thornton, & Stein, 1983), and work stress.

The importance both of underlying diatheses and of recent stress have been recognized for years in illness models, but the two concepts were not unified until the early 1960s, when the diathesis–stress model of schizophrenia was developed (Bleuer, 1963; Meehl, 1962; Rosenthal, 1963). According to the original model, schizophrenia develops as an interaction between a biological or genetic substrate (diathesis) and the expression of that substrate under stressful conditions. Unlike previous disease models that highlighted the operation of stress *or* the influence of underlying genetic factors, the diathesis–stress model asserts that the onset of schizophrenia results from an *interaction* between biological diatheses and environmental stress (Spaulding, 1997). A recent review of more than 200 studies suggests that the diathesis in schizophrenia is an abnormality in dopamine receptors (Walker & Diforio, 1997). One environmental stressor that has been noted in the onset or maintenance of schizophrenia is a communication style known as a *double bind*, a term that refers to situations in which a person receives multiple contradictory messages, most notably from parents, and is unsure how to reconcile them. The confusion that results, along with difficulty expressing emotion, is believed to create (environmental) stress that ultimately can activate the diathesis for schizophrenia (Goldstein & Strachan, 1987). The diathesis–stress model has been applied as well to several medical illnesses, including heart disease (Harshfield & Grim, 1997), asthma (Mullins, Chaney, Pace, & Hartman, 1997), diabetes (Lehman, Rodin, McEwen, & Brinton, 1991), and phenylketonuria (Koch, Graliker, Fishler, & Ragsdale, 1963). It has been applied to psychiatric conditions, including depressive disorders (Spangler, Simons, Monroe, & Thase, 1997) and eating disorders (Joiner, Rudd, Heatherington, & Schmidt, 1997).

The conceptualization of diatheses was first limited to genetic vulnerabilities and physical abnormalities (Falconer, 1965; see also Beard, 1881 and Meehl, 1962 as cited in Monroe & Simmons, 1991). This focus was consistent with the dominant medical model of health and disease. In the late 1970s, the emphasis shifted, however, with the introduction of the biopsychosocial model of illness (Engel, 1977). That model extends the previous reductionistic view of medical illness to one that includes biological, psychological, and social influences. Several aspects of an individual's environment interact with biological factors to produce illness.

Diathesis–Stress Approach to Understanding Chronic Pain

Stress

According to the diathesis–stress model, for personality disorders to develop, the underlying vulnerability or diathesis must be activated by the stress of chronic pain.

Several aspects of the chronic pain experience can be considered stressful enough to serve as activating agents (Banks & Kerns, 1996; Melzack, 1999). The physical sensation of pain can be considered a stressor, given its noxious and aversive nature. The experience of pain also can be stressful; many times the pain is intermittent and difficult to predict. As Banks and Kerns (1996) have indicated, acute pain is purposeful and warns us of potential harm, which can result in anxiety. Unlike acute pain, however, chronic pain is biologically purposeless, although our brain and body respond as if the pain were acute.

Stress in pain also can come from associated secondary losses (Banks & Kerns, 1996): Physical disability, financial strain, hopelessness, and isolation are common among chronic pain patients. Interactions with the health insurance industry for authorization of treatment, and the risk being of being "cut off" from medical or financial support also can be considered stressors. Patients with pain often are involved simultaneously with the legal system, the workers' compensation system, and the medical system. Difficulties with finances, intimacy, and self-esteem attributable to role dysfunction and isolation are common among people experiencing chronic pain. Another issue is whether these physical (pain), emotional, mental, and social stressors contribute to the deterioration of previously adequate personality functioning and defense mechanisms—resulting in personality dysfunction—or whether poor premorbid coping abilities for such stressors and difficulties result in the problems themselves. In the diathesis–stress model, causal attributions can be circular rather than linear: There is a negative-feedback loop.

The diathesis–stress model has already been applied to the development of chronic musculoskeletal pain (Flor & Turk, 1994; Turk & Flor, 1994) and has been proposed as a model for the development of postherpetic neuralgia (Dworkin & Banks, 1999). According to the model, chronic pain disorders are a function of the interaction between an individual's premorbid biological and psychological predispositions (diathesis) and the challenges or stressors (stress) faced as a result of physical impairment and tissue damage (Banks & Kerns, 1996). Patients who have a premorbid diathesis will develop chronic pain attendant to injury; those who lack the diathesis will not (Flor & Turk, 1984; Turk & Salovey, 1984). These authors have suggested, for example, that low back pain occurs when an individual has a predisposition to develop hyperactive back muscles, has inadequate coping strategies, and experiences intense, recurrent unpleasant emotional stimuli, such as family or work problems. These authors are careful to note that the underlying predisposition could include either genetic or early-learning experiences. Once stress and sympathetic arousal activate the factors, the pain cycle begins, with pain acting as a new stressor that causes increased muscle tension, and the cycle is perpetuated (Turk & Salovey, 1984).

Diathesis–Stress Model of Personality Disorders in Chronic Pain

So far, we have discussed early theories of the interaction between genetic vulnerabilities and environmental stressors in medical illness, psychiatric illness, and in chronic pain, including postherpetic neuralgia (Dworkin & Banks, 1999). Diathesis–stress models also have been applied to the development of personality disorders in the general population (Paris, 1998). As first discussed earlier by Cloninger, Martin, and Guze (1990), the diathesis–stress model of personality disorders suggested that "there are, in fact, good reasons to consider biological factors [read genetic vulner-abilities] as having a privileged role in psychopathology. Genetic predispositions determine which kinds of disorder individuals may develop, whereas psychosocial factors function as precipitants to psychopathology" (Paris, 1998, p. 129). In essence, there were biological predispositions that might or might not be expressed in the presence of specific psychosocial stressors. The diathesis was always genetic and the stress was always psychosocial. Paris (1998) believed the diathesis–stress model was applicable to personality disorders, and he considered the diathesis to include un-derlying personality traits. He believed that the disorders represent an intensity of personality traits and, once those traits reached a threshold, the expression of the disorder occurred.

The application of the model to chronic pain is recent. Weisberg and Keefe (1997) proposed the basic premise that, before pain onset, there could be an under-lying predisposition to a given personality disorder or disorders that become activated by the stress of the injury, pain, and other sequelae. Presumably, this predisposition is not activated or actualized as a result of the stress of normal daily life: Under such circumstances, the individual's coping mechanisms work relatively well (Weis-berg & Keefe, 1997). For example, premorbidly, an individual who uses activity when faced with emotional stress might be very productive and therefore receives behaviorally reinforcement for that productivity. If, however, after injury, the indi-vidual attempts to engage in the same amount of (over) activity, pain can increase (Gil, Ross, & Keefe, 1988). When in pain, the sufferer is challenged beyond his or her coping abilities by the physiological stress of the pain and by the cognitive, affective, social, occupational, and legal stress associated with a disability. The ac-cumulation of these stressors might exacerbate personality traits to the extent that a personality disorder is exhibited (Weisberg & Keefe, 1999) and might also result in disabling chronic pain.

For a diathesis–stress model to account sufficiently for personality disorders in patients with chronic pain, it must first be shown that the pain precedes the expression of disorder. This task is difficult: It is often problematic to identify the exact onset both of chronic pain and of a personality disorder. There are also other difficult problems associated with such a model, which are discussed next.

Problems With the Framework

Several criticisms have been leveled against diathesis–stress models in general, and they are perhaps applicable to the diathesis–stress model of personality disorders and chronic pain. First, the models tend to be vague and to lack specific predictions beyond the original data (McFall, Townsend, & Viken, 1995). Although they explain existing patterns adequately, they offer little in terms of predictions that can be tested. Until the models can be used to make specific predictions, their assumptions will be difficult to validate through empirical study. Monroe and Simmons (1991) stated, "together stress and diatheses essentially cover the vistas of explanatory concepts in contemporary psychopathology research" (p. 422), and more specific definitions are needed to advance research on these models. This presents a challenge for research.

Relevant to this criticism is that the term stress tends to be poorly defined. This is less a problem in the case of stress related to the occurrence of pain, but as Monroe and Simmons (1991) have suggested, it is not known what specific qualities of life experience (e.g., severity of stress versus specific characteristics of stress) affect illness. It is also unknown whether there is a threshold effect for stress, such that personality disorders will develop only in patients with chronic pain if they reach a certain level of stress (as hypothesized in O'Banion's total stress load hypothesis, 1981). Alternatively, the effects of stress might be gradual, so that each stressful experience results in a slight increase in personality dysfunction. The timing of stress is seldom made explicit in diathesis–stress models. As a consequence, little is known about the importance of the temporal characteristics of the stressor and their influence on the diatheses. These questions have been raised in work on depression (Monroe & Simmons, 1991), and they will need to be considered in the further development of a diathesis–stress model of personality disorders and chronic pain.

Another criticism of diathesis–stress models is that research has focused almost exclusively on the effects of the stress on the diathesis. Few studies have considered the reverse (Monroe & Simmons, 1991). Rather than a linear model, as implied, diatheses and stressors likely influence each other in a nonlinear way. For example, an underlying predisposition might influence the type of stress a person is exposed to in life. If, for example, the underlying predisposition is adventure-seeking–impulsivity, this trait might increase the individual's proclivity to engage in risky behaviors that are likely to result in injury and pain. Not only might a diathesis affect the probability of being exposed to stress, diatheses might also influence the types of events an individual perceives as stressful (Monroe & Simmons, 1991). Applying this to the diathesis–stress model of personality disorders and chronic pain, it is possible that some patients who have an underlying vulnerability for developing a disorder diathesis will be more likely to perceive an injury as stressful than would someone without the diathesis.

Diatheses also could influence an individual's response to stress. For instance, Daley, Hammen, Davila, and Burge (1998) investigated the relationship among personality, psychopathology, stress, and depression. Their data suggest that, when persons are faced with stress, their personality disorders act as vulnerability factors for developing depression. Specifically, people with personality disorders have fewer psychological and social resources to help them deal with stress, so they are more likely to demonstrate depressive symptomatology. Moreover, Daley et al. (1998) have reported that individuals with personality disorders, particularly those with Cluster A or Cluster B symptoms, were more likely to generate episodic–dependent stress when faced with a negative event, again increasing their risk for depression. Applying these findings to the diathesis–stress model for chronic pain, it is quite possible that pain patients have preexisting personality dysfunction that increases the likelihood of their developing chronic pain after an injury.

Clinical Implications

Viewed within the diathesis–stress framework, personality disorders in patients with chronic pain could be the result of underlying biological (and perhaps psychosocial) vulnerabilities *and* environmental stressors brought on by pain and the difficulties that often ensue. In taking this view, clinicians might be less likely to attribute personality deficits to the individual and more likely to see the maladaptive personality in a situational context. In fact, one study (Weisberg, Gallagher, & Gorin, 1996) demonstrated a much lower prevalence of personality disorders assessed longitudinally in the context of a multidisciplinary pain program than was found in studies that used cross-sectional clinical or structured-interview approaches (Fishbain, Goldberg, Meagher, Steele, & Rosomoff, 1986; Gatchel et al., 1996; Large, 1986; Polatin, Kinney, Gatchel, Lillo, & Mayer, 1993; Reich, Tupin, & Abramowitz, 1983). Longitudinal evaluation of an individual could provide more contextual references to explain behaviors. This has advantages and disadvantages. The paradigm of viewing each person's strengths rather than deficits is a premise of mental health practitioners, and it would do well in the chronic pain population. However, a personality disorder diagnosis is useful when it helps to account for certain behaviors, when it contributes to treatment planning, or when both aims are met. Ignoring a disorder could cause the clinician to miss potentially harmful behaviors that are seen commonly in some personality disorders (e.g., overmedication). In addition, the underlying motivation to engage in both harmful and beneficial behaviors might be better understood within the context of personality.

The goal of chronic pain management is primarily to return individuals to their premorbid level of function. Therefore, assessment of premorbid function is at least as necessary as is the assessment of current function—and it could be more important. Any discrepancies noted between premorbid and current function that cannot be attributed to the pain disability should be accounted for, and these can include personality factors. Livengood and Johnson (1998) and Weisberg and Keefe (1999) noted that patients with personality disorders will have varying needs regarding chronic pain management and will interact with physicians and health professionals in unique ways. Unless clinicians understand possible underlying needs, they risk frustration during the treatment process, and this can result in less-than-optimal care for the patient.

In the next section, we discuss research strategies that could lead to a better explanation of the interaction between personality and pain, with a diathesis–stress model in mind. In the meanwhile, clinicians are encouraged to conduct a thorough assessment of psychosocial factors both before and after the onset of pain. Many of the measures currently in use have been described in earlier chapters, and in the last section of this chapter, research tools and promising clinical measures are summarized again briefly.

Future Research

If, in fact, personality lies on a continuum of function from healthy to pathological and also is under the influence of environmental stress, then some assumptions should be testable. According to Paris (1998), five "scenarios" should result in predictions about the probability that an individual will develop a personality disorder or chronic pain syndrome when there is information about the presence of certain biological markers, stress levels (physiological and psychological), and coping–support mechanisms (mediating factors) to deal with stress. In the first scenario, individuals with a premorbid disorder (as defined in the *DSM-IV*; APA, 1994) should be at greater risk of developing a chronic pain disability when they are under extreme stress. In the second scenario, individuals with a genetic marker for a disorder who are experiencing extreme stress might or might not express that disorder, depending on their coping mechanisms or protective factors. In the third scenario, individuals with low genetic vulnerability and high situational stress might display one or more personality disorders if they are not buffered by protective factors. In the fourth scenario, individuals with specific biological personality traits and premorbid personality factors might solicit negative interactions from health care providers and support systems, thereby resulting in chronic pain disability and perhaps the full expression of one or more disorders. In the final scenario, individuals with underlying personality traits who are faced with the extreme stress of pain and the resulting sequelae might lose their ability to cope and, therefore, display a personality disorder. These scenarios are testable with the biological and psychological measures that currently exist.

Another area for research should include the prospective assessment of large cohorts of individuals for personality disorders either before pain onset, similar to the research of Bigos et al. (1991), or during the acute phase, similar to the study by Gatchel, Polatin, and Kinney (1995), with longitudinal follow-up for the development of chronic pain. This could demonstrate a clearer relationship between the pain and the disorder. Reassessment for changes, both in persons who develop chronic pain and in those who do not, could help us understand predictive risk factors for the development of chronic pain; treatment could then be targeted earlier to minimize personality risk factors. Such studies could be even more ambitious if they were to examine serum physiological–neurochemical markers, such as cortisol, serotonin, and noradrenalin, during each phase in the development of chronic pain, with the premise that there are biological markers for the development of both chronic pain and personality disorders. Indeed, Melzack (1999) suggested a close relationship between biochemical markers of stress, such as cortisol, and chronic pain.

Research also is needed to elucidate the nature and quality of the stress of chronic pain and how they influence the activation of underlying personality disorder diatheses. Once specific qualities or types of stressors are identified as particularly likely to activate personality diatheses, interventions can be targeted to minimize them and, consequently, to reduce the probability that a personality disorder will develop.

The Personality Screening Process

In chapter 1 of this book, the pros and cons of early personality screening were discussed. In terms of actual screening issues, we should again emphasize that pain treatment professionals must be astutely aware that, when evaluating patients with pain, especially those with acute pain, the assessment process has practical drawbacks. It is often lengthy, it can be disturbing for patients to complete personality inventories, and the psychological assessment often reinforces patients' conviction that their physicians believe the pain is imaginary. Patients need to understand that the reason they are asked to take a particular assessment battery is to provide an overall picture of general psychophysiological functioning and not to label them with a disorder. Therefore, it is imperative that patients be properly educated about the function of psychological assessments and services in any treatment program.

We find that using the term *behavioral medicine evaluation* is better than using *psychological evaluation* for our patients and our referral sources alike. We also emphasize that one reason for the behavioral medicine evaluation is that, as with any chronic medical condition, various pain syndromes can lead to pressures and changes of lifestyle that most people find unpleasant at the very least. Unplanned and unwanted lifestyle changes can lead to stress, making patients feel worse than they ever anticipate, and this can actually interfere with physical recovery. We explain this in terms of pain-and-stress cycle (Figure 12.1), and then we point out that it is important to confront the cycle to move toward successful treatment.

We also avoid the terms *psychological problem* and *psychopathology* whenever possible. Rather, we use *stress*, *behavioral medicine*, and other terms that have more neutral connotations. Most patients are relieved and consequently are more open to the evaluation process. A focus on the somatic aspects of evaluation, such as the psychophysiological evaluation (biofeedback) if conducted, and the importance of stress and its physiological counterpart (tension) in pain perception, can help patients engage in the evaluation process more easily. Chapter 11 of this text advocates, a stepwise approach in which the administration of each new assessment battery is predicated on the results of the previous test. In this way, the patient is not completely overwhelmed by massive amounts of psychological testing.

Again, as previously reviewed in chapter 1, one of the important positive aspects of personality screening in the early stages of pain is the potential prevention of a chronic pain disability. Indeed, early detection is recognized as a high-priority area for clinical research (Human Capital Initiative Coordinating Committee, 1996). As Linton and Bradley (1996) have cogently pointed out, although cost reduction is often used as an argument for early intervention, there is a paucity of adequate analyses reported in the literature. Goossens and Evers (1997) have similarly noted this lack of data in the area of low back pain. The few studies that have been reported clearly suggest such savings (cited by Linton & Bradley, 1996). Mitchell and Carmen (1990) presented preliminary findings from a multicenter trial (involving some 3,000

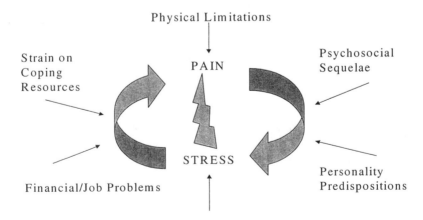

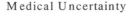

Figure 12.1.   Pain–stress vicious cycle.

patients with acute soft-tissue and back injuries). It was found that there was a savings each month of $1 million to $1.5 million in wage loss and health care costs. In a follow-up of 542 patients, Mitchell and Carmen (1994) reported that early intensive intervention produced savings projected at $5,000 per patient. Linton and Bradley (1992) have also reported cost savings attributable to an early intensive intervention with back pain patients. As Linton and Bradley (1996) concluded in their review of the literature, current data suggest it is possible to prevent the development of chronic disability:

> However, if this goal is to be met, we need to continue to make bold attempts—both clinically and scientifically—to provide effective secondary prevention measures. Research to date has provided a very good beginning, but the details have yet to be worked out. If the promise of prevention is to be fully realized, these details are urgently needed. (p. 454)

What Tools Should We Use to Assess Patients With Chronic Pain?

Gatchel (1991) and many others, including contributors to this text, note that no single psychological device can be used reliably in personality assessment. One cannot assume that any instrument can be used to produce a sole conclusive predictive or descriptive variable. Assessment data should be considered along with other information. The history of social relationships, the presence or absence of social support networks, job and life satisfaction and success, and the history of coping with stressors must be considered to make a probability statement concerning given behavior, such as response to pain. Completely accurate predictions are rare when based on a single psychological or personality assessment instrument. Many of the procedures are discussed in other chapters of this text.

Beck Depression Inventory–II

The BDI–II consists of 21 items with a cumulative scoring system that focuses on physical manifestations. The original inventory was developed (Beck, 1967) to assess the cognitive components of depression, which, like anxiety, is a frequent concomitant of chronic pain and therefore is an important psychosocial variable to evaluate. Although it is unclear whether depression precedes or follows the onset of pain symptoms in most cases, knowledge of its presence can be quite helpful.

The simplicity of the BDI–II makes it attractive to patients, who can complete it in approximately 5 minutes. Clinicians like it, too: Scoring takes less than 1 minute. The BDI–II can be repeated to gauge the progression of depressive symptoms and the effects of treatment. When the inventory is used in conjunction with a psychosocial interview, grossly exaggerated or underplayed scores can provide significant insight about patients' defense mechanisms and approaches to pain, and can suggest more psychiatric or psychological counseling in a comprehensive treatment program.

Minnesota Multiphasic Personality Inventory-2

Ever since Hanvik (1951) first used MMPI scale descriptors to access a chronic pain population, an abundance of research has expanded this form of evaluation of the

10 primary clinical scales by which MMPI-2 responses are classified. Chapters 2 and 5 in this text review research on these profiles and others. For example, patients who exhibit one profile type, the *neurotic triad* (hysteria, depression, and hypochondriasis scales elevated), are more aware that their symptoms have a psychological component, and they usually are better able to express their anxiety and stress.

The Symptom Checklist-90–Revised (SCL-90–R) can be administered as an alternative to the MMPI-2. This test was developed to measure psychopathology in psychiatric and medical outpatients (Derogatis, Lipman, & Covi, 1973), and it has a high degree of convergence with the MMPI-2. It takes only about 20 minutes to complete, and it provides an alternative to the much longer MMPI-2. Unlike the MMPI-2, specific profile patterns that can be useful in a chronic pain patient population have not yet been developed. Clinically, we have found significant elevations on major scales, such as depression, anxiety, fear, somatic distress, can be a general red flag of emotional distress. The SCL-90–R also can be a good measure of overall symptomatology when there is an elevation of the global symptom reporting summary scale (Kinney, Gatchel, & Mayer, 1991).

Multidimensional Pain Inventory

Chapter 11 points out that the MPI can serve as a useful measure of coping displayed by patients with pain. The inventory consists of empirically derived scales designed to assess chronic pain. Its benefits include brevity, its empirical derivation, and its use as providing a normative data base of chronic pain patients. Its 13-scale/factor structure and psychometric properties have been replicated in numerous studies. Cluster analyses on a heterogeneous sample of chronic pain patient responses (Turk & Rudy, 1988) identified three distinct profiles: dysfunctional, interpersonally distressed, and adaptive coper, which can differentiate among patients in various areas, such as observed physical functioning, self-reported pain, depressive mood, quality of interpersonal relationships, and perceived functional limitation. Such behaviors obviously would be extremely important for pain management specialists to consider in any pain management program.

Millon Behavioral Health Inventory

Chapter 4 discusses the MBHI (Millon, Green, & Meagher, 1982), a 150-question true–false test based on 20 clinical scales that reflect medically related concerns. As pointed out in chapter 11, although the MBHI is usually not perceived as a personality assessment, it was intended as an alternative to the MMPI-2 for use in an actual medical population, including pain patients. One advantage of the MBHI over the MMPI-2 is that it can be completed in about 20 minutes. Most patients also find it less threatening than the MMPI-2 because it includes questions related to medical care.

Short Form Health Survey

The SF-36 was developed for various uses, including clinical practice and research (Ware & Sherbourne, 1992). It has good psychometric properties and is becoming popular with third-party payers for outcome monitoring of patients with chronic medical conditions. Its eight scales measure health concepts, such as physical functioning, bodily pain, social functioning, and mental health, and it has two global component scales. Elevated scores on the Mental Component Summary Scale are usually a good index of potential emotional distress in patients. The absolute clinical utility of the SF-36 with individual patients is not well-established because of its psychometric limitations (Gatchel, Polatin, Mayer, Robinson, & Dersh, 1998). The test is brief (10–20 minutes to complete), and it does divide health into distinct physical, social, and mental health components. Thus, as a global index of emotional distress, it can be useful for patients who are not resistant to admitting to such problems.

Schedule for Nonadaptive and Adaptive Personality

The SNAP, a 375-item multiple-choice instrument that assesses 3 dimensions of temperament and 12 dimensions of personality (Clark, 1993), has great potential as an effective assessment instrument for personality disorders. This relatively new inventory is not reviewed extensively elsewhere in this text, so we provide a more detailed discussion here. Table 12.1 shows the various validity, trait, and temperament scales.

The SNAP is a factor analytically derived, self-report measure of trait dimensions important in the domains of normal-range personality and personality disorders. It was developed to provide a means for: (a) assessing personality pathology in terms of trait dimensions as an addition to categorical assessment systems (e.g., *DSM*), (b) exploring relations between personality traits and disorder diagnoses, and (c) investigating whether personality traits are continuous from the normal range to psychopathology (Clark, 1993). The basic content was derived from personality characteristics that comprise the domain of personality disorders. The test was subjected to several rounds of item writing, data collection, and rationally and empirically driven revision of items and scales.

In two initial investigations (Clark, 1990), a total of 34 raters (approximately half counseling or clinical psychology graduate students and half professional psychologists) sorted more than 200 symptoms of personality disorders derived from *DSM-III* (APA, 1980) and *DSM-III-R* (APA, 1987) criteria, as well as symptoms from other conceptualizations of personality and traitlike disorders, into synonym categories. The 22-symptom groupings represented the consensual set of symptom clusters produced by the different raters (see Clark, 1990). The empirically derived symptom clusters formed the basis for the creation of dimensional self-report scales. A broad range of items was written to assess 18 of the 22 clusters, and a prototype test was administered to university students. Scales were identified to assess content for the remaining four clusters, so scale development was not undertaken. Following the method outlined by Tellegen and Waller (in press), factor analysis was used to evaluate items and constructs. In an interactive process of item writing, data collection, and cross-validation using university student and outpatient and inpatient samples, items were revised or eliminated to clarify emerging constructs, to enhance the internal consistency of the scales, and to increase the independence of the scales from one another.

Table 12.1—*Scales of the Schedule for Nonadaptive and Adaptive Personality*

Scale	Low Scorer ($T \leq 35$)	High Scorer ($T \geq 65$)
Validity Scales		
Variable response inconsistency	Responds quite consistently to content-matched items	Responds inconsistently to content-matched items
True response inconsistency	Denies items regardless of content (nay saying)	Admits to items regardless of content (yea saying)
Desirable response inconsistency	Endorses socially undesirable item regardless of content	Endorses socially desirable items regardless of content
Rare virtues	Admits to common faults	Presents self unrealistically; claims rare, highly socially desirable behavior
Deviance	Provides conventional and straightforward responses	Endorses deviant items rarely reported by normal participants
Invalidity index (linear combination of the other 5 validity scores)	Profile with $T < 65$ likely valid; examine other validity scales	Profile likely invalid; interpret only with caution; consider dissimulation, carelessness, and low reading ability
Trait Scales		
Mistrust	Has trustful, even naively positive, attitude toward others	Has pervasively suspicious and cynical attitude toward others
Manipulativeness	Respects others' rights and property; does not bend the truth or use others to advantage	Reports willingness to use people and systems for personal gain without regard for others' rights or feelings
Aggression	Does not become readily angry; easily controls temper; rarely argues or fights	Reports high frequency and intensity of anger and aggression
Exhibitionism	Prefers not to be noticed; dresses and acts to avoid attention	Seeks overt attention through behavior; takes the limelight whenever possible
Entitlement	Self-effacing and humble; does not believe special recognition is deserved	Has unrealistically positive self-regard; feels special treatment is required

Self-harm	Very low self-esteem; engages in self-destructive thoughts and behaviors	Satisfied with self; does not consider suicide as a solution to problems
Eccentric perceptions	Reports odd somatosensory perceptions, cognitions, and beliefs	Denies depersonalization, derealization, and unusual perceptual experiences
Dependency	Expresses little self-reliance and low self-confidence or enjoyment in decision making	Enjoys and is confident in handling own problems and making own decisions
Impulsivity	Acts on a momentary basis without an overall plan; takes chances of all kinds	Acts in a thoughtful, planful, cautious manner; prepares for the future
Propriety	Expresses preference for traditional, conservative morality and proper conduct	Rejects social rules and convention with little concern for traditional right and wrong
Workaholism	Favors work over leisure; perfectionistic; has self-imposed demands for excellence	Does not enjoy hard work; does exhibit ambition; always finds time for fun; enjoys laziness
Detachment	Interpersonally aloof, reserved, expresses a preference for being alone	Open, warm, seeks social contact
Temperament Scales		
Negative temperament	Experiences wide range of negative emotions; overreacts to daily stresses and hassles	Experiences little distress; recovers quickly from negative experiences
Positive temperament	Experiences a wide variety of positive emotions; pleasurably and actively engaged in life	Does not find life exciting; easily fatigued; rarely enthusiastic or interested
Disinhibition	Acts spontaneously with little concern for consequences; seeks stimulating experiences; fails to honor obligations	Serious; conservative values; follows all rules; does things in proper order

Note. Respondents with moderately deviant scores (i.e., $T = 36$–45; 55–64) will exhibit the described characteristics more moderately or in fewer situations. Scale descriptions adapted from schedule for Nonadaptive and Adaptive Personality (SNAP): Manual for Administration, Scoring, and Interpretation by Lee Anna Clark. Copyright © 1993 by the Regents of the University of Minnesota. All rights reserved. "Schedule for Nonadaptive and Adaptive Personality" and "SNAP" are trademarks owned by the University of Minnesota. Reproduced by permission of the University of Minnesota Press.

New items were written to develop validity and diagnostic scales, and three temperament scales from a separate research instrument, the General Temperament Survey (Clark & Watson, 1990), were added to assess the remaining symptom clusters and to complement the trait scales. The result was the 3 temperament, 12 trait, and 5 validity scales shown in Table 12.1.

The SNAP's assessment of personality pathology from a trait-dimensional perspective offers several advantages over categorical representations of personality disorders (e.g., *DSM*). In dimensional models, patients are rated on distinct traits rather than being placed in one or more diagnostic categories. That is, symptomatology is scored on a continuum of graded severity with the SNAP; in traditional medical models, each disorder is coded as either present or absent (Clark, Watson, & Reynolds, 1995). A primary advantage is that many diagnoses can be replaced with a smaller set of basic personality dimensions. On the SNAP, these are positive temperament, negative temperament, and disinhibition versus constraint—convergent with several independently derived representations of personality that are relevant to personality disorders (Watson, Clark, & Harkness, 1994a). If a more detailed analysis is desired, each "supertrait" is related to several narrower dimensions (e.g., exhibitionism, aggression, and impulsivity, respectively) that can be scored as well.

A second advantage is that information about the severity of psychopathology is more readily accessible as relative elevations on the trait dimensions (Widiger & Shea, 1991). Instruments such as the SNAP provide information about individual functioning and dysfunctioning as well as about mild or severe pathology. In contrast, categorical diagnosis does not provide information about subthreshold pathology (missing a diagnosis by a single criterion) or extreme manifestations of a disorder (meeting all criteria).

Beyond simplicity of use and greater information regarding severity, research suggests trait-dimensional approaches are more consistent with the nature of personality and personality disorders. The high comorbidity of personality disorders and the continuity of normal and disordered personalities are difficult to reconcile within a categorical model but are easily explained using trait-dimensional assessment (e.g., Clark, Livesley, & Morey, 1997; Livesley, Schroeder, Jackson, & Jang, 1994). A primary disadvantage of trait-dimensional assessment is clinicians' current unfamiliarity with the use of instruments such as the SNAP.

SNAP and Five-Factor Trait-Dimensional Measures

There are important connections between the SNAP and other popular assessment instruments, including five-factor measures, such as the NEO-PI–R (Neuroticism, Extroversion, Openness-Personality Inventory–Revised; Costa & McCrae, 1992) that have been used with chronic pain patients (see chapter 4). Research suggests that personality measures with three core factors, such as the SNAP, converge in a replicable pattern with five-factor measures (Clark, Vorhies, & McEwen, 1994; Clark & Watson, in press; Watson, Clark, & Harkness, 1994b). Specifically, for the SNAP scales, negative temperament corresponds well with the dimension of neuroticism, positive temperament corresponds well with the dimension of extraversion, and disinhibition versus constraint converges strongly with conscientiousness but also overlaps partly with agreeableness. The fifth factor in instruments such as the NEO-PI–

R, openness, is generally unrelated to the temperament scales on the SNAP but has correlated moderately negatively with propriety and positively with eccentric perceptions and impulsivity (Clark, 1991; Clark et al., 1994).

Clearly, there is reliable overlap between these two assessment systems, but there are also differences in terms of content. Of relevance to assessment of personality in chronic pain, some researchers have expressed concern about the utility of five-factor measures in clinical settings because these measures were developed primarily to assess normal range personality (Ben-Porath & Waller, 1992). The SNAP, in contrast, was designed specifically to assess the full range of traits from normal through extreme personality pathology. Considering this important issue, Clark et al. (1994) compared the ability of the three SNAP temperament scales that were not derived primarily from personality disorder criteria with reliable measures of the five factors (aggregations of two convergent five-factor instruments) to predict the trait scales of the SNAP that were derived primarily from personality disorder criteria. In multiple-regression analyses, each SNAP trait scale was predicted significantly by two or more of the five-factor scales, all of which were entered as a block (accounting for about 35% of the variance on average). After entering the five-factor measures, the SNAP's negative temperament, positive temperament, and disinhibition temperament scales were added to the regression models. One or more of the temperament scales added significantly to the prediction of each of the trait scales after accounting for the five-factor measures (average increment in variance accounted for about 7%). Thus, both the three- and the five-factor models of personality appear to be important predictors of personality pathology, although some three-factor instruments, such as the SNAP, might explain reliable variance in personality pathology beyond that captured by the five-factor model.

Recent and Continuing Improvements

Since its initial publication in 1993, the SNAP has maintained its basic item and scale structure, but it has been improved in several important ways. First, items to score *DSM-III-R* (APA, 1987) personality disorders have been supplemented with a set of 50 items to assess *DSM-IV* (APA, 1994) disorders. Moreover, revisions are under way to fold these additional items into the body of the SNAP and to remove outdated items that were needed only for *DSM-III-R* diagnoses. When these revisions are complete, the 375-item length of the SNAP should be largely unchanged.

Second, consistent with traditional testing practice, the current version of the SNAP provides norms separately by gender. However, this practice is being reconsidered not only by test developers, researchers, and clinicians, but also by the federal government. Specifically, the Civil Rights Act of 1991 (P. L. 102–166) prohibits within-group norming based on race, color, religion, national origin, or gender in employment settings (Bush, "President Bush signs compromise civil rights bill," 1992). To allow use of the instrument in these situations, SNAP materials are being developed that will include non-gender-specific norms.

Third, although templates for hand-scoring of the SNAP are available, an automated scoring and profile-plotting program is now available for personal computers. This could save clinicians and researchers considerable time.

Fourth, another report form of the SNAP has been developed for use with collateral raters, such as a parent, spouse, or friend. Preliminary research supports the internal structure of the other-report form and its reliable convergence with the standard self-report form of the SNAP (Harlan & Clark, in press). In research and in clinical practice, the addition of another informed viewpoint can provide complementary information about individuals' personality functioning.

Finally, and perhaps most important, the SNAP is undergoing a major restandardization. Although the validity of the SNAP has been strongly supported in clinical samples (Clark, 1993; Clark et al., 1994), college students serve as the instrument's normative group. Research suggests that community-dwelling adults typically report somewhat less personality pathology (e.g., Vittengl, Clark, Owen-Salter, & Gatchel, 1999), so existing norms might overestimate the pathology of many nonstudent adult individuals. The restandardization project will involve a large sample of community-dwelling adults at several sites in the United States, and it will include lower-income participants and members of ethnic minorities. For many clinical and research applications, including evaluation of chronic pain patients, this new standardization sample could provide more appropriate norms against which to evaluate personality pathology.

Use With Pain Populations

Researchers have started using the SNAP with patients with pain. For example, in one study (Vittengl et al., 1999), personality pathology was assessed in a group of patients with chronic low back pain. The study group differed significantly from a normal comparison group on 12 of the 15 dimensional temperament scales. Specifically, they described themselves as experiencing more negative emotions, such as anger, guilt, and anxiety; as being untrustful, cynical, easily angered, and provoked to aggression; and as having low self-esteem. The study group also reported being less happy, enthusiastic, and optimistic than did the control group. These characteristics remained relatively stable from pretreatment to posttreatment evaluations. Thus, the characteristics appeared to be enduring personality characteristics, which is in keeping with the definition of personality as enduring and stable over time.

Conclusions: Future Directions

Trait and personality disorder approaches have much to offer the field of chronic pain research. Future studies should compare personality traits in patients with chronic pain who have different personality disorder diagnoses. Research also needs to compare the degree to which personality disorder diagnosis and personality trait measures are useful in explaining assessments of pain and adjustment in chronic pain populations.

Psychological tests can provide a reliable and standardized way to assess personality traits in patients with chronic pain. Although several psychological tests have been used, the Minnesota Multiphasic Personality Inventory (MMPI) has been the most popular. Descriptive studies using the MMPI have identified common profile subtypes in diverse populations of patients with chronic pain. Although there is a large body of predictive research on the MMPI and chronic pain, there is great debate as to its utility. Two factors in particular have contributed to the debate. First, the results of predictive studies of personality traits in patients with chronic pain have been inconsistent. Although some studies have found a relationship between some personality traits (hypochondriasis, hysteria, and depression) and treatment outcome, other studies have not found evidence for such relationships. Second, concerns have been expressed that some patients who have physical findings that result from underlying disease or injury could appear to be neurotic on the MMPI because they score high on items that measure somatic focus (e.g., items on the hysteria and hypochondriasis scales) (Love & Peck, 1987). Future research is needed to resolve this debate.

Several conclusions can be based on the review of the literature presented in this text. First, the assessment of personality can be useful for identifying personality traits and disorders that could influence the course and treatment of chronic pain. Pain treatment programs are more likely to succeed when they account for individual personality differences in treatment decisions. Second, personality disorders occur at a higher rate in the chronic pain population than in the general population. It has long been observed that chronic pain patients have psychiatric comorbidity that includes both clinical symptoms, such as depression and anxiety, and personality traits and disorders; however, a causal relationship between personality traits or disorders and chronic pain has not been established. Many scholars and researchers posit that some personality traits—histrionic, dependent, depressive—predispose the development of chronic pain disorders. More recently, however, there is increasing evidence that the occurrence of an acute episode of pain and the resulting physical, emotional, and psychosocial consequences could account for the various forms of psychopathology often observed in the chronic pain population. These diagnoses include the Axis I depressive and anxiety disorders and the high rate of Axis II personality disorders, most commonly the dependent, histrionic, and passive–aggressive disorders.

Although incompatible with the concept of a "long-standing, lifelong pattern" required for *DSM* diagnosis of personality disorders, a diathesis–stress model (Weisberg & Keefe, 1997) of personality disorders in chronic pain has been proposed. In this model, traits that are normally controlled by the individual's defensive structure become exacerbated by the stress of acute pain and by subsequent psychosocial stressors, and, when poorly managed, can result in a personality disorder. One recently published study (Vittengl et al., 1999) appears to support the diathesis–stress model. In that study, dimensional personality characteristics and categorical personality disorders (*DSM-III-R*) in chronic pain patients were investigated. In a subset, personality was assessed in patients both before and six months after treatment in a functional restoration program. The assessment measures were the MMPI, the SCID II (Structured Clinical Interview for *DSM-III-R*; Spitzer, Williams, Gibbon, & First, 1988), and the SNAP. The SCID II results were similar to those of other structured-interview studies. Compared with the control group, the patients with chronic pain demonstrated a higher frequency of eight disorders. In the subset of patients assessed before and after treatment, paranoid, obsessive–compulsive, passive–aggressive, and self-defeating disorders decreased significantly. Overall, Vittengl and colleagues' results demonstrate greater stability of dimensional personality traits, before-to-after treatment (MMPI and SNAP), than of categorical personality disorders assessed with the SCID II. The authors cited regression to the mean and the "arbitrary nature" of diagnostic threshold points inherent in categorical diagnoses as possible explanations for changes from pre- to posttreatment. A third explanation, not cited in that study, is that of our previously hypothesized diathesis–stress model (Weisberg & Keefe, 1997). After treatment that has increased function and coping as primary goals, stress likely decreases, and individuals who met criteria for personality disorders before treatment continue to have similar traits, although not to the extent necessary for a categorical diagnosis. Only large-scale, prospective studies, similar to those of Bigos and Battie (1987) and Gatchel et al. (1995), will shed more light on the possible causal nature of these difficult conditions. Fortunately, though, we have an array of assessment methods that can be used to identify personality disorders for the purpose of comprehensively treating patients with pain. Also, dealing more effectively with personality disorders in the acute stage of pain could prevent the development of chronicity.

References

Ader, R., Felton, D., & Cohen, N. (Eds.). (1990). *Psychoneuroimmunology*. San Diego: Academic Press.

American Psychiatric Association. (1980). *Diagnostic and statistical manual of mental disorders* (3rd ed.). Washington, DC: Author.

American Psychiatric Association. (1987). *Diagnostic and statistical manual of disorders* (3rd ed., rev.). Washington, DC: Author.

American Psychiatric Association. (1994). *Diagnostic and statistical manual of mental disorders* (4th ed.). Washington, DC: Author.

Banks, S. M., & Kerns, R. D. (1996). Explaining the high rates of depression in chronic pain: A diathesis–stress framework. *Psychological Bulletin, 119*(1), 95–110.

Beck, A. T. (1967). Depression: Clinical, experimental and technical aspects. New York: Harper and Row.

Ben-Porath, Y. S., & Waller, N. G. (1992). "Normal" personality inventories in clinical assessment: General requirements and the potential for using the NEO Personality Inventory. *Psychological Assessment, 4*, 14–19.

Bigos, S. J., & Battie, M. C. (1987). Acute care to prevent back disability. Ten years of progress. *Clinical Orthopaedics and Related Research, 221*, 121–130.

Bigos, S. J., Battie, M. C., Spengler, D. M., Fisher, L. D., Fordyce, W. E., Hansson, T. H., Nachemson, A. L., & Wortley, M. D. (1991). A progressive study of work perceptions and psychosocial factors affecting the report of back injury. *Spine, 16*(1), 1–6.

Bleuer, M. (1963). Conception of schizophrenia within the last 50 years and today. *Proceedings of the Royal Society of Medicine, 56*, 945–952.

Bonica, J. (1990). History of pain concepts and therapies. In J. Bonica (Ed.), *The management of pain* (Vol. I, p. 2). Philadelphia: Lea & Febiger.

Buchsbaum, M., Goodwin, F., & Muscettola, G. (1981). Urinary MHPG stress response, personality factors, and somatosensory evoked potentials in normal controls and affective disordered patients. *Neuropsychobiology, 7*, 212–224.

Bush, G. W. (1992). President Bush signs compromise civil rights bill. *Psychological Science Agenda*, p. 3.

Clark, L. A. (1990). Toward a consensual set of symptom clusters for assessment of personality disorder. In J. N. Butcher & C. D. Spielberger (Eds.), *Advances in personality assessment* (Vol. 8, pp. 243–266). Hillsdale, NJ: Erlbaum.

Clark, L. A. (1991). *Schedule for normal and abnormal personality and its disorders*. Dallas: Author.

Clark, L. A. (1993). *Schedule for nonadaptive and adaptive personality and its disorders.* Dallas: Author.

Clark, L. A., Livesley, W. J., & Morey, L. (1997). Special feature: Personality disorder assessment: The challenge of construct validity. *Journal of Personality Disorders*, *11*, 205–231.

Clark, L. A., Vorhies, L., & McEwen, J. L. (1994). Personality disorder symptomatology from the five-factor model perspective. In P. T. Costa & T. A. Widiger (Eds.), *Personality disorders and the five-factor model of personality* (pp. 95–116). Washington, DC: American Psychological Association.

Clark, L. A., & Watson, D. (1990). The General Temperament Survey. Dallas: Southern Methodist University.

Clark, L. A., & Watson, D. (in press). Temperament: A new paradigm for trait psychology. In L. Pervin & O. John (Eds.), *Handbook of personality* (Vol. 2). New York: Guilford Press.

Clark, L. A., Watson, D., & Reynolds, S. (1995). Diagnosis and classification of psychopathology: Challenges to the current system and future directions. *Annual Review of Psychology*, *46*, 121–153.

Cloninger, C., Martin, R., & Guze, S. (1990). The empirical structure of psychiatric comorbidity and its theoretical influence. In J. Maser & C. Cloninger (Eds.), *Comorbidity of mood and anxiety disorders* (pp. 439–462). Washington, DC: American Psychiatric Press.

Costa, P. T., & McCrea, R. R. (1992). *Revised NEO Personality Inventory (NEO-PI-R), and NEO Five Factor Inventory (NEO-FFI) manual.* Odessa, FL: Psychological Assessment Resources.

Daley, S., Hammen, C., Davila, J., & Burge, D. (1998). Axis II symptomatology, depression and life stress during the transition from adolescence to adulthood. *Journal of Consulting and Clinical Psychology*, *66*(4), 595–603.

Derogatis, L. R., Lipman, R. L., & Covi, L. (1973). SCL-90: An outpatient psychiatric rating scale. *Psychopharmacology Bulletin*, *9*, 13–28.

Dworkin, R., & Banks, S. (1999). A vulnerability–diathesis–stress model of chronic pain: Herpes zoster and the development of postherpetic neuralgia. In R. Gatchel & D. Turk (Eds.), *Psychosocial factors in pain* (pp. 247–269). New York: Guilford Press.

Engel, G. L. (1977). The need for a new medical model: A challenge for biomedicine. *Science*, *196*(4286), 129–136.

Fabrega, H., Ulrich, R., Pilkonis, A., & Mezzich, J. (1993). Personality disorders diagnosed at intake at a public psychiatric facility. *Hospital and Community Psychiatry*, *44*(2), 159–162.

Falconer, D. (1965). The inheritance of liability to certain diseases, estimated from the incidence among relatives. *Annals of Human Genetics*, *29*, 51–71.

Fishbain, D. A., Goldberg, M., Meagher, B. R., Steele, R., & Rosomoff, H. (1986). Male and female chronic pain patients categorized by DSM-III psychiatric diagnostic criteria. *Pain*, *26*, 181–197.

Flick, S., Roy-Byrne, P., Cowley, D., Shores, M., & Dunner, D. (1993). DSM-III-R personality disorders in a mood and anxiety disorders clinic: Prevalence, comorbidity, and clinical correlates. *Journal of Affective Disorders*, *27*, 71–79.

Flor, H., & Turk, D. C. (1984). Etiological theories and treatments for chronic back pain: I. Somatic models and interventions. *Pain*, *19*, 105–121.

Gasser, T., Muller-Myhsok, B., Wszolek, Z., Oehlmann, R., Calne, D., Bonifati, V., & Bereznai, B. (1998). A susceptibility locus for Parkinson's disease maps to chromosome 2p13. *Nature Genetics*, *18*(3), 262–265.

Gatchel, R. J. (1991). Early development of physical and mental deconditioning in painful spinal disorders. In T. G. Mayer, V. Mooney, & R. J. Gatchel (Eds.), *Contemporary conservative care for painful spinal disorders* (pp. 278–289). Philadelphia: Lea & Febiger.

Gatchel, R. J., Garofalo, J. P., Ellis, E., & Holt, C. (1996). Major psychological disorders in acute and chronic TMD: An initial examination. *Journal of the American Dental Association, 127*, 1365–1374.

Gatchel, R. J., Polatin, P. B., & Kinney, R. K. (1995). Predicting outcome of chronic back pain using clinical predictors of psychopathology: A prospective analysis. *Health Psychology, 14*, 415–420.

Gatchel, R., Polatin, P., Mayer, T., & Garcy, P. (1994). Psychopathology and the rehabilitation of patients with chronic low back pain disability. *Archives of Physical Medicine and Rehabilitation, 75*, 666–670.

Gatchel, R. J., Polatin, P. B., Mayer, T. G., Robinson, R., & Dersh, J. (1998). Use of the SF-36 health status survey with a chronically disabled back pain population: Strengths and limitations. *Journal of Occupational Rehabilitation, 8*, 237–246.

Gil, K., Ross, S., & Keefe, F. (1988). Behavioral treatment of chronic pain: Four pain management protocols. In R. France & K. Krishnan (Eds.), *Chronic pain* (pp. 376–413). Washington, DC: American Psychiatric Press.

Goldstein, M., & Strachan, A. (1987). The family and schizophrenia. In T. Jacobs (Ed.), *Family interaction and psychopathology* (pp. 481–507). New York: Plenum Press.

Goossens, M. E. J. B., & Evers, S. M. A. A. (1997). Economic evaluation of back pain interventions. *Journal of Occupational Rehabilitation, 7*, 15–32.

Griesinger, W. (1965). *Mental pathology and therapeutics*. New York: Hafner. (Original work published 1867)

Hanvik, L. J. (1951). MMPI profiles in patients with low back pain. *Journal of Consulting Psychology, 15*, 350–353.

Harlan, E., & Clark, L. A. (in press). Short-forms of the Schedule for Nonadaptive and Adaptive Personality (SNAP) for self and collateral ratings: Development, reliability, and validity. *Assessment.*

Harshfield, G., & Grim, C. (1997). Stress hypertension: The "wrong" genes in the "wrong" environment. *Acta Physiologica Scandinavica, 161*(Suppl. 640), 129–132.

Hathaway, S. R., & McKinley, J. (1943). *Minnesota Multiphasic Personality Inventory*. Minneapolis: University of Minnesota Press.

Human Capital Initiative Coordinating Committee. (1996). *Doing the right thing: A research plan for healthy living*. Washington, DC: American Psychological Association.

Hunt, M. (1993). *The study of psychology*. New York: Doubleday.

Joiner, T. J., Rudd, M., Heatherington, T., & Schmidt, N. (1997). Perfectionism, perceived weight status, and bulimic symptoms: Two studies testing a diathesis–stress model. *Journal of Abnormal Psychology, 106*(1), 145–153.

Kiecolt-Glaser, J., & Glaser, R. (1987). Psychosocial moderators of immune function. *Annals of Behavioral Medicine, 9*, 16–20.

Kinney, R. K., Gatchel, R. J., & Mayer, T. G. (1991). The SCL-90-R: Evaluated as an alternative to the MMPI for psychological screening of chronic low back pain patients. *Spine, 16*, 940–942.

Koch, R., Graliker, B., Fishler, K., & Ragsdale, N. (Eds.). (1963). *Clinical aspects of phenylketonuria*. Philadelphia: Lippincott.

Large, R. G. (1986). DSM-III diagnoses in chronic pain: Confusion or clarity? *Journal of Nervous and Mental Disease, 174*(5), 295–303.

Lazarus, R., & Folkman, J. (1984). *Stress, appraisal, and coping*. New York: Springer.

Lehman, C., Rodin, J., McEwen, B., & Brinton, R. (1991). Impact of environmental stress on the expression of insulin-dependent diabetes mellitus. *Behavioral Neuroscience, 105*(2), 241–245.

Linton, S. J., & Bradley, L. A. (1992). An 18-month follow-up of a secondary prevention program for back pain: Help and hindrance factors related to outcome maintenance. *Clinical Journal of Pain, 8*, 227–236.

Linton, S. J., & Bradley, L. A. (1996). Strategies for the prevention of chronic pain. In R. J. Gatchel & D. C. Turk (Eds.), *Psychological approaches to pain management: A practitioner's handbook.* New York: Guilford Press.

Livengood, J., & Johnson, B. (1998). Personality disorders in chronic pain patients. *Pain Digest, 8,* 292–296.

Livesley, W. J., Schroeder, M. L., Jackson, D. N., & Jang, K. L. (1994). Categorical distinctions in the study of personality disorder: Implications for classification. *Journal of Abnormal Psychology, 103* 6–17.

Love, A., & Peck, C. (1987). The MMPI and psychological factors in chronic low back pain: A review. *Pain, 28,* 1–12.

McFall, R., Townsend, J., & Viken, R. (1995). Diathesis–stress model or "just so" story? *Behavioral and Brain Sciences, 18*(3), 565–566.

Meehl, P. (1962). Schizotaxia, schizotypy, schizophrenia. *American Psychologist, 17,* 827–838.

Melzack, R. (1999). Pain and stress: A new perspective. In R. J. Gatchel & D. C. Turk (Eds.), *Psychological factors in pain: Critical perspectives* (pp. 89–106). New York: Guilford Press.

Millon, T., Green, C. J., & Meagher, R. B. (1982). *Millon Behavioral Health Inventory* (3rd ed.). Minneapolis, MN: Interpretive Scoring System.

Mitchell, R. I., & Carmen, G. M. (1990). Results of a multicenter trial using an intensive active exercise program for the treatment of acute soft tissue and back injuries. *Spine, 15,* 514–521.

Mitchell, R. I., & Carmen, G. M. (1994). The functional restoration approach to the treatment of chronic pain in patients with soft tissue and back injuries. *Spine, 19,* 633–642.

Monroe, S., & Simmons, A. (1991). Diathesis–stress theories in the context of life stress research: Implications for depressive disorders. *Psychological Bulletin, 110*(3), 406–425.

Mullins, L., Chaney, J., Pace, T., & Hartman, V. (1997). Illness uncertainty, attributional style and psychological adjustment in older adolescents and young adults with asthma. *Journal of Pediatric Psychology, 22*(6), 871–880.

Newman, B., & Liu, E. (1998). Perspective on BRCA1. *Breast Disease, 10*(1–2), 3–10.

O'Banion, D. (1981). *The ecological environment and stress: An ecological and nutritional approach to behavioral medicine.* Springfield, IL: Charles C Thomas.

Paris, J. (1998). Significance of biological research for a biopsychosocial model of the personality disorders. In K. Silk (Ed.), *Biology of personality disorders* (Vol. 17, pp. 129–148). Washington, DC: American Psychiatric Press.

Pickar, D., Labarca, R., Doran, A., Wolkowitz, O., Roy, A., Breier, A., Linnoila, M., & Paul, S. (1986). Longitudinal measurement of plasma homovanillic acid levels in schizophrenic patients. Correlation with psychosis and response to neuroleptic treatment. *Archives of General Psychiatry, 43,* 669–676.

Polatin, P. B., Kinney, R. K., Gatchel, R. J., Lillo, E., & Mayer, T. G. (1993). Psychiatric illness and chronic low-back pain. The mind and the spine—Which goes first? *Spine, 18*(1), 66–71.

Reich, J., & Thompson, D. (1987). DSM-III personality disorder clusters in three populations. *British Journal of Psychiatry, 150,* 471–475.

Reich, J., Tupin, J. P., & Abramowitz, S. I. (1983). Psychiatric diagnosis of chronic pain patients. *American Journal of Psychiatry, 140*(11), 1495–1498.

Rosenberg, R., & Iannaccone, S. (1995). The prevention of neurogenetic disease. *Archives of Neurology, 52*(4), 356–362.

Rosenthal, D. (1963). A suggested conceptual framework. In D. Rosenthal (Ed.), *Genian quadruplets* (pp. 505–516). New York: Basic Books.

Schleifer, S., Keller, S., Camerino, M., Thornton, J., & Stein, M. (1983). Suppression of lymphocyte stimulation following bereavement. *Journal of the American Medical Association, 250,* 374–377.

Selye, H. (1956). *The stress of life.* New York: McGraw-Hill.

Siever, L., Amin, F., Coccaro, E., Bernstein, D., Kavoussi, R., Kalus, O., Horvath, T., Warne, P., Davidson, M., & Davis, K. (1991). Plasma homovanillic acid in schizotypal personality disorder. *American Journal of Psychiatry, 148,* 1246–1248.

Silverman, J. M., Siever, L. J., Horvath, T. B., Coccaro, E. F., Klar, H., Davidson, M., Pinkham, L., Apter, S. H., Mohs, R. C., & Davis, K. L. (1993). Schizophrenia-related and affective personality disorder traits in relatives of probands with schizophrenia and personality disorders. *American Journal of Psychiatry, 150*(3), 435–442.

Spangler, D., Simons, A., Monroe, S., & Thase, M. (1997). Comparison of cognitive models of depression: Relationships between cognitive constructs and cognitive diathesis–stress match. *Journal of Abnormal Psychology, 106*(3), 395–403.

Spaulding, W. (1997). Cognitive models in a fuller understanding of schizophrenia. *Psychiatry, 60*(Winter), 341–346.

Spitzer, R. L., Williams, J. B., Gibbon, M., & First, M. B. (1988). *Structured clinical interview for DSM-III-R.* New York: New York State Psychiatric Institute.

Tellegen, A., & Waller, N. (in press). Exploring personality through test construction: Development of the Multidimensional Personality Questionnaire. In S. R. Briggs & J. M. Cheek (Eds.), *Personality measures: Development and evaluation* (Vol. 1). Greenwich, CT: JAI Press.

Turk, D. C., & Flor, H. (1984). Etiological theories and treatment for chronic back pain. II. Psychological models and interventions. *Pain, 19,* 209–233.

Turk, D., & Rudy, T. (1988). Toward an empirically derived taxonomy of chronic pain patients: Integration of psychological assessment data. *Journal of Consulting and Clinical Psychology, 56,* 233–238.

Turk, D., & Salovey, P. (1984). Chronic pain as a variant of depressive disease: A critical reappraisal. *Journal of Nervous and Mental Disease, 172,* 398–404.

Uhl, G. R., Sora, I., & Wang, Z. (1999). The u opiate receptor as a candidate gene for pain: Polymorphisms, variations in expression, nociception, and opiate responses. *Proceedings of the National Academy of Sciences, 96*(14), 7752–7755.

Vittengl, J., Clark, L., Owen-Salter, E., & Gatchel, R. (1999). Diagnostic change and personality stability following functional restoration treatment in a chronic low back pain patient sample. *Assessment, 6,* 79–92.

Walker, E., & Diforio, D. (1997). Schizophrenia: A neural diathesis–stress model. *Psychological Review, 104*(4), 667–685.

Ware, J. E., & Sherbourne, C. D. (1992). The MDS 36-item short form health survey (SF-36). *Medical Care, 30,* 473–483.

Watson, D., Clark, L. A., & Harkness, A. R. (1994a). Negative affectivity: The disposition to experience aversive emotional states. *Psychological Bulletin, 96,* 465–490.

Watson, D., Clark, L. A., & Harkness, A. R. (1994b). Structures of personality and their relevance to psychopathology. *Journal of Abnormal Psychology, 103,* 18–31.

Weisberg, J. N., Gallagher, R. M., & Gorin, A. (1996, November). *Personality disorder in chronic pain: A longitudinal approach to validation of diagnosis.* Paper presented at the 15th Annual Scientific Meeting of the American Pain Society, Washington, DC.

Weisberg, J. N., & Keefe, F. J. (1997). Personality disorders in the chronic pain population: Basic concepts, empirical findings, and clinical implications. *Pain Forum, 6*(1), 1–9.

Weisberg, J. N., & Keefe, F. (1999). Personality, individual differences, and psychopathology in chronic pain. In R. Gatchel & D. Turk (Eds.), *Psychosocial factors in pain: Critical perspectives* (pp. 56–73). New York: Guilford Press.

Widiger, T. A., & Shea, T. (1991). Differentiation of Axis I and Axis II disorders. *Journal of Abnormal Psychology, 100,* 399–406.

Zuckerman, M. (1999). *Vulnerability to psychopathology.* Washington, DC: American Psychological Association.

AUTHOR INDEX

Numbers in italics refer to listings in the chapter reference sections.

Aaron, L. A., 151, *162*
Abashian, S., 167, 168, 170, *175, 175, 176*
Abbot, R., 207, *216*
Abramowitz, S. I., 112, *124,* 229, 232, *238,* 266, *281*
Abrams, M. R., 151, 152, *160, 163*
Abramson, L. Y., 146, *159,* 204, *213*
Abramson, U., 170, *174*
Adams, K. M., 51, *54*
Ader, T., 262, *278*
Adler, N., 207, *214*
Affleck, G., *102,* 141, 145, *159,* 205, 207, 211, *214, 215, 217*
Akeson, W. H., *22, 57*
Akhtar, S., 243, *256*
Alarcon, G. S., 151, *162*
Albers, K. R., 151, *162*
Alexander, J., *257*
Alexander, R. W., 151, *162*
Allport, G. W., *102*
Alterdings, M. D., 246, *254*
American Psychiatric Association, 12, *19,* 77, *84,* 221, 222, 223, 226, *237,* 243, *254,* 260, 271, *278*
American Psychological Association, *254*
Amin, F., 261, *282*
Anderson, G., 9, *22*
Anderson, K. O., 209, *214*
Anderson, S., 134, *162*
Anderson, V. C., 114, *122*
Andreski, P., 96, *103*
Andrew, J. M., 67, *84*
Angst, J., 184, *199*
Antoni, M., 61, 62, 72, *85, 87*
Antoni, M. H., 72, 73, 77, 79, 80, *84, 85, 86, 87, 88*
Apter, S. H., 227, *238,* 261, *282*
Arathuzik, D., 151, *159*
Archer, C. R., 89, 90, 93, 97, 99, *107*
Archer, R. P., *124*
Arena, J. G., 209, *216*
Armentrout, D., *21*
Armentrout, D. P., 52, 53, *54, 57*
Armor, D. A., 205, *217*
Arthur, R. J., 66, *88*
Asmundson, G. J. G., 246, *254*

Aspinwall, L. G., *217*
Asselin, L. A., *124*
Atkinson, J. H., Jr., 53, *54*
August, S., *84*
Aurelius, M., *102*
Ayres, S. Y., 120, *123*
Azariah, R., 207, *214*
Azrin, N. H., *35*

Bagby, R. M., 184, *202*
Baggett, L., *84*
Baggi, L., 82, *85*
Baile, W. F., *103*
Bailey, S. I., 13, *22*
Baker, C., 89, 90, *106*
Bandura, A., 146, *159,* 204, *214*
Banks, S., 263, *279*
Banks, S. M., 263, *278*
Baracco, G., 192, *201*
Barber, T. X., 188, *199*
Bardham, P. N., *33*
Barnes, D., 48, 49, *54, 55*
Barnes, G. E., 188, *199*
Barnett, J., 48, 49, *54,* 250, *255*
Barnett, P., 75, 76, *85*
Barr, J. S., 29, *33*
Barrett, J. F., 8, *19*
Barry, H., 29, *33*
Bartol, C. R., 187, *199*
Bates, M. S., 169, 171, *174*
Battié, M. C., 16, *20,* 50, *55,* 122, *122, 123,* 267, *278, 278*
Baum, A., 4, 8, *19, 20,* 182, 196, 197, 198, *199*
Baumann, U., 184, *199*
Beals, R., 8, *19*
Beals, R. K., *55*
Beaulier, C. L., 150, *160*
Beaupre, P. M., 111, *123*
Bech, P., 183, *200*
Beck, A. T., *159,* 206, *214, 247, 254, 278*
Beck, N., 134, *162*
Becker, J., 134, *164,* 171, *174*
Beckham, J., *256*
Beckham, J. C., 211, *214*
Beecher, H. K., 5, *19,* 182, 183, 188, *199*

Bellissimo, A., 4, *19*
BenDebba, M., 97, 98, *103*
Bending, A. W., *199*
Benjamin, B., 68, *87*
Bennett, R. M., 158, *159*
Ben–Porath, Y. S., 115, 122, *122, 123,* 275, 278
Berenznai, B., 261, *279*
Bergner, M., 92, *104*
Bernstein, D., 261, *282*
Bernstein, I. H., 52, *55*
Bevins, T., 52, *57*
Bibring, G., 236, *237*
Biering-Sorensen, F., *21,* 45, 50, *56*
Bigos, S. J., 16, *20,* 50, *55,* 122, *122, 123,* 267, 278, *278*
Black, R. G., 44, *55*
Blais, M., 221, 222, *237*
Blaney, N. T., 99, *103*
Blaney, P., 72, *86*
Bleuer, M., 262, *278*
Block, A. R., *214*
Blum, N., 226, 227, 233, *238*
Blumberg, H., 93, *103*
Blume, H. G., 48, *56*
Blumer, D., *20,* 49, 51, *54, 55,* 241, *255*
Blumetti, A. E., 47, *55*
Bockian, N., 84, *88*
Bockian, N. R., 81, *85*
Bolstad, B. R., *174*
Bombardier, C. H., 53, *55*
Bond, M. R., *125,* 181, 182, 190, 192, 193, 196, *199*
Bonica, J., 4, *20,* 92, *104,* 261, *278*
Bonifati, V., 261, *279*
Boothby, J. L., 129, 133, 142, 147, 148, *159*
Borchgrevink, G. E., 62, 83, *85*
Borchgrevink, P. C., 62, 83, *85*
Borgatta, E. F., 94, *103*
Borreani, C., 192, *201*
Bossio, L. M., 208, *216*
Bostock, J., 29, *33*
Boyce, P., 96, *103*
Boyd, J. H., 241, *256*
Boyer, S. L., *214*
Bozza, G., 92, *106*
Bradley, L. A., 7, 13, 18, *20, 21,* 51, 52, *55, 57,* 110, 111, 118, *122, 124,* 151, *162,* 209, *214,* 268, 269, *280, 281*
Braith, J., 89, 92, 97, 99, *105*
Brandwin, M. A., 48, *55*

Brant-Zawakzki, M. N., 9, *21*
Brauer, E., *56*
Braverman, B., 249, *255*
Breier, A., 261, *281*
Brenner, C., 29, 30, *33*
Brenner, G. F., 211, *211, 214*
Breslau, N., 96, *103*
Breuer, J., 26, 27, *33*
Breuer, S. R., 75, 76, *88*
Brickman, A. L., 99, *103*
Brimlow, D. L., *103*
Brinker, J., *103*
Brinton, R., 262, *280*
Brooks, W. B., 53, *55*
Brown, G., 97, *105,* 130, 141, 143, *160, 161,* 210, 212, *214, 215*
Brown, J. D., 205, *217*
Brown, R. A., 188, *199*
Brown, T., 29, *33*
Browne, G., 151, *164*
Buch, C. N., *88*
Buchsbaum, M., 261, *278*
Buckelew, S. P., 134, 152, *160, 160, 162,* 168, *174*
Buckingham, B., 89, *106*
Bullinger, M., 62, *87*
Bulman, R. J., 205, *214*
Burchiel, K. J., 114, *122*
Burckhardt, C. S., 158, *159*
Burge, D., 265, *279*
Burke, J. D., 241, *256, 242, 257*
Burker, E. J., 211, *214*
Busch, S. M., 96, *103*
Bush, F. M., 93, *103*
Bush, G. W., *278*
Bush, T., 99, *106*
Bushnell, M. C., 90, *106*
Butcher, J. N., 37, 39, 40, 41, 42, 44, 52, 54, *55, 55, 56,* 109, 111, 112, 113, 114, 115, 117, 118, 119, 120, 122, *122, 123,* 183, *199*
Butler, R. W., 150, *160, 161*
Buzzelli, G., 92, *106*
Byrnes, D., 72, 73, *85*

Caldwell, D., 97, *105,* 141, *161,* 210, *215, 256*
Callahan, L. F., 7, *21,* 110, 111, *124, 175*
Callas, P. W., 235, *237*
Calne, D., 261, *279*
Calsyn, D., 42, *55*
Calsyn, D. A., 41, 43, 51, *55, 56*

Camerino, M., 262, *281*
Camfield, M. R., 209, *216*
Campbell, S. M., 158, *159*
Cantor, N., 206, *216*
Capelli, M., 192, *201*
Capestany, R., *124*
Capra, P., 74, 75, 76, *85,* 250, *255*
Carlton, T. K., 120, 121, *124*
Carmen, G. M., 18, *21,* 269, *281*
Carnrike, C. L., *175*
Carr, J., 134, *164*
Carrier, B., 89, 90, *106*
Carrieri, W., 167, *174*
Carron, H., 169, *175*
Carter, S., *33*
Carver, C. S., 144, 145, *160,* 204, 206, 207,
        208, 210, 212, *214, 216*
Castlebury, R., 221, 222, *237*
Cattell, R. B., 94, 96, 98, *103,* 193, *199*
Caudill, M. A., 157, 158, *162*
Celetano, D. D., 226, *238*
Chamberlain, K., 207, *214*
Chan, C. W., 113, *124*
Chaney, J., 262, *281*
Chapman, C. R., 44, *55*
Chapman, S., 14, *20*
Chapman, W. P., 92, *103*
Chase, T. N., 62, *87*
Chilcoat, H. D., 96, *103*
Chino, A. F., 120, *123,* 129
Choca, J., 80, *85*
Christal, R. E., *107*
Clancy, S., 134, 141, *164,* 210, *217*
Claridge, G. S., 192, *199*
Clark, K. C., 207, 212, *214*
Clark, L. A., 15, 16, *20, 22,* 236, *237,* 241,
        245, 251, *255, 257,* 271, 274, 275,
        276, 277, *278, 279, 280, 282*
Clark, M. R., 152, *161*
Clark, S. R., 158, *159*
Clarkin, J., 228, 229, *239,* 242, *255*
Cloninger, C., 263, *279*
Cloninger, R., 244, *255*
Cobb, S., *85*
Coccaro, E., 226, 227, *237, 238,* 261, *282*
Cochrane, K., 226, *237*
Cohen, M. J., 51, *57,* 111, *124*
Cohen, N., 118, 119, *123,* 262, *278*
Cole, R., 182, *199*
Coleman, P., 151, *163,* 207, *216*
Collard, L., 245, *255*
Collen, M. F., 92, *107*

Colligan, R., 113, *124,* 205, 206, *214, 216*
Collins, W., *201*
Comstock, G. W., 68, *85*
Conlon, M. F., *35*
Cook, D. B., 89, 90, 99, *107,* 184, *202*
Cooper, T., 226, *237*
Coryell, W., 99, *105,* 242, 243, *257*
Costa, P. T., 66, *85,* 94, 96, 97, 98, 100,
        103, 104, 105, 184, *199,* 236, *237,*
        245, *255, 279*
Costantini, M., 192, *201*
Costello, N., 73, *88,* 187, *199*
Costello, R. M., 53, *55,* 118, 119, *123,* 206,
        209, *214*
Courbasson, C. M. A., *160*
Coventry, M. B., 29, *33*
Covi, L., 248, *255,* 270, *279*
Covington, E., 169, 171, 172, *175*
Cowley, D., 260, *279*
Cox, G. B., 44, *55*
Craig, R. J., 80, *85*
Crews, F., 26, *33*
Crinean, J., 207, *215*
Crissom, J. E., 141, *161,* 168, 170, 171,
        174, 256
Cronbach, L., 110, *123*
Crown, J. M., 171, *174*
Crown, S., 171, *174*
Curtis, J. L., *33*
Curtis, K., 167, *175*
Cushman, D., 29, *35*
Custer, R., 96, *106*
Cutler, R., 170, 171, *174*

Daeschner, C. D., *160*
Dahlstrom, L. E., 42, *55*
Dahlstrom, W. G., 42, *55,* 114, 115, 121,
        123, 183, *199*
Daley, S., 265, *279*
Dallenbach, K. M., 25, *33*
Dalrymple, D. G., 188, *200*
Damarin, F. L., 150, *160*
Davidson, M., 227, *238,* 261, *282*
Davidson, P. O., 184, 187, 188, *200*
Davies, M., 226, *238*
Davila, J., 265, *279*
Davis, K. L., 222, 226, 227, 229, *237, 238,*
        261, *282*
Davis, R. D., 62, 67, 72, 77, 78, 80, 84, *87*
Dawson, E., 6, 13, *21,* 44, 45, 51, *57*
Deardorff, W. W., 120, *123,* 129
DeAvila, M., 208, *216*

Deckel, A. W., *85,* 250, *255*
DeClemente, C. C., 157, *162*
DeGood, D., 140, 142, 156, 157, 158, *160,*
    163, 164, 169, *175*
Della Corte, M., 92, *106*
Dembroski, T. M., 66, *85*
Denison, D. B., 114, *122*
Dennis, N., 28, *33*
De-Nour, A. K., 99, *103*
D'Eon, J. L., 142, 151, *163*
DeRidder, D. T., 132, *162*
Derogatis, L. R., 142, *160,* 248, *255,* 270,
    279
Dersh, J., 251, *256,* 271, *280*
DeVellis, R., 134, *164,* 166, *176*
DeVilder, J., 93, *103*
Diamond, P., 75, 76, *85,* 250, *255*
Dickson, A. C., 167, *174*
Diforio, D., 262, *282*
Digman, J. M., 94, 95, 101, *103, 104,* 184,
    200
Dimsdale, J. E., 92, *107*
Dishman, R. K., 171, *174*
Divine, G. W., 53, *55*
Dobson, K. S., 152, *160*
Dodd, M. J., 167, *174*
Donham, G. W., 197, *200*
Doran, A., 261, *281*
Dougherty, L. M., 89, 90, 93, 97, 98, 99,
    107, 184, *202*
Dowdly, S. W., 143, 144, 145, 149, 151,
    163
Dozois, D. J. A., 152, *160*
Draugelis, R., 48, *58*
Drummond, R., 183, *200*
Dubner, R., 97, *104*
Dubreuil, D., 92, *104*
Duncan, G. H., 90, *106*
Dunner, D., 260, *279*
Durand, E. J., 135, *164*
Dush, D. M., 120, *123*
Dworkin, R. H., *21,* 203, 209, *214,* 263,
    279
Dworkin, S. F., 151, *164,* 252, *255*
Dwyer, J., 208, *215*
Dwyer, K. A., 143, 144, 145, 149, 151, *163*

Eber, H. W., 94, 96, 98, *103*
Edelmann, R. J., 193, *201*
Edman, G., 184, 197, *201*
Edwin, D., 114, *124*
Efantis-Potter, J., 72, 73, *85*

Egan, K., 203, *215*
Eisenbud, J., 29, 30, *33*
Ellermeier, W., 92, *104*
Elliott, T. R., 62, 82, 83, *85*
Ellis, A., 138, 147, *160*
Ellis, E., 203, *215,* 234, *237,* 242, 245, *255,*
    259, 266, *280*
Ellman, P., 29, 30, *33*
Endicott, J., 78, *88,* 226, 227, *238*
Endler, N. S., 132, 135, 136, 137, *160*
Engel, B. T., *103*
Engel, G. L., *20,* 28, 29, 30, 31, *33,* 48, *55,*
    67, *85, 87,* 261, 262, *279*
Engstrom, D., 167, *174*
Epker, J. T., 7, 11, 12, *20*
Esterling, B., 73, *84*
Esterson, A., 26, *33*
Estlander, A., 169, *174,* 206, 207, 208, 209,
    210, *214, 215*
Etscheidt, M. A., 249, *255*
Evers, S. M. A. A., 18, *20,* 268, *280*
Exton-Smith, A. N., 181, *200*
Eysenck, H. J., 96, *104,* 182, 183, 184, 187,
    188, 192, *200, 201,* 244, *255*
Eysenck, S. B. G., 96, *104,* 183, *200*

Fabrega, H., 260, *279*
Fader, K., 188, *199*
Fagan, P. J., 100, *104*
Fahey, J. L., 208, *216*
Falconer, D., 261, 262, *279*
Fan, A. Y., *200*
Feifel, H., 151, *163*
Felton, B. J., *162,* 210, *214*
Felton, D., 134, *162,* 262, *278*
Feltz, C., *54*
Fernandez, E., 125, 212, *214*
Ferrante, F. M., 208, *215*
Fibel, B., 206, *215*
Fillingim, R. B., 169, *175*
Fillion, L., 136, *160*
Finneran, J., 170, *175*
First, M., 12, *22,* 78, *88,* 226, 233, *238,*
    242, *257* 277, *282*
Fishbain, D., 14, *20,* 74, *86,* 109, *123,* 170,
    171, *174,* 232, *237,* 242, *255,* 266,
    279
Fisher, L. D., *20,* 50, *55,* 122, *123,* 267,
    278
Fisher, R., 111, 112, *125,* 188, *200*
Fishler, K., 262, *280*
Fitzgerald, R. G., 68, *87*

Fitzgerald, T., 207, *215*
Fleck, S., 68, *87*
Flescher, J., *33*
Fletcher, M. A., 73, *84, 87*
Flick, S., 260, *279*
Flor, H., 263, *279, 282*
Folkman, J., 261, *280*
Folkman, S., 130, 132, 133, *160, 162,* 165, *174*
Folstein, M. F., 112, *125*
Fordyce, W. E., *20, 56,* 120, 121, 122, *123,* 170, *174,* 267, *278*
Forrer, S., 29, *33*
Fowler-Kerry, S., 93, *105*
Frances, A., 228, 229, *239,* 242, 244, *255,* 257
Frank, R., 134, *160, 162,* 166, 168, *174, 176*
Freeman, C., 41, 42, 51, 53, *55, 56*
Fremouw, W. J., 212, *215*
Freud, S., 4, *20,* 25, 26, 27, 28, *33*
Friedman, A. F., 183, *200*
Friedman, A. P., *33*
Friedman, G. D., 92, *107*
Friedman, H. S., *86*
Friedman, M., 66, *85*
Frieze, I. H., 205, *215*
Frye, R. F., 193, *201*
Frymoyer, J., 9, *22,* 52, *57,* 235, *237*
Furmanski, A. R., *33*
Fyer, M. R., 242, *255*

Gafni, A., 151, *164*
Gallagher, R. M., 233, 235, *237, 239,* 257, 266, *282*
Gallinek, A., 28, *33*
Galton, F., 94, 98, *104*
Gamberale, F., 151, *161*
Gano, D., 212, *215*
Garbin, C. P., 52, *55*
Garcia, A., 207, *214*
Garcy, P., *20,* 259, *280*
Garcy, P. D., 242, *256,* 259, *280*
Garofalo, J. P., 203, *215,* 234, *237,* 242, 245, *255,* 259, 266, *280*
Garron, D., 92, *104*
Garron, D. C., 49, 52, *55, 56*
Gasser, T., 261, *279*
Gatchel, R. J., 3, 4, 5, 7, 8, 9, 11, 12, 14, 15, 16, *19, 20, 21, 22,* 48, 49, *54, 55, 56,* 74, 75, 80, 83, *85,* 112, *123, 124,* 182, 198, *199,* 203, *215, 216,* 223,

227, 233, 234, 235, *237, 238,* 242, 244, 245, 246, 248, 250, 251, *255, 256, 257,* 259, 266, 267, 269, 270, 271, 276, 277, 278, *279, 282*
Gazendam, B., 168, *175*
Geisser, M. E., 113, 118, 119, 120, *124,* 140, 142, 149, *163*
Genest, M., 165, *176*
Gentry, W. D., 13, *20,* 47, 51, 52, *55, 56, 57,* 193, *202*
George, L. K., 241, *256*
Gertrudis, I. J. M., 97, 99, *104*
Getto, C. J., *56,* 84, 91, 95, *104*
Gibbon, M., 78, *88,* 226, 233, *238,* 242 *257,* 277, *282*
Gibbons, M., 12, *22*
Gidro-Frank, L., 28, *33*
Gil, K., 138, 141, 151, 152, *160, 163,* 181, *200, 256,* 264, *280*
Gilberstadt, H., 44, *56*
Ginsberg, B., 181, *200*
Gitlin, M. J., 203, 209, *214*
Glaser, R., 262, *280*
Goldberg, L. R., 94, *104, 106*
Goldberg, M., 14, *20,* 74, *86,* 232, *237,* 242, *255,* 266, *279*
Golden, C. J., 48, *56*
Goldie, I., 151, *161*
Goldman, S., 113, *124*
Goldner, J. L., 47, *56*
Goldstein, D., 73, *86*
Goldstein, M., 262, *280*
Goodkin, K., 72, 73, *84, 86*
Goodwin, F., 261, *278*
Goosens, M. E. J. B., 18, *20*
Gordon, A., 98, *104*
Gordon, T., 28, *33*
Gorin, A., 233, *239, 257,* 266, *282*
Gorsuch, R. L., 132, *163*
Gorton, G., 243, *256*
Gossens, M. E. J. B., 268, *280*
Gottschalk, L., 29, *34*
Gough, H. G., *86*
Gracely, R., 89, 97, *104*
Graham, J. R., 37, 38, 39, 40, 41, 42, 46, *55, 56,* 114, 115, 121, 122, *123,* 183, *199, 200,* 209, *215*
Graliker, B., 262, *280*
Grant, J., 167, 168, *175, 176*
Graven, P. S., 29, *33*
Gray, M. G., 29, *35*
Green, C., 68, 73, *86, 87,* 184, 192, *201,* 236, *238,* 249, *256,* 270, *281*

Greenacre, P., 29, *34*
Greene, D., *104*
Greene, R. L., 121, *123*
Greer, S., 205, *215*
Greewald, H. P., 92, *104*
Griesinger, W., 261, *280*
Griesser, H. J., 95, *103*
Griffith, P., 99, *105*
Grim, C., 262, *280*
Grinker, R. R., 29, *34*
Groban, S. E., *56*
Grove, K. S., 82, *86*
Grove, R. N., 82, *86*
Grubman, J. A., 52, *57*
Gruen, W., *215*
Gruenberg, E., 242, *257*
Grzeiak, R. C., 4, *21*
Gu, R., *200*
Guck, T. P., *56, 123*
Guze, S., 263, *279*
Gwadry, F. G., 140, 141, *163*

Haazen, I. W. C., 148, *164*
Haddox, J. D., 93, *105*
Haile, J. M., 111, *122*
Hale, S. L., 96, *106*
Hale, W. D., 206, *215*
Halliday, J. L., 29, 30, *34*
Hamer, R. M., *107*
Hamilton, M., 247, *256*
Hammen, C., 265, *279*
Hanlon, R. B., *107*
Hannson, T. H., *20,* 50, *55*
Hansen, F. R., 11, *21,* 45, 50, *56*
Hansson, T. H., 267, *278*
Hanvik, L. J., 6, 11, 13, *21,* 42, 43–44, *56,*
   248, *256,* 269, *280*
Hargreaves, A., 93, *105*
Harkapaa, K., 168, 171, *174,* 207, 208, 209,
   215
Harkins, S. W., 89, 90, 92, 93, 97, 99, *103,*
   105, 106
Harkness, A. R., 274, *282*
Harlan, E., *280*
Harlow, T., 116, *123*
Harper, D. C., 74, *86*
Harrington, W. G., 93, *103*
Harris, S. D., 145, *160,* 207, *214*
Harshfield, G., 262, *280*
Hart, H., 29, *34*
Hart, R. P., 89, 90, 99, *107,* 184, *202*
Hart, R. R., *56*

Hartman, V., 262, *281*
Harvey, M., 84, *88*
Haslam, D. R., 184, 187, *200*
Hathaway, S. R., 37, *57,* 109, *123,* 205,
   215, 226, *237, 280*
Haugh, L. D., 235, *237*
Haybittle, J. L., 205, *215*
Haythornthwaite, J., 152, 157, 158, *161,*
   162
Hazlewood, L. A., 75, 76, *88*
Heatherington, T., 262, *280*
Heaton, R., 56, 84, 91, 95, *104*
Heiden, L., 212, *215*
Heilbronn, M., *20,* 49, 51, *54, 55,* 241, *255*
Heinberg, L. J., 152, *161*
Helgeson, V. S., 205, *215*
Helmes, E., 109, 110, *123*
Helms, M., *256*
Helzer, J. E., 242, *257*
Hendler, N. H., 49, *56*
Henriques, F., 28, *33*
Herbert, M., *175, 217*
Hernandez, J. T., *175*
Herring, C., 234, 235, *238*
Herron, L. D., 46, *56, 83, 88*
Herz, G., 76, *88*
Heslegrave, R., 222, *238*
Hetzel, R. D., 208, 211, *216*
Hewett, J., *160,* 168, *174*
Hewett, J. E., *54,* 134, 152, *160, 162*
Heyneman, N. E., 212, *215*
Hickman, N. W., *55*
Hickok, L., 245, *255*
Higgins, P., 97, *102,* 141, *159, 217*
Hill, A., 151, *161,* 210, *215*
Hilsenroth, M., 221, 222, *237*
Hirschmuller, A., 26, *34*
Hirshfield, R. M. A., 99, *105*
Hislop, I. G., 67, *87*
Hitchcock, E. R., 98, *104*
Hobbs-Hardee, B., 206, 209, *214*
Hofbauer, R. K., 90, *106*
Hogan, R., 94, 95, *105*
Holdwick, D. J., 221, 222, *237*
Holland, M. A., 76, *88*
Holm, J., 167, *175*
Holman, C., 111, *124*
Holmes, T. H., 29, *34, 67, 86*
Holroyd, K. A., 150, *163, 167, 175*
Holt, C., 203, *215,* 234, *237,* 242, 245, *255,*
   259, 266, *280*
Holzman, A. D., 209, 212, *217*

Honor, L. F., 76, *88*
Hopkin, K., 9, *21*
Hopson, L., 51, *55*
Hornyak, M., 95, *103*
Horowitz, M., 207, *214*
Horvath, T., 226, 227, *237, 238,* 261, *282*
Hstrup, D. M., 113, *124*
Hsu, *82*
Huger, R., 157, 158, *161*
Hughes, D., 152, *160*
Hulsey, T. L., 53, *55,* 118, 119, *123*
Human Capital Initiative Coordinating
    Committee, 18, *21, 280*
Huncke, B., 193, *200*
Hunt, M., 261, *280*
Hunter, M., 196, *201*
Hurri, H., 168, 171, *174*
Hurt, S., 228, 229, *239,* 242, 244, *255, 257*
Huskisson, E. C., 188, *200*
Hutchinson, P. R., 32, *35*
Hyler, S., 226, *238*

Iannaccone, S., 261, *281*
Ickes, W., 171, *174*
Inglis, J., 188, *201*
Ingram, F., *86*
Ingram, R. E., 53, *54*
Inouye, J., 94, 101, *103*
Ironson, G., 73, *84, 87, 88*

Jackson, D. N., 67, 70, *86,* 274, *281*
Jackson, W. T., 62, 83, *85*
Jacobs, M., 130, *161*
Jacobsen, P. B., *161*
Jahanshahi, M., 96, *106,* 196, *201*
James, L. D., 148, 152, 158, *161*
Jamison, R. N., 129, 157, 158, *161, 162,*
    208, *215*
Jancis, M., 44, *56*
Jang, K. L., 274, *281*
Janoff-Bulman, R., 205, *215*
Jarvikoski, A., 168, 171, *174,* 207, 208,
    209, *215*
Jaworski, T. M., *122*
Jay, G. W., 82, *86*
Jayson, M. I. V., 246, *256*
Jeans, M. E., 188, 190, *202*
Jenkins, C. D., 66, *86,* 207, 208, *215*
Jensen, M. C., 9, *21*
Jensen, M. P., 129, 130, 133, 141, 142, 146,
    147, 148, 151, 152, 156, 157, 158,
    159, 161, 203, *215, 256*

Jess, P., 183, *200*
Joffe, R. T., 242, *256*
Johnson, B., 259, 266, *281*
Johnson, C., *57*
Johnson, J. C., 152, *162*
Johnson, J. H., 67, *88*
Johnson, J. L., 97, *105*
Joiner, T. J., 262, *280*
Jones, C. M., 92, *103*
Jones, D., 48, *58*
Jordan, J. S., 53, *55*
Joreskog, K., *105, 161*

Kaemmer, B., *55,* 114, 115, 121, *123,* 183,
    199
Kahana, R., 236, *237*
Kalton, W., 203, *215*
Kalus, O., 261, *282*
Kamen-Siegel, L., 208, *215*
Kaplan, G., 166, *176*
Karno, M., 241, *256*
Karoly, P., 129, 142, 146, 150, 151, 155,
    157, 158, *161,* 203, *215*
Karr, K. M., 207, *216*
Kato, W., 99, *106*
Kavoussi, R., 261, *282*
Keefe, F., 11, 15, 16, *22,* 97, *105, 106,* 111,
    112, 113, 120, *123, 125,* 138, 140,
    141, 142, 149, 151, *162, 163, 164,*
    168, 170, 171, *174,* 206 *214,* 210,
    211, *215, 216,* 223, 229, 233, 235,
    239, 243, *256, 257,* 259, 264, 266,
    277, 278, *280, 282*
Keefe, P., 130, 141, 142, *161*
Keefe, R. S. E., 227, *238*
Keith, B. R., 138, 152, *160*
Keller, L. S., 37, 40, 42, 44, 51, 54, *55, 56,*
    109, 111, 112, 113, 114, 115, 117,
    118, 119, 120, 122, *123*
Keller, M. B., 99, *105*
Keller, S., 262, *281*
Kellman, H., 226, *238*
Kelly, G. A., 150, *161*
Kemeny, M. E., 205, 208, *216, 217*
Kempen, M. H., 97, 99, *104*
Kendall, D., 62, 83, *85*
Kennard, M., 182, *200*
Kennington, M., 208, 211, *216*
Kerenyi, A. B., *201*
Kernberg, O., 222, *237*
Kerns, R. D., 157, 158, *162,* 168, *175,* 235,
    237, 246, *256,* 263, *278*

Ketcham, A. S., 207, *214*
Kewman, D. G., 48, *55*
Kidd, D. H., 114, *124*
Kiecolt-Glaser, J., 262, *280*
Kiernan, B. D., 156, 157, 158, *160*
Kilgore, R. B., 40, 47, *57*
Kinney, R., *22,* 50, *56,* 112, *124,* 203, *216,* 227, 233, 234, *238,* 242, *256,* 266, 267, 268, 270, 278, *280, 281*
Kinney, T. R., 138, 151, 152, *160*
Kinsler, B. L., 184, 193, *201*
Kirk, R. F., Jr., 193, *201*
Kirkland, F., 212, *215*
Kivlahan, D., 21, 53, *57, 124*
Kiyak, H. A., 207, *215*
Klar, H., 226, 227, *237, 238,* 261, *282*
Kleinke, C. L., 112, *123,* 246, *256*
Klerman, G. L., *19,* 99, *105*
Klimas, N., *84, 87*
Kloff, H., 43, 46, *58*
Knopf, O., 29, 30, *34*
Knowlton, G., 167, *175*
Knussen, C., 151, *160,* 210, *215*
Koch, R., 262, *280*
Kohn, P., 92, *104*
Kokan, P., 43, 46, *58*
Kolb, L. C., 29, 30, *34*
Kole-Snijders, A. M. J., 148, *164*
Kolitz, S., 73, *86*
Korff, M. V., 226, *238*
Kramer, M., 241, *256*
Kramer, S., 226, *238*
Krantz, D., 4, 8, *19, 20*
Krantz, D. S., 182, 196, 197, 198, *199*
Kreindler, M. L., 92, *107*
Kremer, E. F., 53, *54*
Krupp, N. E., 40, 41, 44, 45, *57*
Kulik, J. A., 208, *215*
Kummel, E., 114, *125*
Kunselman, A. R., 113, *124*
Kuperman, S. K., 48, *56*
Kvaal, S. A., 140, 142, 149, *163*

Labarca, R., 261, *281*
Labbe, E. E., 74, *86*
Lair, C. V., 44, *56*
Lancaster, N. P., 29, *34*
Lander, J., 93, *105*
Landon, T., 134, *160,* 168, *174*
Lane, R. D., *200*
Langelier, R., 235, *237*
LaPerriere, A., 73, *84, 86*

Large, R. G., 62, *86,* 150, 151, 154, *162,* 232, *237, 280*
Larsen, R. J., 97, *105*
Lauver, S. C., 97, *105*
Lavori, P., 99, *105*
Lawlis, G. F., 52, *57,* 118, *124*
Lawson, K. C., 140, 141, *162*
Layfield, M., 62, 83, *85*
Lazarus, A., 165, *174*
Lazarus, R., 130, 132, 133, 134, 145, *160, 162,* 261, *280*
Le Resche, L., 252, *255*
Leavitt, F., 44, 45, 49, 52, *55, 56, 104*
Lecci, L., 150, 151, 155, *161*
Lefcourt, H., 165, *174*
Lefebvre, J. C., 111, *123*
Lefebvre, R., 207, *216*
Lehman, C., 262, *280*
Lehman, R. A., *56*
Lehman-Susman, V., 226, *238*
Leon, B., 92, *105*
Lereim, I., 62, 83, *85*
LeResche, L., 226, *238*
Lester, D., 206, *214*
Levander, S., 188, *201*
Levenson, H., 165, 167, *174*
Leventhal, H., 132, 147, 150, *162*
Levine, F. M., 188, *201*
Levine, R., 67, *86*
Lillo, E., *22,* 112, *124,* 203, *216,* 227, 233, 234, *238,* 242, *256,* 266, *281*
Lin, E., 99, *106*
Lindström, K., 96, *106*
Links, P., 222, *238*
Linnoila, M., 96, *106,* 261, *281*
Linssen, A., 148, 158, *163,* 167, 168, *175*
Linton, S. J., 18, *21,* 268, 269, *280, 281*
Lipchik, G., 169, 171, 172, *175*
Lipman, R. L., 270, *279*
Lipman, R. S., 248, *255*
Lipsitt, D. R., 68, *86*
Lipton, J. A., 92, *105,* 169, *175*
Lipton, R. B., 226, *238*
Liu, E., 261, *281*
Livengood, J., 259, 266, *281*
Livesley, W. J., 274, *279, 281*
Locke, B. Z., 241, *256*
Loevinger, J., 62, 70, *86*
Long, A., 152, *160*
Long, B. C., 210, *215*
Long, C. J., *56*
Long, D. M., 97, 98, *103*

Lopez, S., 170, *175*
Loranger, A., 226, *238,* 244, *256*
Lorenz, V., 96, *106*
Lorig, K., *162*
Losonczy, M. P., 226, 227, *238*
Lott, J. S., *88*
Louks, J., 41, 42, 43, 51, *55, 56*
Love, A., 15, *21,* 42, 44, *56,* 109, 113, 120, *124,* 196, *201,* 209, *216,* 277, *281*
Low, W. Y., 193, *201*
Lowry, F. H., 68, *86*
Lubin, B., 83, 84, 102, *106*
Lucente, F. E., 68, *87*
Lumley, M. A., *124*
Luoma, J., 168, *174*
Lushene, R. E., 132, *163*
Lutgendorf, S., 73, *84, 87, 88, 104*
Lynch, M. E., 93, *105*
Lynn, R., 183, 184, 187, *201*

Maes, S., 132, *162*
Magni, G., 111, *124*
Magovern, G., 207, *216*
Mahler, H. I., 208, *215*
Maides, S. A., 166, *176*
Main, C. J., 7, 8, 9, *21, 22,* 109, *124,* 173, *175*
Maiuro, R., 134, *164*
Malinchoc, M., 205, 206, *214, 216*
Malkasian, D., 9, *21*
Mann, J. D., 167, 168, 170, 172, *175, 176*
Manne, S. L., 134, *162,* 207, 210, *217*
Marbach, J. J., 92, *105,* 169, *175*
Marchcutti, M., 111, *124*
Marchese, M., 234, 235, *238*
Marcussen, R. M., 29, *34*
Margolis, R., 13, *20,* 51, 52, *55, 57*
Marks, D. F., *163*
Marshall, R. D., 100, *104*
Martelli, M., 90, *105*
Martignoni, M., 82, *85*
Martin, J. E., 188, *201*
Martin, M. Y., 151, *162*
Martin, N. J., 167, *175*
Martin, R., 263, *279*
Martinez, S., 141, *161, 256*
Marvish, 82
Maruta, T., 113, *124*
Masson, A. H. B., *201*
Massoth, D., 151, *164*
Matthews, K., 207, *216*
Maurer, G., 226, *237*

Mausner, J., 226, *238*
Mayer, T. G., 9, *20, 21, 22,* 48, 49, *54, 55,* 74, 75, 76, *85,* 112, *124,* 203, *216,* 227, 233, 234, *238,* 242, 248, 250, 251, *255, 256,* 259, 266, 270, 271, *280, 281*
McCall, R., 193, *200*
McCallum, S., 111, *124*
McClallen, J. M., 235, *237*
McCoy, C. E., 52, *57,* 118, *124*
McCrae, R. R., 94, 95, 96, 98, 100, *103, 105,* 184, *199,* 236, *237,* 245, *255,* 279
McCreary, C., 6, 13, *21,* 44, 45, 51, *57*
McCulloch, B. J., 135, *164*
McCulloch, J., 114, *125*
McDaniel, L. K., 209, *214*
McDougall, C. E. A., 184, 187, 188, *200*
McEwen, B., 262, *280*
McEwen, J., 245, *255,* 274, *279*
McFadden, S. H., 154, *162*
McFall, M. E., *124*
McFall, R., 264, *281*
McGill, J. C., 52, *57,* 118, *124*
McGrath, P. A., 89, 97, *104, 106*
McGrath, R. E., 120, 121, *124*
McHugh, P. R., 112, *125*
McKinley, J., 37, *57,* 109, *123,* 205, *215,* 226, *237, 280*
McMillan, S. C., 92, *105*
McRae, C., 134, *162*
Meagher, R., 14, 20, 68, *85, 87,* 184, 192, *201,* 232, 236, *237, 238* 242, 249, *255, 256,* 266, 270, *279, 281*
Mears, F., *20*
Mechanic, D., 68, *87*
Meehl, P., 63, *87,* 262, *281*
Meichenbaum, D., 165, *176*
Meilman, P. W., *56, 123*
Mei-Tal, V., 67, *87*
Melamed, B., 211, 212, *214, 217*
Mellin, G., 168, *174*
Melzack, R., 3, 4, 5, *21,* 42, *57,* 89, *106,* 109, 112, *125,* 188, 190, *201, 202,* 252, *257,* 263, 267, *281*
Mendola, R., *217*
Menefee, L. S., 152, *161*
Meniah, J. C., 29, *33*
Menninger, K. A., 29, *34*
Merskey, H., 31, 32, *34,* 49, *57,* 181, 192, 193, *201, 202*

Messick, S., 67, *86*
Meyerowitz, S., 67, *87*
Meyers, R., 197, *200*
Mezzich, J., 260, *279*
Mikail, R., 111, 112, *125*
Mikhail, S. F., 197, *200*
Milhous, R., 235, *237*
Millard, R. W., 184, 193, *201*
Miller, D., 203, *215*
Miller, H. R., 245, *257*
Miller, T. R., 99, 100, 101, *106*
Milles, K., 169, 171, 172, *175*
Millon, C., 61, 62, 77, 79, 80, *85, 87*
Millon, T., 47, *57,* 61, 62, 67, 68, 77, 78, 79, 80, 82, 84, *85, 86, 87,* 184, 192, *201,* 236, *238,* 241, 245, 249, *256,* 270, *281*
Mitchell, D., *256*
Mitchell, R. I., 269, *281*
Modedsti, L. M., 47, *55*
Modic, M. T., 9, *21*
Moffat, F. L., 207, *214*
Mohs, R., 226, 227, *237, 238,* 261, *282*
Monroe, S., 261, 262, 264, 265, *281, 282*
Monti, D., 234, 235, *238*
Mooney, V., 52, *57,* 118, *124*
Moore, J., *21,* 53, 54, *57,* 111, *124*
Moore, M., *35*
Morasso, G., 192, *201*
Moreschi, C., 111, *124*
Morey, L., 245, *256,* 274, *279*
Morgan, W. P., 171, *174*
Morris, D. B., 129, *162*
Morris, E. W., 9, *22*
Morris, R., 252, *257*
Morris, T., 205, *215*
Morrow, K., 134, *160,* 168, *174*
Moseley, T., 167, *175*
Mosley, T. H., 129, *161*
Moss, E., 68, *87*
Moyer, A., 207, *214*
Muir, M., 181, *200*
Muller-Myhsok, B., 261, *279*
Mullins, L., 262, *281*
Mumford, J. M., *106*
Munaij, J., 72, 73, *85*
Murphy, J. K., 74, 76, *87*
Murphy, R. W., *22, 57*
Muscettola, G., 261, *278*
Muten, E., 99, *106*
Myers, C. D., 140, 142, 149, *163,* 169, *175*
Myers, I. B., 183, *201*

Myers, J. K., 241, *256*

Naber, D., 62, *87*
Nachemson, A. L., 50, *55,* 267, *278*
Nagelberg, D. B., 96, *106*
Naliboff, B. D., 51, *57,* 111, *124*
Naring, G., 210, *217*
Nathan, P. W., 5, *21*
Nation, P. C., 120, *123*
Neelon, F. A., 53, *55*
Nelson, D. V., 208, 211, *216*
Nelson, E. S., 207, *216*
Nemiah, J., 29, *34*
Nestadt, M. D., 112, *125*
Newman, B., 261, *281*
Newman, M. C., 47, *56*
Newman, S. P., *162*
Nicassio, P., 130, 143, 151, *160, 162, 175,* 212, *214*
Nichols, D. C., 188, *201*
Niven, C. A., 151, *160,* 210, *215*
Noll, S., 138, 152, *160*
Norem, J. K., 206, *216*
Noriega, V., 145, *160,* 207, *214*
Norman, S., *124*
Norman, W. T., 94, *106*
Norris, M. P., 143, *163*
North, R. B., 114, *124*
Norton, G. R., 246, *254*
Novy, D. M., 208, 211, *216*
Nunley, J., 141, *161, 256*
Nygren, A., 151, *161*

O'Banion, D., 265, *281*
O'Brien, J. P., 48, *58*
O'Brien, S., 111, *124*
Obuchowski, N., 9, *21*
O'Connell, J. K., 171, *175*
O'Connor, P. J., 196, *202*
Odbert, H. S., *102*
Oehlmann, R., 261, *279*
Offord, K., 205, 206, *214, 216*
Ogden, W., 141, *161*
O'Hara, J. P., 208, *215*
O'Hearn, P., 73, *86*
O'Kelley, L. E., 32, *34*
Okifuji, A., 235, *239,* 246, 249, 252, *257*
Oldham, J., 226, *238,* 244, *256*
Olson, K. A., 114, *122*
O'Malley, W. B., 120, 121, *124*
O'Reilly, C. A., 158, *159*
Ormel, J., 97, 99, *104*

Orvaschel, D. A., 242, *257*
Osborne, D., *57*
Owens, J., 207, *216*
Owen-Salters, E., 15, 16, *22, 257,* 276, 277, *282*

Pace, T., 262, *281*
Pancoast, D. L., *124*
Panush, R. S., 211, *211, 214*
Paolo, A. M., *202*
Parbrook, G. D., 188, *200*
Paris, J., 263, 264, 266, *281*
Pariser, R. F., 76, *87*
Parker, G., 96, *103*
Parker, J., *21,* 53, *54, 57,* 134, 152, *162*
Parker, J. D. A., 132, 135, 136, 137, *160*
Parkes, C. M., 29, *34*
Parkes, M., 68, *87*
Partridge, K. B., 68, *85*
Pascual, E., 170, *175*
Pastor, M., 170, *175*
Paul, S., 261, *281*
Paull, A., 67, *87*
Pawl, R. P., 75, 76, *88*
Peabody, D., 94, *106*
Pearson, I. B., 182, 190, 192, 193, *199*
Pearson, J. S., *57*
Peck, C., 15, *21,* 42, 44, *56,* 109, 113, 120, *124,* 196, *201,* 209, *216,* 277, *281*
Peck, J. R., 211, *216*
Pemberton, J., 14, *20*
Penedo, F., 73, *88*
Penzien, D., 129, *161,* 167, *175*
Pepitone-Arreola-Rockwell, F., *57*
Peterson, C., 208, *216*
Peterson, P. J., 82, *88,* 193, *202*
Petrie, A., *201*
Petrie, K., 207, *214*
Petrovich, D. V., 193, *201*
Pettingale, K. W., 205, *215*
Pfohl, B., 226, 227, 233, *238,* 244, *256*
Pheasant, H. C., 46, *56*
Philips, C., 196, *201*
Philips, H. C., 96, *106,* 196, *201*
Phillips, G., 151, *160, 163*
Pickar, D., 261, *281*
Pietri-Taleb, F., 96, *106*
Pilkonis, A., 260, *279*
Pilowsky, I., 8, *21, 125,* 181, 196, *199*
Pincus, T., 7, *21,* 110, 111, *124, 175*
Pinkham, L., 227, *238,* 261, *282*
Piotrowski, C., 83, 84, 102, *106*

Platt, M., 120, *123*
Polatin, P. B., 9, 14, *20, 22, 56,* 112, *124,* 203, *216,* 227, 233, 234, *238,* 242, 251, *256,* 259, 266, 267, 268, 278, *280, 280, 281*
Poloni, L. D., *56, 123*
Polsby, M., 62, *87*
Ponticas, Y., 100, *104*
Pope, M., 9, *22*
Poser, E., *201*
Pozo, C., 145, *160,* 207, *214*
Pransky, G., 207, *215*
Price, D. D., 89, 90, 92, 93, 97, 98, 99, *103, 105, 106, 107,* 184, *202*
Price, J. H., 171, *175*
Prieto, E. J., 51, *55*
Procacci, P., 92, *106*
Prochaska, J. O., 157, *162*
Prokop, C. K., 13, *20,* 51, 52, *55, 57,* 111, *124*

Queen, K. T., 141, *161*

Rabkin, J. G., *87*
Radojevic, V., 151, *162*
Rae, D. S., 241, *256*
Raezer, L. B., 138, 152, *160*
Rafii, A., 89, 90, 98, 99, *106, 107,* 184, *202*
Ragsdale, N., 262, *280*
Rahe, R. H., 67, *86, 88*
Rainville, P., 90, *106*
Ramamurthy, S., 53, *55,* 118, 119, *123,* 206, 209, *214*
Rankin-Hill, L., 169, 171, *174*
Raugh, V., 235, *237*
Reddon, J. R., 110, *123*
Reed, G. M., 205, *216*
Reed, M. L., 226, *238*
Reesor, S., 111, 112, *125*
Regan, C. A., *162*
Regan, J. J., 242, *256*
Regier, D. A., 242, *257*
Reich, J., 112, *124,* 227, 229, 232, *238,* 250, *256,* 259, 266, *281*
Reider, E., *54*
Reiger, D. A., 241, *256*
Reik, T., 28, *34*
Reinhardt, L., 48, *57*
Ressor, K. A., 140, 141, *162*
Reuter, E. K., 96, *106*
Revenson, T. A., 134, *162,* 210, *214*
Reynolds, R. V., 150, *163*

Reynolds, S., 274, *279*
Rice, J. R., 211, *214*
Richardson, M. W., *86*
Richman, L. C., 74, *86*
Riihimaki, H., 96, *106*
Riley, J. L., 113, 118, 119, 120, *124,* 139, 140, 141, 142, 149, *162, 163,* 169, *175*
Rinaldi, P., 227, *238*
Rissler, A., 184, 187, *201*
Roberts, A. H., 48, *57*
Roberts, J., 151, *164*
Robertson, C., *256*
Robertson, J. T., 193, *201*
Robillard, E., 92, *107*
Robins, L. N., 241, *256,* 242, *257*
Robinson, D. S., 207, *214*
Robinson, H., 193, *201*
Robinson, M. E., 113, 118, 119, 120, *124,* 139, 140, 141, 142, 149, *162, 163,* 169, *175,* 212, *217*
Robinson, R., 251, *256,* 271, *280*
Rocchio, P. D., *22,* 46, *58*
Rodger, T. F., 28, 29, *33, 35*
Rodin, J., 208, *215,* 262, *280*
Rodriguez, J., 170, *175*
Rodriguez, R., *217*
Roland, M., 252, *257*
Roll, M., 97, *106*
Romano, J. M., 8, *22,* 129, 133, 141, 146, 147, 148, 149, 152, 157, 158, *161,* 203, *215*
Romanoski, A. J., 112, *125*
Rome, H. P., 29, *34*
Romm, S., 84, *88*
Rose, R. M., *19*
Rosen, A., 63, *87*
Rosen, J. C., 44, *57*
Rosenberg, R., 157, 158, *162,* 261, *281*
Rosenblatt, R., 222, 232, *238,* 250, *256*
Rosenman, R. H., 66, *85*
Rosenstiel, A. K., 106, 138, 140, 141, *163,* 210, 211, *216*
Rosenthal, D., 262, *281*
Rosnick, L., 226, *238*
Rosomoff, H., 14, *20,* 74, *86,* 170, 171, *174,* 232, *237,* 242, *255,* 266, *279*
Rosomoff, R. S., 170, 171, *174*
Ross, J. S., 9, *21*
Ross, S., 264, *280*
Rothberg, S. T., *103*
Rotter, J. B., 147, *163,* 165, 171, *175,* 204, *216*

Roy, A., 96, *106,* 261, *281*
Roy-Byrne, P., 260, *279*
Rozensky, R. H., 76, *88*
Rubino, I. A., 82, *85*
Rudd, M., 262, *280*
Rudy, T., *22, 107, 125,* 129, *161, 163,* 168, *175,* 203, 210, *217,* 235, *237, 239,* 246, 249, *256, 257,* 270, *282*
Ruehlman, L. S., 150, *161*
Russakoff, M., 226, *238,* 244, *256*
Russo, J., 99, *106,* 134, *164*
Ruth, J. E., 151, *163*
Ryan, D., 184, *202*

Sacuzzo, D. P., 53, *54*
Sadigh, M. R., 62, *88*
Sadler, I. J., 140, 142, 149, *163*
Salas, E., 170, *175*
Salovey, P., 8, *22,* 241, *257,* 263, *282*
Samuels, J. F., 112, *125*
Sanchez, S., 170, *175*
Sanders, S. H., 111, 113, *125*
Sanderson, C., 245, *257*
Sandler, I. N., *164*
Sangster, J. I., 210, *215*
Sarason, I. G., 67, *88*
Saul, L. J., 29, *34*
Savage, O. A., 29, *33*
Scarborough, W., 170, *175*
Schachat, R., 92, *107*
Schalling, D., 184, 187, 188, *201*
Scheier, M., 144, *160,* 204, 206, 207, 208, 210, *214, 216*
Schilder, P., 29, 30, *34*
Schleifer, S., 262, *281*
Schmale, A. H., 67, *88*
Schmidt, C. W., 100, *104*
Schmidt, J. P., 119, 120, *125*
Schmidt, N., 262, *280*
Schmidt, R. F., 5, *22*
Schneider, S. C., *217*
Schneiderman, N., 73, *84, 87, 88*
Schoenfeld, L. S., 53, *55,* 118, 119, *123,* 206, 209, *214*
Schoenfeld-Smith, K., 151, *162*
Schroeder, M. L., 274, *281*
Schroll, M., *21,* 45, 50, *56*
Schuerman, J. A., 148, *164*
Schulman, P., 205, *214*
Schultz, W. H., *160*
Schuman, C., 151, *162*
Schwartz, G. E., *200*

Schwartz, J. E., 98, *104*
Schwartz, M. S., 40, 41, 44, 45, *57*
Schwartzman, R., 234, 235, *238*
Schwarzer, C., 132, *163*
Schwarzer, R., 132, *163,* 204, 205, 208, *216*
Schwebel, A. I., 150, *160*
Scott, D. W., 120, *123,* 129
Scott, W. C. M., *35*
Segerstrom, S. C., 208, *216*
Seidenberg, R., *35*
Selby, D., 52, *57,* 118, *124*
Seligman, M. E. P., 146, *159, 163,* 170,
    171, *174, 175,* 204, 205, 206, 208,
    213, *214, 215, 216*
Selinsky, H., *35*
Selye, H., 262, *282*
Seville, J. L., 167, 168, 170, 172, *175, 176*
Shagass, C., *201*
Shanely, L. A., 80, *85*
Shapiro, A. P., 140, 141, *163*
Shatin, D., 114, *122*
Shea, T., 274, *282*
Sheets, V. L., *164*
Sherbourne, C. D., 251, *257,* 270, *282*
Sherman, E. D., 92, *107*
Sherman, R. A., 209, *216*
Shores, M., 260, *279*
Shutty, M. S., 134, 140, 142, 157, *160, 163,*
    164, 168, *174*
Siegal, J. M., 67, *88*
Siegelaub, A. B., 92, *107*
Siever, L., 222, 226, 227, *237, 238,* 261,
    282
Sifneos, P. E., *35*
Silk, S. D., *54*
Silverman, J. M., 226, 227, *237,* 261, *282*
Silverman, J. P., 222, 226, 227, *238*
Simmel, M. L., 29, *35*
Simmons, A., 261, 262, 264, 265, *281, 282*
Simon, G., 99, *106*
Simon, T., 72, 73, *85*
Simoneau, J., *86*
Simons, L. E., 120, *123*
Sivik, T. M., 62, *88*
Skevington, S., 171, *175*
Skodol, A., 226, *238*
Skultety, F. M., *56*
Skultety, M., *123*
Slaughter, C., 28, *33*
Slipman, C., 167, *175*
Smarr, K., 134, 152, *162*
Smith, A. G., 113, *124*

Smith, C. A., 143, 144, 145, 149, 151, 152,
    163, 210, 211, *216*
Smith, D., *55*
Smith, G. M., 94, *107*
Smith, J. E., *103,* 250, *255*
Smith, T. W., *107,* 211, *216*
Snibbe, J. R., 82, *88,* 193, *202*
Snow-Turek, A. L., 143, *163*
Snyder, D. K., 37, 40, 46, *57*
Solomon, P., *201*
Sora, I., 261, *282*
Sorbom, D., *105, 161*
Sorkin, B. A., 92, *107*
Sosner, B., 82, *88,* 193, *202*
Spangler, D., 262, *282*
Spanswick, C. C., 7, 8, *21,* 109, *124*
Spaulding, W., 262, *282*
Spear, F. G., 25, *34, 35,* 181, 192, *201*
Spengler, D. M., 20, *50, 55,* 122, *122,* 267,
    278
Sperling, M., 29, *35*
Sperr, E. V., *87*
Sperr, S. J., *87*
Spielberger, C. D., 132, *163*
Spinhoven, P., 148, 158, *163,* 167, 168, *175*
Spitzer, R., 12, *22,* 78, *88,* 226, 227, 233,
    238, 242, 244, *257,* 277, *282*
Squitieri, P., 208, 211, *216*
Stangl, D., 226, 227, 233, *238,* 244, *256*
Starr, K., 73, *87, 104*
Stavraky, K. M., *88*
Steckley, L. C., 32, *34*
Steel, D. F., 188, *200*
Steele, R., 14, *20,* 242, *255,* 266, *279*
Steele-Rosomoff, R., 74, *86*
Steiger, H. G., 249, *255*
Stein, M., 262, *281*
Stengel, E., 26, 28, 29, *34*
Sternbach, R. A., 6, 7, *22,* 43, 45, 49, 51,
    57, 92, *107,* 120, *125,* 188, 197, *202*
Stewart, W. F., 226, *238*
Stieg, R. L., *107*
Stiles, T. C., 62, 83, *85*
Stone, M., 182, 183, *202*
Stone, R. K., Jr., *57*
Strachan, A., 262, *280*
Strack, S., 151, *163*
Streiner, D. L., 245, *257*
Streuning, E. L., 68, *87*
Strom, S. E., 130, 156, *161*
Strong, J., 150, 151, 154, *162*
Stroud, M. W., 129, 133, 142, 147, 148,
    159

Stucky-Ropp, R. C., 152, *162*
Sullivan, F., 181, *200*
Sullivan, M. J. L., 111, 112, *125,* 142, 151, *163*
Sullivan, T., 242, *255*
Summerfeldt, L. J., 132, 135, 137, *160*
Susman, V. L., 244, *256*
Sutton, C., 193, *201*
Swartzman, L. C., 140, 141, *163*
Sweeney, M., 120, 121, *124*
Sweet, J. J., 75, 76, *88*
Swenson, W. M., *57*
Szaz, T. S., 29, 30, 31, *35*

Taenzer, P., 188, 190, *202*
Taft, K., 208, *215*
Tait, R., 169, *175*
Takemoto-Chock, N. K., 94, 95, *104*
Talton, S. L., 211, *214*
Tan, G., 143, *163*
Tan, S.-Y., *202*
Tatsuoka, M. M., 98, *103*
Taylor, G. J., 184, *202*
Taylor, S. E., 205, 208, 209, *215, 216, 217*
Teasdale, J., 146, *159,* 170, *174,* 204, *213*
Teasell, R. W., 140, 141, *163*
Tellegen, A., *55,* 114, 115, 121, *123,* 183, *199,* 271, *282*
Tennen, H., *102,* 141, 145, *159,* 205, 207, 211, *214, 215, 217*
ter Kuile, M. M., 148, 158, *163,* 167, 168, *175*
Thase, M., 262, *282*
Theorell, T., 97, *106*
Thomas, S. F., *163*
Thompson, D., 229, *238,* 259, *281*
Thompson, R. J., 138, 151, 152, *160, 163*
Thompson-Pope, S., 170, *175*
Thoresen, C. E., *162*
Thorn, B. E., 129, 133, 142, 147, 148, 150, 152, 158, *159, 160, 161*
Thornton, J., 262, *281*
Thurstone, L. L., 94, *107*
Tobin, D. L., 150, *163*
Togerson, W. S., 97, 98, *103*
Tomlinson-Keasey, C., 98, *104*
Toomey, T. C., 167, 168, 170, 172, *175, 176*
Tosi, D. J., 74, 76, *87*
Tota-Faucette, M., 138, 152, *160*
Tovian, S. M., 76, *88*
Towne, W. S., 42, 43, *57*

Townsend, J., 264, *281*
Toye, R., 75, 76, *88*
Trapp, E. P., 44, *56*
Trethowan, W. H., *35*
Trexler, L., 206, *214*
Triana-Alexander, M., 151, *162*
Trimboli, F., 40, 47, *57*
Trowbridge, L. S., 29, *35*
Trull, T. J., 228, 229, *239,* 244, *257*
Tsushima, W. T., 42, 43, *57*
Tucker, J. S., 98, *104*
Tunks, E., *19, 33,* 151, *164*
Tupes, E. C., 94, *107*
Tupin, J., 112, *124,* 222, 232, *238,* 250, *256, 259, 281*
Turk, D. C., 5, 7, *22, 58, 107,* 109, 112, *125,* 129, *163,* 165, 168, *175, 176,* 182, *202,* 203, 208, 209, 210, 212, *214, 217,* 235, *237, 239,* 241, 245, 246, 249, 252, *256, 257,* 263, 270, *279, 282*
Turner, J., 6, 8, 13, *21, 22, 56, 57,* 83, *88,* 129, 130, 133, 134, 140, 141, 146, 147, 148, 149, 151, 152, 156, 157, 158, *161, 162, 163, 164,* 165, 166, *176,* 203, 210, *215, 217*
Tursky, B., 92, *107,* 188, *201*
Tuttle, D. H., 140, 142, 157, *163, 164*
Tyrer, P., *257*

Uhl, G. R., 261, *282*
Ulrich, R., 32, *35,* 260, *279*
Umlauf, R. L., 166, *176*
Underwood-Gordon, L., 130, *161*
Uomoto, J. M., 83, *88*
Urrows, S., *102,* 141, *159, 217*
Ury, G., *21*

Vakkari, T., *174*
Van de Putte, L., 210, *217*
Van Denburg, E., 80, *85*
Van der Heide, L. H., 51, *55*
Van der Staak, C., 210, *217*
van Eck, H., 148, *164*
van Houwelingen, H. C., 148, 158, *163*
Van Lankveld, W., 210, *217*
Vando, A., *202*
Van't Pad Bosch, P., 210, *217*
Vaughn, W. K., 7, *21,* 110, 111, *124*
Venner, R. M., 114, *125*
Vikar-Juntura, E., 96, *106*
Viken, R., 264, *281*

Villela, J., 222, *238*
Visscher, B. R., 205, *216*
Vitaliano, P. P., *164,* 207, *215*
Vittengl, J., 15, 16, *22,* 257, 276, 277, *282*
Vlaeyen, J. W. S., 148, *164*
Volkart, E. H., *87*
Von Korff, Sc. D., 99, *106*
VonBaeyer, C., 47, *56*
Vorhies, L., 274, *279*

Waddell, G., 9, *22,* 114, *125,* 173, *175*
Wade, J. B., 89, 90, 93, 97, 98, 99, *107,*
    184, *202*
Walker, E., 99, *106,* 262, *282*
Walker, S., 134, *162*
Wall, P., 3, 4, 5, *21, 22,* 42, *57,* 109, *125*
Wallace, R. W., 119, 120, *125*
Wallbrown, F. H., 96, *106*
Wallbrown, J. D., 96, *106*
Waller, N. G., 134, *164,* 271, 275, *278, 282*
Wallson, K., 97, *105*
Wallston, B. S., 134, *164*
Wallston, K. A., 134, 141, 143, 152, *160,*
    161, 163, 164, 166, *175, 176,* 210,
    211, *215, 216*
Wallston, R. F., 166, *176*
Wang, H. Y. J., 205, *216*
Wang, Z., 261, *282*
Ward, J. R., 211, *216*
Ware, J. E., 251, *257,* 270, *282*
Ware, S. L., 96, *106*
Waring, E. M., 13, *22*
Warne, P., 261, *282*
Waters, W. E., 196, *202*
Watkins, R. G., 48, *58*
Watson, D., *58,* 111, *125,* 274, *279, 282*
Weinberg, N., *85,* 250, *255*
Weinberger, D. R., 62, *87*
Weiner, P., 47, 48, *56*
Weintraub, J. K., 144, *160,* 204, 207, *214,*
    216
Weir, R., 151, *164*
Weisberg, J., 222, 227, *239*
Weisberg, J. N., 11, 15, 16, *22,* 112, 113,
    120, *125,* 229, 233, 235, *239,* 243,
    257, 259, 264, 266, 277, 278, *282*
Weisenberg, M., 92, *107*
Weisman, A., 206 *214,* 223, 229, 233, 235,
    239
Weiss, E., *35*
Weissman, M. M., 242, *257*
Weisz, G. M., 13, *22*

Welsh, G. S., 42, *55*
Werboff, J., 92, *107*
Westerholm, P., 151, *161*
Westphal, W., 92, *104*
Whiskin, F., 29, *35*
Whitney, C., 151, *164*
Widiger, T. A., 228, 229, *239,* 244, 245,
    255, 257, 274, *282*
Wiens, A. N., 158, *159*
Wigal, J. K., 150, *163*
Wilcoxson, M. A., 75, 76, *88*
Wilfling, F. J., 43, 46, *58*
Wilkie, D. J., 151, *164*
Williams, C. L., 39, 40, 41, *55,* 115, 122,
    123
Williams, D. A., 142, 148, 151, 152, 158,
    160, 161, 181, *200, 202, 256*
Williams, J. B., 12, *22,* 78, *88,* 226, 233,
    238, 242, *257,* 277, *282*
Williams, P. G., *107*
Williamson, D., 212, *217*
Wilson, A. T. M., 29, *35*
Wilson, B. J., 114, *122*
Wilson, J. J., *160*
Wilson, L., 151, *164*
Wiltse, L. L., *22,* 46, *58*
Wimberly, R. L., 114, *124*
Wineman, N. M., 135, *164*
Wingard, D. L., 98, *104*
Wise, C. M., 209, *214*
Wise, E. A., 169, *175*
Wise, T. N., 100, *104*
Wittkower, E., 29, *33, 35*
Wittmer, V. T., 113, 118, 119, 120, *124*
Wolf, S. R., *22, 57*
Wolfe, F., 7, *21*
Wolfe, R., 110, 111, *124*
Wolff, H. G., 29, *34*
Wolkowitz, O., 261, *281*
Wong, M., 152, *160*
Wonklin, J. M., *88*
Woodforde, J. M., 193, *202*
Woodrow, K. M., 92, *107*
Wortley, M. D., 50, *55,* 267, *278*
Wortman, C. B., 205, *214*
Wright, B. A., 67, *88*
Wright, G. E., 152, *162*
Wright, H. P., 29, *35*
Wszolek, Z., 261, *279*

Yellen, A. N., 51, *57,* 111, *124*
Young, L. D., 209, *214*

Young, S. E., 99, *103*
Yunik, S., 67, *88*

Zaki, H. S., 235, *239*
Zanna, V., 82, *85*
Zarski, J. J., 75, 76, *88*
Zatzick, D. F., 92, *107*
Zautra, A. J., 134, *162, 164,* 207, 210, *217*
Zborowski, M., 169, *176*

Zhou, A., *200*
Ziegler, D. K., *202*
Ziesat, H. A., Jr., 193, *202*
Zimmerman, M., 226, 227, 233, *238,* 242, 243, 244, *256, 257*
Zinbarg, R. E., *174*
Zonderman, A. B., 96, *103*
Zook, A., 75, 76, *88*
Zuckerman, M., 260, *282*

SUBJECT INDEX

Acupuncture, 3
Acute postoperative pain
  and personality, 188, 189t, 190
Adaptive coping profile, 129
Adjustment
  coping research in, 146–148
  Coping Strategies Questionnaire and,
    141–142
  optimism and, 211
Age
  pain processing and, 92, 93
  research in, 150, 151
Aggression
  chronic pain and, 32
  pain defense against, 28, 29
Agreeableness
  in five-factor model of normal personal-
    ity, 94
  treatment outcome and, 101
Alexithymia
  definition of, 4
  Minnesota Multiphasic Personality
    Inventory-2 correlated with, 112
Allergic inclination scale, on Millon Behav-
    ioral Health Inventory, 68
Anxiety
  in pain processing, 98
  Somatic Anxiety Scale and, 68
Anxious cluster, of personality disorders,
    232, 292
Aristotle, 25, 261
Arthritis, optimism and, 210–211
Artificial complexes, 30
Asymbolia, and phantom limb pain, 28–29
Attributional Style Questionnaire, in opti-
    mism measurement, 206

Beck Depression Inventory-II (BDI-II)
  in assessment of chronic pain patient, 269
  description of, 247, 252
Behavioral characteristics, Minnesota Multi-
    phasic Personality Inventory-2
    assessment of, 113
Behavioral medicine evaluation, vs. psycho-
    logical evaluation, 16–18, 267–268
Belief
  locus of control and, 165–166

Beliefs
  health-related
    Multidimensional Health Locus of
      Control measurement of, 166–167
  measurement of, 156–157
  moderator variables and, 157–158
  vs. coping strategies in adjustment, 157
Big-Five Factor model of personality
  assessment instruments for, 94–95
  critics of, 94
  factors in, 94
  treatment implications of, 99–101
Biomedical reductionism, 3
Biopsychosocial, to personality disorders, 4,
    5
Biopsychosocial model of illness, 42, 262
Body image, phantom pain and, 29
Borderline personality disorder, 233
Breast cancer, Millon Behavioral Health In-
    ventory assessment of personality—
    coping styles and, 73

Cancer pain
  neuroticism and, 192–193, 194t–195t
  pain and personality factors in, 190, 191t,
    192
Cardiovascular tendency scale, on Millon
    Behavioral Health Inventory, 69
Caregiver, dispositional optimism in, 211–
    212
Catastrophizing
  adjustment and, 146
  Coping Strategies Questionnaire and, 141,
    142
  neuroticism and, 97
  outcome with cognitive-behavioral treat-
    ment, 147–148
  pain and, 212
  in research studies, 153, 155
Chance, as locus of control, 166
CHIP. See Coping with Health Injuries and
    Problems (CHIP) scale
Chronic pain
  behavioral-psychological problems in, 8
  development of
    course of, 7–11
    four-stage model of, 49–50

Chronic pain (*continued*)
  Minnesota Multiphasic Personality In-
    ventory and, 48–50
  prospective prediction of, 11–12
  three-stage progression in, 50
  and personality, 190, 191t, 192–193,
    194t–195t
  personality disorders in
    diathesis-stress model of, 259–262
    prevalence of, 235, 242
  personality factors and, 243–244
    Minnesota Multiphasic Personality In-
      ventory and, 49
  physiologic basis of, 8–9
  prediction of, 11–12
  premorbid, assessment of, 266
  prevention of
    personality disorder screening in, 14–
      18, 18
  sick role in, 8
  as stressor, 262–263
  three-stage model of, 7–8
Chronic pain assessment
  goals of, 109
  Minnesota Multiphasic Personality
    Inventory-2 in
    utility of, 111–114
  Minnesota Multiphasic Personality Inven-
    tory or Minnesota Multiphasic Per-
    sonality Inventory-2 in
    criticisms of, 109–111
    support of, 110–111
Chronic Pain Coping Inventory (CPCI),
    149–150
Chronic pain disability
  prevention of, 268–269
  psychosocial factor in, 9
Chronic pain patient, assessment tools for,
    269–276
Chronic Tension Scale, in Millon Behav-
    ioral Health Inventory, 66
CISS. *See* Coping Inventory for Stressful
    Situations (CISS)
Cluster analysis
  of Minnesota Multiphasic Personality In-
    ventory profiles, 52–53, 118–119
Code types
  Minnesota Multiphasic Personality Inven-
    tory, 117–118
  in Minnesota Multiphasic Personality
    Inventory-2, 117–118, 121
Cognitive-behavioral therapy

coping with pain and, 130
format of, 130
Cognitive Coping Strategies Inventory
    (CCSI), 140
Cognitive Predictors of Pain Treatment Out-
    come, 158
Communication style, in Millon Behavioral
    Medicine Diagnostic, 77
Complaint behavior, introversion-
    extraversion and, 192
Complex regional pain syndrome (CRPS),
    93
Complex Regional Pain syndrome (CRPS)
    Type I
    SCID and SCID-II in, 234–235
Confident coping style, 64–65
Conscientiousness
  in five-factor model of normal personal-
    ity, 94
  health outcomes and, 99
  treatment outcome and, 101
Content scales, in Minnesota Multiphasic
    Personality Inventory-2, 116, 122
Conversion V patients, optimism in, 209
Conversion V profile, 40–41, 41f, 248
  functional *vs.* organic pain and, 44–45
Cooperative coping syle, 64
Coping
  meanings of, 129
  and personality disorders, 246
  process-oriented approach to, 131
Coping construct
  addressing problems with, 154–155
  assessment of beliefs and appraisals *vs.*,
    153
  causation studies, 155
  limitations of, 154
  and need for unique external criterion
    measures, 154
  and nontreatment seekers, 155
Coping Inventory for Stressful Situations
    (CISS), 136
Coping measure(s)
  beliefs and appraisals in, 156–157
  cognitive *vs.* behavioral, 156
  composite or individual, 132–133
  Coping Inventory for Stressful Situations,
    136
  Coping Strategies Questionnaire, 138–
    143
  Coping with Health Injuries and Prob-
    lems scale, 135–137

dispositional *vs.* situational, 132
future development and research in, 149–150, 155–156
Vanderbilt Multidimensional Pain Coping Inventory, 143–146
Ways of Coping Checklist, 133–135
Coping research
  in adjustment, 146–148
  clinician needs and, 155–156
  in laboratory model, 151–152
  longitudinal studies, new, 152
  in moderating factors, 150–151, 152
  in moderator variables, 152
  new designs, 151–153
  psychometric improvements in measures, 149–150
  reading of, 152–153
  recent trends in, 148–151
  recommendations for improving, 146
  relationship to adjustment measures, 146
Coping scales, Millon Behavioral Health Inventory
  confident, 64–65
  cooperative, 64
  forceful, 65
  inhibited, 64
  introversive, 63–64
  respectful, 65
  sensitive, 65–66
  sociable, 64
Coping skills, in personality disorder, 112
Coping Strategies Questionnaire (CSQ)
  and adjustment to chronic pain, 141–142
  behavioral coping strategy scales in, 138, 140
  cognitive subscales in, 138
  factor analyses of, 140–141
  factor loading, mean, and standard deviation in, 138, 139t
  limitations of, 142–143
Coping Strategies Questionnaire (CSQ), psychometric improvements in, 149
Coping strategy(ies)
  beliefs and adjustment and treatment response, 157
  dispositional optimism and, 210–211
  emotion-focused, 131, 132
  illness-focused, 132
  optimists' use of, 207–208
  problem-focused, 131, 132
  as research tools, 158
  use of and optimism, 212

Coping styles
  effect on treatment management and outcome
    Millon Behavioral Health Inventory and, 72
    Millon Behavioral Health Inventory-2 and, 112
  locus of control and, 168
  pain and, 210
Coping with Health Injuries and Problems (CHIP) scale
  description of, 135–136
  principal-components factor analysis of, 136, 137t
  relationships with Coping Inventory for Stressful Situations, 136
Coping with pain
  adjustment and, 146–148
  assessment measures for, 132–133
  cognitive–behavioral therapy in, 130
  coping theory and, 131–132
  developmental–motivational perspective on, 140
  external locus of control and, 170
  research literature on, 129–130
  strategies in, 131–132
Cost reduction, with prevention of chronic pain, 268–269
Couvade, 28
CPCI. *See* Chronic Pain Coping Inventory (CPCI)
CSQ. *See* Coping Strategies Questionnaire (CSQ)
Culture, in five-factor model of normal personality, 94

Deconditioning syndrome, 8
Dependent personality disorder, 232, 233
Depression. *See also* Major depression
  in chronic back pain, 111
  in chronic pain, 8
  in complex regional pain syndrome, 234
  learned helplessness and, 170
  in Minnesota Multiphasic Personality Inventory, 39
  in pain processing, 98
Depressive reaction, to pain, 51
Descartes, René, 3
Diagnostic and Statistical Manual, ed. 3 (DSM-III-R), 221–222
Diagnostic and Statistical Manual, ed. 4 (DSM-IV), 223, 224t–225t

Diathesis–stress model
  application to medical illness, 261–262
  in chronic pain, 15, 235, 259–262
    study support of, 277–278
  clinical implications of, 265–266
  criticisms of, 264–265
  diathesis component of, 261, 265
  history of, 261–262
  stress component of, 261–262
Dispositional optimism
  in caregiver, 211–212
  coping strategies and, 210–211
  defined, 204
  measure of, 206
Dorsalles Functionalles (DOR) scale
  functional vs. organic pain, 42–43

Egyptian papyri, 3
Emotional stability vs. neuroticism, in five-
    factor model of normal personality,
    94
Emotional state, pain response and, 181–
    182
Emotional Vulnerability Scale, on Millon
    Behavioral Health Inventory, 69
Endometriosis, personality factors and pain
    in, 193, 195t
Epidemiology
  incidence in, 223
  of personality disorders, 223, 226
  prevalence in, 223, 226
Ethnicity, pain processing and, 92
Expectations and stress, 204
External locus of control, 165, 166
Extraversion
  chronic pain and, 190
  in five-factor model of normal personal-
    ity, 94
  pain sensation intensity and, 97
  postoperative pain and, 188, 189t, 190
  psychotherapy and, 100
  relationship with neuroticism, 98
  suffering and, 98
Extraversion-introversion
  covariates of and chronic pain, 197–198,
    198f
  Eysenck self-report inventories of, 183–
    184
  in Eysenck's personality theory, 182–183
Eysenck Personality Inventory (EPI), 183
  postoperative pain and, 188, 189t, 190
Eysenck Personality Questionnaire (EPQ),
    183

Factor analysis, in Minnesota Multiphasic
    Personality Inventory and Minnesota
    Multiphasic Personality Inventory-2,
    118, 119
Five Factor Inventory (FFI), 95
Five-factor trait-dimensional measures
    SNAP and, 274
Flamboyant cluster of personality disorders,
    232, 292
Forceful coping style, 65
Four-humor theory, 3
Four-stage model of pain, 49–50
Freud, Sigmund, 4
  and psychogenesis of pain, 26–27
  view about pain, 27–28
F Scale, in Minnesota Multiphasic Personal-
    ity Inventory, 38
Functional Efficacy Scale
  in Millon Behavioral Medicine Diagnostic
    health maintenance and health care
    delivery and, 79
Functional pain
  as continuum, 46
  Dorsalles Functionalles and, 42–43
  Low Back Scale and, 42, 43
  Minnesota Multiphasic Personality Inven-
    tory and, 42–46
  vs. organic pain, 6–7
Future Despair Scale, in Millon Behavioral
    Health Inventory, 67
Future Outlook Scale, in Millon Behavioral
    Medicine Diagnostic, 79

Galen, 3
Gastrointestinal susceptibility scale, in Mil-
    lon Behavioral Health Inventory, 68
Gate-control theory of pain, 5, 42
Gender
  Millon Behavioral Health Inventory psy-
    chogenic attitude scales and, 74
  and pain locus of control, 169
  pain threshold and, 92–93
  research in, 151
General adaptation syndrome, 261–262
Generalized Expectancy for Success, in op-
    timism measurement, 206
Genetic predisposition
  to disease, 261
  to psychopathology, 264
Greeks, psychological approach of, 25
Grieving, phantom pain and, 29
Guilt, pain and, 29–30

Hamilton Rating Scale for Depression, 247

Headache, extraversion and neuroticism and, 195t, 196–197

Headache-Specific Locus of Control (HSLC) scale, 167

Health Concerns (HEA) Scale, in Minnesota Multiphasic Personality Inventory-2, 122

Health Moderators Domain, of Millon Behavioral Medicine Diagnostic, and medical outcomes, 78–79

Health Optimism Scale, 206, 210

Helplessness, in pain patient, 211

Hippocrates, 3, 261

Histrionic personality disorder, 232

HIV-positive diagnosis, Millon Behavioral Health Inventory assessment of personality–coping styles and, 73

Hogan Personality Inventory (HPI)
  in assessment of five-factor model of personality, 94–95
  description of, 94–95

Hopelessness Scale, 206

Hostility
  in genesis of pain, 30
  pain and, 29–30

HSLC. See Headache-Specific Locus of Control (HSLC)

Humors theory of personality and health, 3, 261

Hypochondriasis
  in Minnesota Multiphasic Personality Inventory, 39
  reaction to pain in, 51

Hypomania, in Minnesota Multiphasic Personality Inventory, 40

Hysteria
  in Minnesota Multiphasic Personality Inventory, 39
  pain and, 26–28

Illness behavior, personality factor influence on, 99

Illness Concerns Scale, in Millon Behavioral Medicine Diagnostic, health maintenance and health care delivery and, 79

Incidence, 223

Infirmary patients, definition of, 209

Inhibited coping style, 64

Intensity, in pain processing, 89, 90

Internal locus of control, 165, 166, 167–168

treatment response prediction and, 168–169

Introversive coping style, 63–64

Jeremiah (Lamentations), 25

K Scale, in Minnesota Multiphasic Personality Inventory, 38, 120–121

Laboratory-induced pain
  and personality, 184, 185t–186t, 187–188
  studies of, 185t–186t
  threshold and tolerance focus in, 187

Laminectomy, MCMI outcome prediction in, 83

Learned helplessness
  depression and, 170
  detrimental effects of, 171

Length of treatment, personality disorders and, 83

Life Orientation Test (LOT), in dispositional optimism measurement, 206

Lifestyle Behaviors Domain, of Millon Behavioral Medicine Diagnostic, 80

Life-Threat Reactivity Scale, on Millon Behavioral Health Inventory, 69

Locus of control (LOC). See also Multidimensional Health Locus of Control (MHLC)
  change with multidisciplinary interventions, 171–172
  clinical practice implications, 173–174
  as construct, 165–166
  coping style and, 168
  culture differences and, 169–170
  experience-based mediating factors and, 172
  external, 165, 166, 170
  gender differences and, 169–170
  internal, 165, 166, 167–168
  naturalistic and longitudinal change in, 171–172
  quality of care and, 172–173
  research implications, 173–174
  stability of, 171–173

Low Back (Lb) Scale, for functional vs. organic pain, 42, 43

Low-back loser
  defined, 45
  Minnesota Multiphasic Personality Inventory scores for, 45

Low-back pain
  configurational subgrouping in, 51–53
  introversion-extraversion and, 193, 194t–
    195t, 196
  Millon Behavioral Health Inventory study
    of, 74
  Minnesota Multiphasic Personality Inven-
    tory and treatment outcomes in, 46–
    48
  optimism and treatment outcome in, 209–
    210
  SCID and SCID II interviews in, 233–
    234
  treatment outcomes in
    Minnesota Multiphasic Personality In-
      ventory and, 46–48
Low-back surgery, Minnesota Multiphasic
  Personality Inventory outcome predic-
  tion for, 12–13
L Scale, in Minnesota Multiphasic Personal-
  ity Inventory, 38

Major depression. *See also* Depression
Major depression, in chronic pain, 170–171
Manipulative reaction, to pain, 51
Marke–Nyman Temperament (MNT) inven-
  tory, 184
  pain threshold and tolerance and person-
    ality in, 187
Masculinity–Femininity, in Minnesota Mul-
  tiphasic Personality Inventory, 40
Maudsley Personality Inventory (MPI), pain
  threshold and tolerance in, 183, 187
MBHI. *See* Millon Behavioral Health Inven-
  tory (MBHI)
MBMD. *See* Millon Behavioral Medicine
  Diagnostic (MBMD)
McAndrew scale, for alcoholism and drug
  addiction, 248
MCMI. *See* Millon Clinical Multiaxial In-
  ventory (MCMI)
Medical diagnosis, pain processing and, 93
Medical outcomes measures, health modera-
  tors of Millon Behavioral Medicine
  Diagnostic and, 78–79
MHLC. *See* Multidimensional Health Locus
  of Control (MHLC)
Millon Behavioral Health Inventory
  (MBHI), 184, 249–250
  in assessment of chronic pain patient, 270
  basis of, 63
  and chronic pain populations

  descriptive studies, 73–74
    in prediction of outcome, 74–76
    coping scales in, 63–66
    psychogenic attitude scales and, 74
    reliability of, 72
  goal of, 62
  limitations of, 76–77
  Millon Behavioral Medicine Diagnostic
    and, 76–80
  prognostic indices scales, 69
    uses of, 69
  psychogenic attitude scales and
    gender and, 74
  Psychogenic Attitude scales in, 63, 66–68
    reliability of, 72
  psychosomatic correlates scales in, 68–69
    allergic inclination, 68
    cardiovascular tendency, 69
    gastrointestinal susceptibility, 68
  reliability of, 72
  research and clinical uses of, 72–73
  validation of, 69–70
    external–criterion, 71–72
    internal–structural, 70–71
    theoretical–substantive, 70
Millon Behavioral Medicine Diagnostic
  (MBMD)
  cognitive appraisal characteristics in, 79
  domains in, 77–80
Millon Clinical Multiaxial Inventory-III
  (MCMI-III)
  of personality disorders and acute dis-
    tress, 80
  scales in, 80, 81t
Millon Clinical Multiaxial Inventory
  (MCMI)
  in dimensional approach to personality
    disorders, 245
  outcome prediction studies and, 82–83
  studies of personality disorder in patients
    with pain, 82
Minnesota Multiphasic Personality
  Inventory-2, 41–42
  in assessment of personality and behav-
    ioral characteristics, 113
  chronic pain assessment controversy and,
    109–111
  comparisons with Minnesota Multiphasic
    Personality Inventory
    in cluster analysis, 118–119
    in code type subgrouping, 117–118
    in factor analysis, 119–120

in patient profile height, 116–117

content scales in, 116, 122

development of, 114–116

in identification of psychopathology, 111–112

interpretative strategies for, 120–122

item changes in, 114–115

items reflective of both psychiatric and chronic illness, 110

norms in, 115–116

in outcome prediction, 113–114

overlap across clinical and validity scales, 110

psychiatric sample comparison group in, 115

standardized scores in, 113

theories of psychopathology in, 110

in treatment planning, 113–114

validity scales in, 116

Minnesota Multiphasic Personality Inventory and MMPI-2

in chronic pain assessment

correlation of patient characteristics with pain variables in, 111

Minnesota Multiphasic Personality Inventory (MMPI)

clinical scales in, 37, 38t, 39–40

views of, 40

cluster types, 53f, 53–54

configurational profiles

subgouping of, 51–54

description of, 37–38

development of chronic pain and, 48–50

personality factors and, 50

in dimensional approach to personality disorders, 245

in examination of psychological functioning, 44–45

and functional vs. organic pain, 42–46

introversion-extraversion in chronic pain, 193, 194t–195t, 196

low-back pain treatment outcomes and, 46–48

with chemonucleolysis, 46

electrical spinal epidural stimulation, 48

with lumbar intervertebral fusions, 46

with lumbar laminectomy, 47–48

pain management programs, 48

with surgical interventions, 47

optimism measurement with, 205–206

in outcome prediction, 46–48, 113–114

pain profile studies, 6–7

P-A-I-N typology in, 53, 53f

prediction studies for chronic pain, 11–12

score configurations in, 40–41, 41f

Social Introversion scale of, 183–184

in treatment planning, 113–114

utility of, 276–277

validity scales in, 37–38, 38t

Minnesota Multiphasic Personality Inventory-2 (MMPI-2), 252

alternatives to, 248, 250

in assessment of chronic pain patient, 269–270

MLPC. See Multidimensional Health Locus Control (MLPC)

MMPI. See Minnesota Multiphasic Personality Inventory (MMPI)

Moderator variables

beliefs vs., 157–158

research in, 150–151, 152

Multidimensional Health Locus of Control (MHLC). See also Locus of control (LOC)

gender and, 169

for health-related beliefs, 166–167

Ways of Coping Checklist relationship with, 134

Multidimensional Pain Inventory (MPI)

in assessment of chronic pain patient, 270

description of, 249

personality and coping in, 246

National Institute of Mental Health (NIMH) study, prevalence of psychopathology, 241–242

Negative emotions, in pain processing, 90

Negative Treatment Indicators (TRT) Scale, in Minnesota Multiphasic Personality Inventory-2, 122

Neuroticism

causal relationship to pain disorders, 96–97

extroversion relationship with, 98

health outcomes and, 99

psychological distress and, 97

psychotherapy and, 100

sensation intensity and, 98

unplesantness and, 98

Neuroticism, Extraversion, Openness–Personality Inventory–Revised (NEO-PI-R), 184

Neuroticism, Extraversion, Openness–
    Revised (NEO-PI-R) (*continued*)
  in personality assessment, 94–95
  Schedule of Nonadaptive and Adaptive
    Personality and, 274
Neurotic triad, 6, 40, 41, 41f
  functional *vs.* organic pain and, 44–45
Normal personality
  big-five factor model of, 94–95
  personality trait theory and, 94
  structure of, application to chronic pain
    and illness, 96–99
    neuroticism and, 96–97

Obsessive–Compulsive personality disorder,
    complex regional pain syndrome and,
    234–235
Openness to Experience (culture)
  in five-factor model of normal personal-
    ity, 94
  treatment outcome and, 100–101
Optimism
  constructs related to, 204
  defensive, 204–205
  definitions of, 203–204
  dispositional, 204
  functional, 204
  and health, 207–208
  measures of, 205–206, 210
  and pain, 208–212, 213f
  and psychosocial adjustment, 211
  unrealistic, 205
Optimism model in pain, 212–213, 213f
Optimism–Pessimism Prescreening Ques-
    tionnaire, 206
Optimism–Pessimism Scale, of Minnesota
    Multiphasic Personality Inventory,
    205–206
Outcome
  with cognitive-behavioral treatment for
    catastrophizing, 147–148
  coping styles and, 72
  internal locus of control and, 167–170
  Millon Behavioral Health Inventory rela-
    tionship to, 72, 76
  openness and, 100–101
  optimism and, 209–210
  personality and, 277
  personality diagnosis and, 228, 236
  personality disorder in chronic pain and,
    235–236
  personality style and, 236

psychopathology effect on, 242–243
  SF-36 monitoring of, 270–271
Outcome prediction
  belief and, 157
  comparison of Millon Behavioral Health
    Inventory and Minnesota Multiphasic
    Personality Inventory, 74–76
  Millon Clinical Multiaxial Inventory and,
    82–83
  Minnesota Multiphasic Personality Inven-
    tory in, 113–114
  Minnesota Multiphasic Personality
    Inventory-2 in, 113–114, 119
  in multidisciplinary chronic pain and
    headache treatment center, 75
  in outpatient rehabilitation program, 75
  toleration of physical discomfort in medi-
    cal procedure and, 75–76
Outcomes. *See also* Treatment response pre-
    diction
  Millon Behavioral Medical Diagnosis
    health moderator scales and, 78–79
  Millon Clinical Medical Inventory predic-
    tive studies of, 82–83
  Minnesota Multiphasic Personality Inven-
    tory and, 46–48

Pain. *See also* Acute postoperative pain;
    Chronic pain
  assessment goal of, 101
  as biopsychosocial process, 182
  early research in, 181–182
  symbolic significance of, 29, 31
P-A-I-N cluster analysis, 118, 119
Pain Locus of Control (PLOC)
  description of, 167
  gender and, 169
  scores before and after treatment, 172t
Pain patient, types of, 209
Pain processing
  anxiety and depression and, 98
  demographic factors in, 92–93
  four-stage model of, 89–90, 91f
    behavioral expression in, 90
    sensation intensity in, 89, 90
    structured interview in, 91
    suffering in, 90, 91
    unplesantness in, 89, 90
    validity of, 91–92
    visual analog scale assessment of, 89,
      90–91
  normal personality structure and, 93–99

psychopathology and
  Minnesota Multiphasic Personality
    Inventory-2 assessment of, 94, 102
  stages of, Medical College of Virginia
    Pain Questionnaire assessment of, 102
Pain puzzle, 9–10, 10f
Pain Reactivity Scale, in Millon Behavioral
    Health Inventory, health maintenance
    and health care delivery and, 79
Pain–stress cycle, 17, 17f, 268, 268f
Pain threshold
  definition of, 187
  gender and, 92–93
Pain tolerance, definition of, 187
Pain Treatment Responsivity Scale, on Mil-
    lon Behavioral Health Inventory, 69
P-A-I-N typology
  for chronic pain, 53f, 53–54
Patient profiles, on Minnesota Multiphasic
    Personality Inventory and Minnesota
    Multiphasic Personality Inventory-2,
    116–117
Pattern theory of pain, 4
Period prevalence, 226
Personality. *See also* Normal personality
  and cancer pain, 190, 191t, 192
  definition of, 260
  and laboratory-induced pain, 184, 185t–
    186t, 187–188
Personality assessment
  Millon Behavioral Health Inventory, 61,
    62–76
  Millon Behavioral Medicine Diagnostic
    in, 76–80
  Millon Clinical Multiaxial Inventory in,
    61, 62, 80–83, 81t
Personality Assessment Schedule (PAS), in
    dimensional approach to personality
    disorders, 245
Personality characteristics, Minnesota Multi-
    phasic Personality Inventory-2 assess-
    ment of, 113
Personality clusters, 229
Personality/Coping Style scales, of Millon
    Behavioral Medicine Diagnostic, 78
Personality disorder diagnosis
  benefits of, 228
  clinical application of, 235–236
  clinical interview in, 229, 230t–231t,
    232–233
  in Diagnostic and Statistical Manual, ed.
    4 (DSM-IV) in, 223, 224t–225t

in Diagnostic and Statistical Manual of
    Personality Disorders, ed. 3 (DSM-
    III-R), 221–222
  dimensional *vs.* categorical, 228–229
  epidemiological factors in, 223, 226
  methods of, 226–228
    issues in, 221–222
  rationale for, 222–223
  semi-structured interview studies in, 227,
    229, 230t–231t, 232–233
  stepwise approach to, 251–254, 253f
  structured interview studies in, 226, 227,
    233–235
Personality disorders
  assessment instruments for, 244–246
    selection of, 246–251
  assessment of
    categorical *vs.* dimensional, 244–245
    longitudinal *vs.* cross-sectional, 266
  characteristics of individuals with, 241
  clusters of, 231–232, 244, 260
  coping and, 246
  definition of, 260
  dimensional approach to, 245–246
  DSM-IV definition of, 246
  and pain, future research in, 266–267
  premorbid and postmorbid function and,
    260–261
  prevalence of, 243–244
    in chronic pain patient, 81–82, 111–
    112, 259–260
  severity of and outcome, 84
  type of and outcome, 84
Personality disorder screening
  in chronic pain population, 14–18
  diathesis–stress model of, 15
  in early stages of pain, 16–18
Personality factors, influence on pain pro-
    cessing, 99
Personality Interview Questionnaire (PIQ),
    in dimensional approach to personal-
    ity disorders, 245
Personality measures, in prediction of treat-
    ment response, 12–14
Personality screening
  and prevention of chronic pain disability,
    267–269
  terms used in, 267–268
Personality theory
  of Eysenck, 182–183
  of Millon, 78
Personality traits, in chronic pain research,
    15

Personality trait theory, normal personality
    and, 94
Personality types, *vs.* personality disorders,
    236
Pessimism, premorbid, 67
Pessimists, optimists *vs.,* 207–208, 212–213
Phantom pain
    asymbolia for, 28–29
    psychogenesis theory of, 28
Pittsburgh Scale of Social Extraversion-
    Introversion and Emotionality for pain
    threshold and tolerance, 184, 187–188
Plato, 25, 261
PLOC. *See* Pain Locus of Control (PLOC)
Point prevalence, 223
Powerful others, as locus of control, 166
Praying and hoping, adjustment and, 148
Premorbid Pessimism Scale, in Millon Be-
    havioral Health Inventory, 67
Profile types, in prediction of treatment re-
    sponse, 51–53
Psychiatric Indicators Domain, of Millon
    Behavioral Medicine Diagnostic, 77–
    78
Psychoanalysis, hysteria and pain in, 26–28
Psychoanalytic ideas
    Freud, 25–28
    Greeks, 25
    Jeremiah, 25
Psychoanalytic theories
    Engel, 31, 48–49
    Freud, 26–28
    Szasz, 30, 31
Psychodynamic theory of pain, 4
Psychogenic Attitude scales, Millon Behav-
    ioral Health Inventory, 66–67
Psychological distress
    neuroticism and, 97
    psychopathology and, 112
Psychoneuroimmunology, 262
Psychopathology
    base rates of, National Institute of Mental
        Health prevalence study, 241–242
    National Institute of Mental Health preva-
        lence study of, 241–242
    psychopathic deviate, 40
    temperament and trait factors in, 243
Psychosomatic V. *See* Conversion V

Readiness for change, prediction of treat-
    ment response and, 157
Recent Stress Scale, in Millon Behavioral
    Health Inventory, 66–67

Renaissance, 3
Repertory grid measures, new uses of, 150
Resentment
    chronic pain and, 29, 32
    pain and, 29–30
Respectful coping style, 65

Schedule for Nonadaptive and Adaptive
    Personality (SNAP)
    application of, 245–246
    in assessment of chronic pain patient,
        271
    description of, 235
    in dimensional approach to personality
        disorders, 245–246
    dimensions of temperament and personal-
        ity in, 251, 252
    and five-factor trait-dimensional mea-
        sures, 274–276
    improvements in, recent and continuing,
        275–276
    restandardization of, 276
    temperament scales of, 273t, 274
    trait scales of, 272t–273t, 274
    use with pain populations, 276
    validity scales, 272t, 274
Schizophrenia, in Minnesota Multiphasic
    Personality Inventory, 40
Self-reports, of coping, 132
Self-statements, positive-coping and adjust-
    ment, 148
Selye, Hans, 261–262
Semi-structured interview
    in dimensional approach to personality
        disorders, 245
    in personality disorder diagnosis, 226–
        228
Sensitive coping style, 65–66
Severity of pain, research in, 151
Short Form Health Survey (SF–36), 251,
    252, 270–271
Sixteen Personality Factor (16 PF) Ques-
    tionnaire, 193
SNAP. *See* Schedule for Nonadaptive and
    Adaptive Personality (SNAP)
Sociable coping style, 64
Social Alienation Scale, in Millon Behav-
    ioral Health Inventory, 67–68
Social cluster, of personality disorders
Social Introversion Scale, comparison with
    Eysenck Personality Questionnaire,
    183–184

Social Support Scale, in Millon Behavioral Medicine Diagnostic, medical outcomes and, 79

Somatic Anxiety Scale, in Millon Behavioral Health Inventory, 68

SOPA. *See* Survey of Pain Attitudes (SOPA)

Specificity theory of pain, 3–4

Spiritual Faith Scale, in Millon Behavioral Medicine Diagnostic, medical outcomes and, 79

State scales, in Minnesota Multiphasic Personality Inventory, 40

Stress
  in behavioral medicine, 17
  Chronic Tension Scale measurement of, 66
  definition of, 261, 264–265
  in development of chronic pain, 262–263
  in diathesis-stress model of personality and chronic pain, 262–263
  Millon Behavioral Health Inventory Recent Stress Scale measurement of, 66–67
  optimism and health and, 207–208
  transactional adaptation to, 131

Stress-coping research, pain-coping research and, 155

Structured clinical interview for DMS III-R (SCID and SCID II)
  for personality disorders in chronic pain, 242

Structured Clinical Interview for DSM-III-R (SCID), 226, 227
  to predict chronic pain, 12

Structured Clinical Interview for DSM-IV (SCID), 250, 252

Structured interview
  in pain processing, 91
  in personality disorder diagnosis, 226, 227
  for treatment response prediction, 14

Structured Interview for DSM-III (SCID I and SCID II), 244–245

Structured Interview for DSM Personality Disorders (SIDP), 226, 227

Structured Interview for DSM Personality Disorders (SIDP-R), 226, 227

Suffering
  extraversion and, 98
  neuroticism and, 96–97
  in pain processing, 90, 91

personality factor influence on, 99

Survey of Pain Attitudes (SOPA), 157, 158

Symbolization, in Szasz, T. S., 31

Symptom scales, in Minnesota Multiphasic Personality Inventory, 40

System Check List 90 Revised (SCL-90-R), as alternative to Minnesota Multiphasic Personality Inventory-2, 248

Temporomandibular joint disorders, SCID and SCID II interviews in, 234

Toronto Alexithymia Scale (TAS)
  chronic pain and, 193
  social introversion and, 184

Total stress load hypothesis, 265

Trait scales, in Minnesota Multiphasic Personality Inventory, 40

Treatment Prognostics Domain, of Millon Behavioral Medicine Diagnostic, 79–80

Treatment response prediction. *See also* Outcomes
  locus of control and, 168–169
  Minnesota Multiphasic Personality Inventory and, 12–14
  structured interviews in, 14

Unpleasantness
  neuroticism and, 98
  in pain processing, 89, 90

Validation, of Millon Behavioral Health Inventory, 69–70

Validity, of Ways of Coping Checklist, 135

Validity scales
  in Minnesota Multiphasic Personality Inventory, 37–38, 38t
  in Minnesota Multiphasic Personality Inventory-2, 116, 121
  assessment of, 120–121

Vanderbilt Multidimensional Pain Coping Inventory (VMPCI)
  correlation with general impairment measures, 145
  correlation with Vanderbilt Pain Management Inventory subscales, 144–145
  goal in, 143–144
  limitations of, 145–146
  and prediction of adjustment changes, 145
  psychometric improvements in, 149

Vanderbilt Multidimensional Pain Coping
    Inventory (VMPCI) (*continued*)
  studies of, 143
  subscales of, 144t
Vanderbilt Pain Management Inventory
    (VPMI), studies of, 143
Visual analog scale (VAS) measurement, of
    pain processing, 89, 90–91
VPMI. *See* Vanderbilt Pain Management In-
    ventory (VPMI)

Ways of Coping Checklist (WOC)
  description of, 133–134
  problem-focused and emotion-focused

    scales in, 133
  relationship with Multidimensional Health
    Locus of Control, 134
  validity of, 135
West Haven-Yale Multidimensional Pain In-
    ventory. *See* Multidimensional Pain
    Inventory (MPI)
Wishful thinking, 210–211
WOC. *See* Ways of Coping Checklist
    (WOC)
Work Interference (WRK) Scale, in Minne-
    sota Multiphasic Personality
    Inventory-2, 122

ABOUT THE EDITORS

Robert J. Gatchel, PhD, received his BA in Psychology from the State University of New York at Stony Brook in 1969 and his PhD in Clinical Psychology from the University of Wisconsin in 1973. Dr. Gatchel is currently the Elizabeth H. Penn Professor of Clinical Psychology and professor in the Departments of Psychiatry and Rehabilitation Science at the University of Texas, Southwestern Medical Center at Dallas. He is also the program director of the Eugene McDermott Center for Pain Management at the Medical School, and is the research director at the Productive Rehabilitation Institute of Dallas for Ergonomics (PRIDE). He is a diplomate of the American Board of Professional Psychology and is a director of the American Board of Clinical Health Psychology.

Dr. Gatchel has conducted extensive clinical research on the psychophysiology of stress and emotion, the comorbidity of psychological and physical health problems, and the assessment/treatment of chronic stress and pain behavior. Much of this research was supported by grants from the National Institutes of Health. He is the recipient of consecutive Research Scientist Development Awards from the National Institute of Mental Health.

Dr. Gatchel has published over 150 scientific articles and 50 book chapters, and has authored or edited 16 other books, including *Psychosocial Factors in Pain: Critical Perspectives* (with Dennis C. Turk). He is also on the editorial board of numerous psychological and medical journals, such as the *Clinical Journal of Pain*, the *Journal of Occupational Rehabilitation,* and *Spine*.

James N. Weisberg, PhD, is an assistant professor of Clinical Psychiatry and Behavioral Sciences in the Department of Psychiatry and Behavioral Sciences, State University of New York at Stony Brook (Long Island), where he maintains an active clinical practice, conducts research, and trains medical students, psychiatry residents and clinical psychology students.

Dr. Weisberg received his PhD in Clinical Psychology in 1992 from the Ferkauf Graduate School of Psychology at the Albert Einstein College of Medicine, of Yeshiva University in New York. He completed his psychology residency at the University of North Carolina School of Medicine and a fellowship in Pain Management in the Department of Psychiatry at Duke University Medical Center. He has authored or co-authored a number of articles and chapters on personality and pain as well as coping with pain. He is currently collaborating in the development of an interactive media program for low-back pain-management funded by the National Institutes of Health. He speaks nationally on the topics of personality disorders and chronic pain, as well as cognitive–behavioral pain management, stress management, and biofeedback.

Dr. Weisberg lives in Setauket, New York with his wife and their two sons. He is an avid pilot and enjoys sailing and kayaking in the bays of Long Island.